Clinical Neuropsychological Assessment

A Cognitive Approach

CRITICAL ISSUES IN NEUROPSYCHOLOGY

Series Editors

Antonio E. Puente
University of North Carolina, Wilmington

Cecil R. Reynolds
Texas A&M University

Current Volumes in this Series

BEHAVIORAL INTERVENTIONS WITH BRAIN-INJURED CHILDREN
A. MacNeill Horton, Jr.

CLINICAL NEUROPSYCHOLOGICAL ASSESSMENT:
A Cognitive Approach
Edited by Robert L. Mapou and Jack Spector

FAMILY SUPPORT PROGRAMS AND REHABILITATION:
A Cognitive–Behavioral Approach to Traumatic Brain Injury
Louise Margaret Smith and Hamish P. D. Godfrey

NEUROPSYCHOLOGICAL EVALUATION OF THE
SPANISH SPEAKER
Alfredo Ardila, Monica Rosselli, and Antonio E. Puente

NEUROPSYCHOLOGICAL EXPLORATIONS OF
MEMORY AND COGNITION:
Essays in Honor of Nelson Butters
Edited by Laird S. Cermak

NEUROPSYCHOLOGICAL TOXICOLOGY:
Identification and Assessment of Human Neurotoxic Syndromes,
Second Edition
David E. Hartman

THE NEUROPSYCHOLOGY OF ATTENTION
Ronald A. Cohen

A PRACTICAL GUIDE TO HEAD INJURY REHABILITATION:
A Focus on Postacute Residential Treatment
Michael D. Wesolowski and Arnie H. Zencius

PRACTITIONER'S GUIDE TO CLINICAL NEUROPSYCHOLOGY
Robert M. Anderson, Jr.

A Continuation Order Plan is available for this series. A continuation order will bring delivery of each new volume immediately upon publication. Volumes are billed only upon actual shipment. For further information please contact the publisher.

Clinical Neuropsychological Assessment

A Cognitive Approach

Edited by

Robert L. Mapou

Henry M. Jackson Foundation for the Advancement of Military Medicine
Washington, D.C.

and

Jack Spector

Walter Reed Army Medical Center
Washington, D.C.

Plenum Press • New York and London

Library of Congress Cataloging-in-Publication Data

On file

ISBN 0-306-44869-6

A Division of Plenum Publishing Corporation
233 Spring Street, New York, N. Y. 10013

10 9 8 7 6 5 4 3 2 1

Printed in the United States of America

Contributors

Arthur L. Benton • Departments of Neurology and Psychology, University of Iowa, Iowa City, Iowa 52242

David Caplan • Neuropsychology Laboratory, Massachusetts General Hospital, Boston, Massachusetts 02114

Daniel X. Capruso • Department of Neurology, State University of New York at Buffalo, Buffalo, New York 14203

Anne-Lise Christensen • Center for Rehabilitation of Brain Injury, University of Copenhagen, 2300 Copenhagen S, Denmark

Thomas H. Crook III • Memory Assessment Clinics, Inc., 8311 Wisconsin Avenue, Suite B8, Bethesda, Maryland 20814

Bryan D. Fantie • Human Neuropsychology Laboratory, The American University, Washington, DC 20016-8062

Sue Franklin • Department of Psychology, University of York, York YO1 5DD, England

Rhonda B. Friedman • Department of Neurology, Georgetown University Medical Center, Washington, DC 20007

Guila Glosser • Department of Neurology, The Graduate Hospital, Philadelphia, Pennsylvania 19146

Felicia C. Goldstein • Neurobehavioral Program, Department of Neurology, Emory University School of Medicine and Wesley Woods Center, Atlanta, Georgia 30329

Robert C. Green • Neurobehavioral Program, Department of Neurology, Emory University School of Medicine and Wesley Woods Center, Atlanta, Georgia 30329

Kerry deS. Hamsher • Department of Neurology, University of Wisconsin Medical School, Milwaukee, Wisconsin 53233-1325

Kasper Jørgensen • Department of Neurology, Bispebjerg Hospital, 2400 Copenhagen NV, Denmark

Janice Kay • Department of Psychology, University of Exeter, Exeter EX4 4QG, England

Glenn J. Larrabee • 630 South Orange, Suite 202, Sarasota, Florida 34236

Robert L. Mapou • Henry M. Jackson Foundation for the Advancement of Military Medicine, Walter Reed Army Medical Center, Washington, DC 20307-5001

Allan F. Mirsky • Laboratory of Psychology and Psychopathology, National Institute of Mental Health, Bethesda, Maryland 20892-1366

Jack Spector • Division of Neurosurgery and Department of Psychology, Walter Reed Army Medical Center, Washington, DC 20307-5001

Janet E. Tatman • Human Neuropsychology Laboratory, The American University, Washington, DC 20016-8062

Kevin W. Walsh • Austin Hospital, Heidelberg 3084, Melbourne, Australia

Foreword

Practicing neuropsychologists and students in clinical neuropsychology must increasingly cross disciplinary boundaries to understand and appreciate the neuroanatomical, neurophysiological, and neuropharmacological bases of cognition and behavior, current cognitive theory in many different domains of functioning, and the nature and tools of clinical assessment. Although the cognitive functions and abilities of interest are often the same, each of these fields has grappled with them from sometimes very different perspectives. Terminology is often specific to a particular discipline or approach, methods are diverse, and the goals or outcomes of study or investigation are usually very different. This book poises itself to provide a largely missing link between traditional approaches to assessment and the growing area of cognitive neuropsychology.

Historically, neuropsychology had as its central core the consideration of evidence from clinical cases. It was the early work of neurologists such as Broca, Wernicke, Hughlings-Jackson, and Liepmann, who evaluated and described the behavioral correlates of prescribed lesions in individual patients and focused investigation on the lateralization and localization of cognitive abilities in humans. An outgrowth of those approaches was the systematic development of experimental tasks that could be used to elucidate the nature of cognitive changes in individuals with well-described brain lesions. Although that tradition continued in some centers, other researchers interested in brain and behavior relationships began a psychometric tradition, developing tests that could be applied to large numbers of individuals to evaluate levels of cognitive functioning in many different domains and to serve as markers of "organicity." Cognitive psychologists, meanwhile, largely confining their work to studies with unimpaired subjects within university research centers, developed theories of cognitive organization quite separate from theories of brain function.

Over the course of the last two decades, cognitive psychologists have increasingly drawn upon not only cognitive theory, but upon empirical evidence in individual patients with well-described neurological damage, for insights into the cerebral organization of cognitive skills and abilities. Investigations of individual cases not only served to support or refute theories of cognition, but greatly enhanced an understanding of the neurological underpinnings of many cognitive functions. At the same time, clinical neuropsychologists looked to their colleagues in cognitive psychology to provide a greater understanding of the dimensions of cognitive abilities.

The studies of leading cognitive neuropsychologists such as Allport, Baddeley, Berndt, Caramazza, Cermak, Coltheart, Marshall, McCarthy, Newcombe, Posner, Shallice, Squire, Warrington, and many others have provided exciting, sometimes breathtaking insights into the architecture of specific cognitive abilities. It is with admiration and appreciation that I read studies that literally cleave the components of cognitive skills, such as single-word reading, spelling, or object recognition. Yet, such studies have often seemed somewhat removed, and difficult to integrate with the task of clinical assessment I may have at hand. The core work of cognitive neuropsychology has involved exquisite, highly individualized analyses of different types of very selective impairments of cognitive function that may be observed in a small group of individual patients following brain damage. Or, they have involved repeated, in-depth studies of larger samples of well-defined and controlled clinical cases such as may be seen in a large clinical research center. Such studies often involve development of very prescribed stimuli, and are by nature not standardized or normed for some general noninvolved population. They often require multiple examinations to titrate the specific nature of deficits or spared functions through analysis of performance on skillfully designed tasks that delineate the core features of a specific cognitive deficit. Although such detailed functional analyses of particular cognitive skills in patients with very discrete lesions or very defined syndromes may provide a clearer window through which to observe the organization and structure of normal cognition, problems often emerge when the clinician attempts to use these same tools in the clinic. Many, if not most, patients seen in clinical practice have large, diffuse, and/or multifocal lesions that result in involvement of multiple cognitive systems. They also need to be seen in a restricted time frame in a setting with limited tools and human resources.

As a clinician working primarily within a rehabilitation setting, I rarely needed to address whether brain damage had occurred and the issue of localization was often moot. Although it can be argued that the localization and extent of lesions can provide valuable prognosticative information and should have relevance with regard to issues of resource allocation, at our present state of knowledge such relationships are dependent on many factors and have not been sufficiently clarified. Evaluation in that context usually needs to focus on functional capacities, on identification of preserved skills that could be used in the development of compensatory approaches, on issues of safety and potential for independence in activities of daily life, and on identifying the most important deficits on which to focus treatment efforts, whether of a restorative or compensatory nature. The tools clinicians usually bring to bear are those that have been most widely standardized, have the strongest data base with regard to localizing potential, and provide the most discrete information relative to different domains of cognitive function. Yet they still often do little more than identify domains of deficit and shed some light upon severity. Most currently used clinical neuropsychological tests still require many different abilities or skills and still provide quite gross estimates of dysfunction in specific cognitive domains within a controlled context. Flexible approaches to traditional testing, such as those described by Edith Kaplan, Muriel Lezak, and Kevin Walsh, push the limits of those tests, but often still are bound by the limited theory on which many tests are based. Another problem in providing timely, cost-effective, and useful assessments is the large number of different domains in which there are likely to be deficits. In cases of traumatic brain injury, dementia, multiple sclerosis, acquired immune deficiency syndrome, or cerebrovascular accidents of moderate dimension, lesions will likely involve multiple functional systems. The detailed analysis of those functional systems in such patients is time consuming, complicated, and necessarily imprecise.

In this text, the editors have recognized the need for detailed assessment of cognitive functions, and have gathered together a group of authors who provide practical tools for doing so within the context of truly clinically based evaluation. Their approach and the work described by their contributing authors embody the scientist-practitioner model that is so widely heralded yet so rarely observed. The introductory and overview chapters outline important issues in the assessment of cognitive abilities in clinical populations and provide valuable historical perspectives. The chapters focusing on specific cognitive functions will provide the practicing clinician with powerful tools needed to conduct evaluations that both rely and build upon what is known about the neural organization of those same cognitive skills. Armed with such tools, the clinical neuropsychologist should be in a better position to evaluate and understand the specific nature of cognitive deficits with which his or her patients present.

As a field, we still have a long way to go in understanding how any of these deficits, however interesting or discrete, impacts the everyday adaptive functioning of individuals. Although it seems that a greater understanding of a deficit could lead to more effective intervention strategies, there is as yet little information in this area. Indeed, even the finest grained analysis of a deficit will not necessarily point to strategies or techniques that will restore or help ameliorate the deficit. A significant challenge of the next decade will be to utilize the information derived from increasingly theory-based and cognitively oriented neuropsychological assessment to refine our clinical interventions and ultimate practical utility. Although it is easy to say that a greater understanding of a phenomenon will lead to a more effective treatment, the development and articulation of treatment approaches and studies of their efficacy still are largely undeveloped.

This book takes an important step in mapping important findings in "cognitive neuropsychology" onto clinically useful assessment tools. It is written in such a way that those coming to the topic for the first time can gain both a broad overview of issues and a great deal of specific application. For those already in the field, clinical experience will enhance the applicability of the procedures and many will find new clinical tools or new ways to use or interpret findings on familiar tools. This book does more than fill a gap; it provides a needed link between a rich and growing cognitive neuropsychology literature and the practice of clinical neuropsychology. It should challenge individuals at both ends of the applied spectrum of neuropsychology to think about the scope and limits of what they do and should encourage the growing dialogue between experimentalists and practitioners.

Catherine A. Mateer

University of Victoria
Victoria, British Columbia, Canada

Preface

The roles taken by clinical neuropsychologists today are diverse and go beyond the need for detection, lateralization, and localization of brain lesions. Clinical neuropsychologists are now employed in a variety of settings, including neurology and neurosurgery units, psychiatric hospitals, rehabilitation facilities, and outpatient medical and mental health clinics. Within these settings, neuropsychologists are asked to describe a patient's neurobehavioral competencies, to apply these findings to diagnosis, to make predictions for recovery and for daily functioning, to make treatment recommendations, and to implement treatment plans. Neuropsychologists also are asked to justify their findings with respect to reliability and validity of test performances, especially as related to the different goals of assessment, and they may be called on to discuss the efficacy of recommended treatments.

To accomplish each of these tasks, it is essential that today's practicing clinical neuropsychologists and new students of clinical neuropsychology understand the empirical relationships between human cognition and brain function. In the past, it may have been sufficient to understand the relation between a test score and gross indices of brain damage, including lesion presence, type, and location. Today, however, clinical neuropsychologists must understand how neurobehavioral disorder disrupts different brain systems and what the impact of disruption is on test performances. The neuropsychologist's task is one of understanding how a patient's behavior, manifested by neuropsychological test performances, reflects the functioning of different cognitive and motor systems, and how this, in turn, relates to the presence or absence of a particular type of brain disorder.

To gain this knowledge, clinical neuropsychologists must consult and keep up with primary sources of data, such as journal articles and meeting presentations, and secondary summaries of data, such as focused review articles and textbooks. When this book was first conceptualized in the late 1980s, three types of textbooks were readily available: (1) those devoted to specific neuropsychological batteries (e.g., Halstead-Reitan Neuropsychological Test Battery; Luria-Nebraska Neuropsychological Battery); (2) those devoted to neurobehavioral syndromes (e.g., *Clinical Neuropsychology,* edited by Heilman and Valenstein, *Neuropsychological Assessment of Neuropsychiatric Disorders,* edited by Grant and Adams, *Neurobehavioral Consequences of Closed Head Injury,* by Levin, Benton, and Grossman); and (3) those that were a compilation of test procedures and normative data, with introductory neuropsychological principles (e.g., *Neuropsychological Assessment,* by Lezak). There was less information available on non-battery-based approaches to assessment and on approaches that emphasized the relation between cognitive function and the diagnosis and treatment of neurobehavioral disorder. Thus, this book was developed to add to the literature on cognitively oriented approaches to clinical neuropsychological assessment. Since we began the book, we have seen an increased emphasis in the literature on understanding the specific patterns of cognitive and motor difficulties associated with particular neurobehavioral disorders. We also have seen textbooks that discuss the application of cognitive neuropsychological research to clinical practice. We hope that this book will contribute to the growing literature in this area.

Chapter contributors reflect a scientist-practitioner model. All do research on the areas of cognition about which they have written, and most are practicing clinical neuropsychologists. The book is divided into three parts. In the first part, contributors describe approaches to assessment of specific aspects of cognition. These chapters include the empirical basis for the models and instruments described and case illustrations of the methods presented. In the second part, contributors describe broader approaches to assessment, each of which has a basis in understanding the patient's cognitive strengths and weaknesses and how this relates to neurobehavioral disorder. Again, each chapter provides empirical support for the methods described and includes case examples. We conclude the book with a final part consisting of two chapters that integrate many of the ideas presented and suggest future directions for the field.

Preparation of this book has taken a great deal of time and effort. We would like to acknowledge the support and patience of our colleagues and contributors over the last several years. We would also like to thank our students, for challenging some of our ideas and making us think more carefully about how we justify what we do clinically. Finally, of course, we would like to thank our families for their support, particularly during those times when we were working feverishly to meet publication deadlines.

We also wish to make a special acknowledgment of the work of Nelson Butters. Dr. Butters has been a key force and player in the field of neuropsychology for more than 20 years. He pioneered studies of memory and amnesia in the 1970s, and in the 1980s he expanded his work to understanding the differences in cognitive patterns associated with different types of dementia. Dr. Butters can be credited with first documenting many of the cognitive differences between cortical and subcortical dementias. He always has been at the front of developments in the field, including the application of new test instruments, such as the Wechsler Memory Scale-Revised and the California Verbal Learning Test. Dr. Butters is also a clinician. He has been instrumental in the birth and growth of the American Board of Clinical Neuropsychology and served as its vice president from 1991 to 1993. In sum, Nelson Butters truly personifies the scientist-practitioner model of the clinical neuropsychologist. Because his work embodies the spirit in which this book was developed and represents the type of approach to assessment that we advocate, it is in his honor that we dedicate this book.

Robert L. Mapou
Jack Spector

Contents

Clinical Neuropsychological Assessment

A Cognitive Approach

1

Introduction

ROBERT L. MAPOU

Changes in the role of the neuropsychologist over the past decade have been accompanied by a shift in the goals of neuropsychological assessment. Historically, clinical neuropsychological assessment has been used to evaluate brain–behavior relationships in individuals who have suffered or are believed to have suffered brain dysfunction. Results have been used largely for diagnosis, including lateralization and localization of lesions. Increasingly, however, neuropsychologists have been asked to answer additional questions regarding a patient's prognosis for further recovery, ability to complete functional tasks, and need for treatment. Although clinical neuropsychology has not lost its fundamental grounding in scientific knowledge of brain–behavior relationships, these changes in the role of the neuropsychologist and the goals of assessment have necessitated a rethinking regarding the emphasis of assessment.

THE HISTORICAL ROOTS OF CLINICAL NEUROPSYCHOLOGY

Neuropsychological textbooks can be consulted for a comprehensive review of the historical roots of neuropsychology (Kolb & Whishaw, 1990; Walsh, 1987). By the nineteenth century, clinicians and experimentalists, who tended to be the same people at that time, debated the nature of brain functioning. Some, such as Flourens, argued that the brain functioned *holistically,* while others, with roots in Gall and Spurzheim's phrenology, believed that brain functions were *differentiated and localized.* Dax, Broca, and Wernicke, for example, provided the first evidence for localization of language to the left hemisphere. From the last half of the nineteenth century to the early twentieth century, the debate between holistic versus localized functioning of the brain continued, with those such as Goltz, Head, and Lashley arguing for a holistic

---

ROBERT L. MAPOU • Henry M. Jackson Foundation for the Advancement of Military Medicine, Walter Reed Army Medical Center, Washington, DC 20307-5001.

Clinical Neuropsychological Assessment: A Cognitive Approach, edited by Robert L. Mapou and Jack Spector. Plenum Press, New York, 1995.

view, and others, including Lichtheim, Dejerine, and Fritsch and Hitzig, taking the side of localization.

Recent articles have traced the roots of modern neuropsychology and neuropsychological techniques to several different disciplines and areas of research including behavioral neurology, clinical psychology, experimental psychology, cognitive psychology, and psychometric testing (Benton, 1992; Hartman, 1991; Meier, 1992; Mirsky & Duncan, 1987). Hartman (1991), in particular, has outlined some of the diverse and less well-known roots of our discipline, including early work in mental testing at the turn of the century. He reviewed studies from the mental testing movement and concluded that the movement made four contributions to neuropsychology: (1) the investigation of individual differences in cognitive and motor function, (2) the application of statistical methods to these studies, (3) the development of test equipment and assessment techniques, and (4) the recognition that there are multiple influences on cognitive and motor function. Hartman then reviewed early experimental and clinical psychological studies of cognition, such as those that examined the effects of different physiological manipulations on cognition. Many measures of different aspects of cognition (attention, language, visuospatial skills, abstraction, learning, and memory) emerged from this work, and a number of these researchers were among the first to apply psychological methods to diagnosis of neurological and psychiatric patients.

In the 1940s, Halstead did his pioneering work on a battery of tests designed to verify his theory of "biological intelligence." Around the same time, Goldstein was developing a battery to assess abstract thinking, and Luria was using a set of measures to evaluate impairment in different functional systems of the brain. Many of our modern neuropsychological methods have been derived from the work of these "clinical scientists" (Mirsky & Duncan, 1987). Credit must also be given to the "basic brain scientists," such as Lashley, Köhler, Hebb, and others, whose work has contributed to current knowledge of brain–behavior relationships. Thus, there is no single root of modern clinical neuropsychology.

SCHOOLS OF NEUROPSYCHOLOGY

As neuropsychological methods began to be applied increasingly to clinical assessment in the 1970s and early 1980s, clinicians came to identify themselves with one of three "schools" of neuropsychology: *Lurian, psychometric,* and *process-oriented.* The *Lurian* tradition emphasizes the bedside, clinical examination of higher cognitive functioning. The Lurian investigation is theory-driven and unstructured, or rather, structured by the unique demands of the patient and his or her circumstances. Psychometric rigor is sacrificed for richness of clinical data. The Lurian investigation is neither replicable nor easily scored; efforts at standardizing the Lurian investigation have been opposed on the grounds that aggregating patient data results in a loss of clinically relevant information (Christensen, 1979; Luria, 1980).

In the *psychometric* tradition, there are those who use the Halstead-Reitan Neuropsychological Test Battery (HRNTB), as developed and researched by Reitan and colleagues (Reitan & Davison, 1974; Reitan & Wolfson, 1985). This approach emphasizes the use of a standardized, fixed group of measures and actuarial interpretation. The approach is atheoretical and very much influenced by the psychometrically valued qualities of standardization, replicability, and discriminative power.

In contrast to the Lurian and psychometric traditions, a third school of assessment, referred to as *process-oriented, patient-centered,* or *qualitative* (Benton, Hamsher, Varney, & Spreen, 1983; Kaplan, 1988; Lezak, 1983), serves as a bridge between the Lurian and psychometric traditions and emphasizes the use of a flexible battery of procedures, consisting of a core set of tests and additional circumstance-specific procedures. Most of the tests composing the process-oriented battery are psychometrically reliable and valid, although the expressed purpose of the battery is clinical description and syndrome analysis.

In the early to mid-1980s, a series of articles debated the merits of these different techniques (Adams, 1980, 1984; Delis & Kaplan, 1983; Golden, 1980; Golden et al., 1982; Hutchinson, 1984; Spiers, 1984; Stambrook, 1983). The primary focus of these articles was on the Luria-Nebraska Neuropsychological Battery (LNNB; Golden, Hammeke, Purisch, & Moses, 1984; Golden & Maruish, 1986), Golden's standardization of portions of Luria's investigation, as compared to the HRNTB and process-oriented approaches. Underlying these debates, however, was a debate between battery-based or psychometric approaches to assessment versus more flexible approaches. Describing this debate, Goodglass (1994), in his Distinguished Award address at the 1993 American Board of Professional Psychology Convocation, stated:

> Given that both the first [battery-based] School of investigators and second [process-oriented school] were asking questions about brain injury and psychology in humans, their focus could hardly be more different. For the first, the question was whether there is evidence of brain damage. The implication, in the application of tests, was that one kind of evidence is as good as another, and all the bits could be pooled to give a general level of overall probability. In the second approach the question as to *whether* there is brain damage is rarely an issue; in most cases the subject is known to have suffered damage. Rather the issue is to define the deficit and to determine whether there is a selective relationship between lesion site and deficit symptoms—particularly whether such relationships are replicable across patients with similar deficit patterns. Tests that are developed within this framework, understandably, are targeted at a particular cognitive or perceptual ability. (p. 6)

Goodglass (1994) then continued:

> Clearly, cross-fertilization among the two approaches could only enrich the test repertory available to the psychologist confronted with a patient with known or suspected brain damage, because now one could choose from tests that were non-specific in their sensitivity to brain injury and supplement them with others that might point to a focus of injury. Such a blending was not uniformly accepted by all practitioners in what was beginning to be called neuropsychology. Differences in philosophy and approach persisted for a time. . . . (p. 6)

It seems, however, that debates regarding battery selection and approach to testing have largely faded into the past, perhaps indicative of a growth process for the field. Although neuropsychologists today can trace their training to one of these "schools," the clinical practice of most neuropsychologists is now more similar than different. Few would disagree that a certain measure of psychometric rigor is necessary in assessment, especially as neuropsychologists are called to task for the reliability and validity of their findings in forensic and other settings. At the same time, few would argue against observing and noting what the patient does as he or she solves tasks during evaluation. The same final score on a task can reflect many different paths to completion, and each of these different paths can have a different implication for the way in which the brain is functioning. Thus, although it is important to develop conclusions using the strict, psychometric rigor of battery-based approaches, such as those of Reitan (Reitan & Davison, 1974; Reitan & Wolfson, 1985), we cannot ignore the interactive nature of brain functioning, in the tradition of Luria (1980), and must also attend to how the patient completes the neuropsychological tasks.

ADVANCES IN NEUROSCIENCE RESEARCH

In addition to the changes in the field of clinical neuropsychology, there has been a growth of research on brain functioning over the past decade. Advances in neuroimaging technology, including magnetic resonance imaging (MRI), positron emission tomography (PET), and single photon emission computed tomography (SPECT), have made it possible for scientists to map brain regions associated with different aspects of cognitive, motor, and affective functioning (e.g., Andreasen, 1988; Belliveau et al., 1991; Crease, 1993; Kim et al., 1993; Sergent, Zuck, Terriah, & MacDonald, 1992; Talbot et al., 1991; Turkheimer, Yeo, Jones, & Bigler, 1990; Zatorre, Evans, Meyer, & Gjedde, 1992). Older neurodiagnostic methods, such as computerized axial tomography and electrophysiological studies, have markedly improved in their sensitivity to brain dysfunction. Topographic brain mapping has emerged as a useful tool for understanding and characterizing brain dysfunction (e.g., Duffy, 1986; John, Prichep, Fridman, & Easton, 1988), although not without controversy (Asbury, 1986; Duffy, Bartels, & Neff, 1986; Oken & Chiappa, 1986). Cognitive event-related potential (ERP) indices, such as the P-300, have been applied to research on a variety of disorders (e.g., Duncan, 1990; Duncan-Johnson, 1981; Halliday, Callaway, & Rosenthal, 1984; Handelsman et al., 1992; Harter, Diering, & Wood, 1988; Ollo, Johnson, & Grafman, 1991). Indeed, recognition of the explosion of research in the neurosciences led to the designation of the 1990s as "The Decade of the Brain."

With these advances in neurodiagnostic technology, the focus of neuropsychological assessment can now shift to its basis in behavior and cognition. Instead of being used primarily to detect and localize brain lesions, the data from assessment can be used to understand a patient's neurobehavioral competencies. This, in turn, can be applied to differential diagnosis of specific disorders and to treatment planning (Leonberger, 1989; Mapou, 1988b). It is this *behavioral* and, ultimately, *cognitive* nature of neuropsychological assessment that distinguishes it from more medically based neurodiagnostic technologies. Although such sophisticated technologies can provide valuable information on brain structure, metabolic activity, and electrophysiological activity, for the most part, these methods cannot provide information about a patient's *thinking, affect, or behavior.* Neuroimaging and electrophysiological studies are very useful diagnostically, but they cannot tell the clinician *what the patient is capable of doing*. Additionally, these methods cannot be viewed as "ecologically valid," as they provide no information on everyday functioning. Hence, it is clear that neuropsychological assessment still has an important role in the diagnosis and treatment of individuals with neurobehavioral disorders

SHIFTS IN THE DIRECTION OF NEUROPSYCHOLOGICAL RESEARCH

At the same time that there have been improvements in neurodiagnostic technology, there also have been advances in knowledge of the neuropsychological sequelae of different neurological and psychiatric disorders. Today, much more is known about the specific cognitive sequelae of neurobehavioral disorders seen in the clinic. Research has illustrated, for example, the types of cognitive profiles associated with (1) dementing disorders including Alzheimer's disease, Parkinson's disease, and Huntington's disease (Bondi & Kaszniak, 1991; Brandt, Corwin, & Krafft, 1992; Cummings, 1990; Monsch et al., 1994; Randolph, Braun, Goldberg, & Chase, 1993; Tröster et al., 1993); (2) traumatic brain injury (Levin, Benton, & Grossman, 1982; Levin, Grafman, & Eisenberg, 1987); (3) multiple sclerosis (Heaton, Nelson, Thompson, Burks, & Franklin, 1985; Huber et al., 1992; Rao et al., 1993; Ryan, Clark, Klonoff, & Paty, 1993); (4) HIV disease and AIDS (Grant & Heaton, 1990; Mapou & Law, 1994; Martin et al., 1992; Martin, Heyes, Salazar, Law, & Williams, 1993; Van Gorp et al., 1993); and (5) depression (Cassens, Wolfe, & Zola, 1990; Hill et al., 1992; Massman, Delis, Butters, Dupont, & Gillin, 1992), among others. Recent reserach also has provided new ways to detect malingering of neuropsychological deficits (Binder, 1993; Binder & Willis, 1991). Such information can be applied directly to differential diagnosis in the clinic. Because of this advancing knowledge, consultation requests have become more sophisticated, asking for increasingly focused responses to informed and specific questions.

As an indication of the explosion of knowledge regarding the cognitive sequelae of neurobehavioral disorders, consider that 10 years ago, there were, perhaps, only five journals solely devoted to clinical and experimental neuropsychology. Today, in comparison, there are probably close to 20 neuropsychological journals. In addition to the well-established journals, such as the *Journal of Clinical and Experimental Neuropsychology, Brain, Brain and Language,* and *Brain and Cognition,* there are many new journals including those published by major psychological (*Neuropsychology,* American Psychological Association) and neuropsychological (*Archives of Clinical Neuropsychology,* National Academy of Neuropsychology) organizations. Neurology and psychiatry journals now devote much space to neuropsychological research. There are also new topical journals (e.g., *Journal of Head Trauma Rehabilitation, Brain Injury*) that devote a substantial proportion of space to neuropsychological studies. One must also note the growing number of neuropsychology textbooks that are available. Six years ago, for example, the series of which this textbook is a part included only four volumes. Today, as this volume goes to press, there are more than 20 published textbooks in the series, and many more under review or in preparation. The dilemma, then, for today's research or clinical neuropsychologist, is not where to find information but, rather, how to keep up!

And what is the content of most of these publications? As suggested several years ago, there is no longer a need to evaluate the sensitivity of neuropsychological tests to brain damage per se (Leonberger, 1989; Mapou, 1988b). Rather, it was proposed that research should focus on developing tests sensitive to different aspects of cognitive function, as associated with different types of brain disorders. A review of the tables of contents of recent journal issues and textbooks confirms that this is the direction that most researchers have taken. Studies that solely evaluate the sensitivity of tests or test batteries to brain damage are now quite rare, but studies examining the cognitive sequelae of neurobehavioral disorders are frequent and constitute much of what is published.

This book was developed to add to the literature on clinical neuropsychological assessment. It was designed as a textbook that would introduce the reader to (1) how to assess various realms of cognition and (2) nonbattery-based approaches that applied these techniques. It was designed to be accessible to the clinician, while being grounded in empirical research on brain–behavior relationships. Most of the contributors do some combination of research and clinical practice. Many will be well known to the reader from the research arena, and many are Diplomates in Clinical Neuropsychology. Therefore, these contributors bring a unique perspective to clinical neuropsychological assessment of cognitive function.

OVERVIEW OF CHAPTERS

Assessment of Specific Aspects of Cognition

A comprehensive neuropsychological evaluation should combine information on sensory and motor functions with assessment of each of the following cognitive domains: arousal and attention; executive, problem-solving, and reasoning abilities; language functions; visuospatial abilities; and learning and memory. Although the depth of assessment in a particular area is often determined by the referral question, when complete, the evaluation should provide at least some information about each of these realms. Part I of the book provides guidelines on the clinical assessment of these cognitive domains.

Understanding deficits in attention is critical to understanding observed difficulties in other aspects of cognition. Learning and memory deficits, for example, can be due primarily to impairment in attention and initial processing of information. Thus, Chapter 2 is devoted to assessment of attention across the lifespan. Allan Mirsky's contributions to research on attention are well known. In 1987, Mirsky outlined an "attention battery" that illustrated the multifaceted nature of attention and, at the same time, provided a model of attention that clinicians could apply to assessment, using available, standardized measures (Mirksy, 1987). In Chapter 2, Mirsky and his research collaborators, Bryan Fantie and Janet Tatman, review the elements of attention and the attention battery, describe empirical support for the model, provide normative data for the measures across the lifespan, and illustrate application of the battery to clinical practice.

The assessment of executive, reasoning, and problem-solving abilities is often difficult (Lezak, 1982; Shallice & Burgess, 1991). The structure of the neuropsychological laboratory frequently makes it hard to elicit deficits that are observed under less-structured and more novel conditions, such as those faced by a patient at work or at home. Yet, these deficits can be profoundly disabling to patients and their significant others. Similar to deficits in attention, deficits in executive, reasoning, and problem-solving abilities have the potential to affect expression of other cognitive skills. Felicia Goldstein and Robert Green have researched the effects of various neurobehavioral disorders, including traumatic brain injury, dementia, and focal brain lesions, on these skills. In Chapter 3, they summarize several models of executive, reasoning, and problem-solving abilities. These authors illustrate the difficulties of assessment in this realm, but cogently and convincingly show that a range of instruments are available for clinical assessment and can provide a wealth of information on a patient's functioning.

It has become increasingly apparent that the traditional syndromes of language disorder, based largely on the Wernicke-Lichtheim model of the late nineteenth century, fail to capture the subtlety of language dysfunction following neurological insult. To address these limitations, cognitive neuropsychologists, in collaboration with psycholinguists and speech/language pathologists, have developed new models of language functioning, which break language into a number of processing steps and modules, each of which can be impaired selectively. They have developed experimental assessment measures to evaluate each of these processing steps and modules. David Caplan has been a pioneer of research in this area. In Chapter 4, Caplan summarizes current thinking on the cognitive neuropsychology of language. He provides an introduction to the *Psycholinguistic Assessment of Language,* which he developed in collaboration with Daniel Bub, and includes a case illustration of its clinical application.

Disorders of written language, too, have been conceptualized using cognitive neuropsychological models. Perhaps one of the earliest cognitive neuropsychological models was the model of reading, developed by Max Coltheart and colleagues in the 1970s (Coltheart, 1985). Using principles of double dissociation, these researchers demonstrated that there were two different paths for reading single words, each of which could be selectively impaired. In one path, words are sounded out phonetically, but in the second path, the visual form of a word is recognized automatically, without reference to its phonetic structure. In the years that have followed, the model has been investigated further and refined. Guila Glosser and Rhonda Friedman have collaborated on studies of reading and writing in patients with focal brain lesions. In Chapter 5, Glosser and Friedman summarize current thinking regarding the cognitive neuropsychology of reading. They further the clinical application of a cognitive neuropsychological model of reading by showing how widely available clinical instruments can be used to test the different modules in the model. In their case illustrations, they also show how a cognitive neuropsychological model can contribute to treatment of a reading disorder.

It was originally thought that disorders of visuospatial, visuoperceptual, and visuoconstructional skills were due solely to dysfunction of the right cerebral hemisphere, in contrast to lateralization of language to the left hemisphere. Over the past 30 years, research has shown that disruption of visuocognitive disorders is more complex than originally thought and that both the right and left hemispheres make different contributions to visuocognitive skills. Furthermore, impairment of attention and executive functions can affect the expression of visuocognitive abilities, even in the absence of a frank deficit in visuospatial perception. Daniel Capruso, Kerry Hamsher, and Arthur Benton have collaborated on studies of visuocognitive disorders in patients with focal and diffuse brain disorder. Hamsher and Benton also have developed several measures of these skills, described in Benton et al. (1983). In their chapter, Capruso, Hamsher, and Benton provide a comprehensive, empirically based framework for assessment of visuocognitive disorders, illustrating the different ways in which visual processing can be impaired by brain dysfunction.

Difficulty with learning and memory is, perhaps, the most frequent complaint presented by patients seen for neuropsychological evaluation. Yet, what is reported as a "memory" problem often turns out to reflect a deficit in another aspect of cognition. Hence, learning and memory must be viewed as requiring the intact functioning of several different cognitive systems. For this reason, assessment of learning and memory incorporates results not only from direct measures of these skills, but from measures of all other cognitive skills. Glenn Larrabee and Thomas Crook have collaborated on research on state-of-the-art tools for clinical assessment of learning and memory. In Chapter 7, Larrabee and Crook outline a framework for assessment of learning and memory and review instruments available for assessment of the different components. They conclude, as do the other contributors, with an illustration of their approach.

Specific Approaches to Neuropsychological Assessment

In Part II, attention is turned to several assessment approaches, the primary emphases of which are on assessment of cognition. In contrast to battery-based approaches, all of these approaches do not use a fixed set of measures, but, rather, select measures that are most applicable to the task at hand. Although the particular measures and techniques may differ among approaches, all have several factors in common that include (1) delineating the cognitive strengths and weaknesses of the patient, (2) supplementing quantitative data with information on the process by which the patient completes neuropsychological tasks, (3) analyzing the types of errors the patient makes, and (4) using this information to draw conclusions about diagnosis and to make recommendations for treatment. Without exception, all are well grounded in current knowledge of brain–behavior relationships.

The work of A. R. Luria has heavily influenced the conceptualization and clinical assessment of brain disorders in the twentieth century. Most clinicians today use some of Luria's techniques as part of their clinical evaluations, and some of these measures have found their way into standardized measures of intellectual functioning (e.g., Kaufman Assessment Battery for Children; Kaufman & Kaufman, 1983). Kasper Jørgensen and Anne-Lise Christensen collaborate on the application of Luria's framework and methods to clinical practice and research. Christensen was the first to make many of Luria's techniques and stimuli available to Western neuropsychologists. In Chapter 8, Jørgensen and Christensen provide a succinct introduction to Luria's model of brain function. They place Luria's model in context, by illustrating how it grew out of the *zeitgeist* of the times in the former Soviet Union. The emphasis of the approach is on understanding how neurological disorder affects the functional systems of the brain, and this is accomplished through careful examination of different cognitive and motor systems. In contrast to other described approaches, there is little emphasis on normative comparisons; each patient is seen as an "individual" experiment. Jørgensen and Christensen provide several excellent illustrations of how Luria's methods are applied in modern clinical neuropsychological assessment.

With an emphasis on the development of processing models of brain function, cognitive neuropsychology has developed somewhat separately from more clinically based approaches, with the latter's roots in psychometric methods, clinical psychology, and behavioral neurology. The influence of cognitive neuropsychology on clinical assessment, diagnosis, and treatment, however, is expanding rapidly. Although its emphasis has been on the development of cognitive models of brain dysfunction, in an effort to understand the individual patient, increasing attention is being given to the development of more standardized and psychometrically based methods of assessment. Janice Kay and Sue Franklin have conducted research on the cognitive neuropsychology of spoken and written language disorders. Recently, they have developed the *Psycholinguistic Assessments of Language Processing in Aphasia*, a standardized cognitive neuropsychological battery for the assessment of aphasia. In Chapter 9, Kay and Franklin outline the origins and basic principles of cognitive neuropsychology and the application of these principles to clinical assessment. They use assessment of word-retrieval difficulties as a specific illustration of the technique, but note that the principles apply to assessment of other cognitive disorders. Their chapter provides the reader with an introduction to the cognitive neuropsychological method and its application to clinical assessment.

All of the approaches in Part II have in common the use of hypothesis testing. In each, the clinical neuropsychologist begins evaluation with hypotheses about the patient's deficits, based on history and initial presentation, then administers measures to test these hypotheses, and finally administers additional measures or tests limits to assess hypotheses developed during initial testing. Kevin Walsh is largely credited with the development of the field of clinical neuropsychology in Australia and has described the application of hypothesis testing to standardized, clinical instruments. His approach has been likened, in many ways, to the Boston Process Approach of Edith Kaplan, because of its emphasis on how the patient solves the particular task, in addition to the final score achieved. In Chapter 10, Walsh outlines the principles and methods of his approach, showing how, similar to the Boston Process Approach, it is more a philosophy of assessment rather than a method strictly based in specific instruments. Throughout the chapter, he uses case illustrations to show how the techniques apply to assessment of very different disorders of brain function.

Integration

How does one integrate process-oriented models with those emphasizing the development of models of cognition? Although the former emphasize an understanding of cognitive functioning as a goal of assessment, they are based less on empirically derived models of cognitive functioning. Cognitive neuropsychological models, although empirically based, have, until recently, offered less to the practicing clinician, because methods were not widely available and most were not standardized. Previously, I described an integration of the Boston Process and cognitive neuropsychological approaches (Mapou, 1988a). In Part III, Chapter 11, I describe a framework for assessment that expands on the original work and also integrates the work of contributors from Parts I and II. I hope to demonstrate how many standardized and readily available instruments fit into the framework and how they can be used to provide a comprehensive undersatnding of a patient's strengths and weaknesses.

Where are we going as a field, particularly now that neurodiagnostic technology has rendered the need for assessment of "brain damage" less necessary? Along with cognitive neuropsychology, is there now a basis for cognitive neuropsychiatry or cognitive neurology that can be applied to clinical assessment? What might the face of clinical neuropsychological assessment be in 5 or 10 years? In Chapter 12, Jack Spector discusses the application of cognitive neuropsychology to clincal neuropsychology and the implications for clinical practice.

In summary, the reader will find here what are believed to be state-of-the-art reviews of current approaches to assessment that are cognitively based, by leaders in the fields of experimental and clinical neuropsychology who, as Goodglass (1994) noted, *still* tend to be the same individuals even in the twentieth century. It is hoped that this work will be useful both to those just beginning their training and to seasoned clinicians looking to expand or to enhance their current methods of assessment. It is believed that these methods offer much to the clinician treating individuals with brain disorders, as an understanding of cognitive strengths and weaknesses better lends itself to the development of compensatory strategies to deal with difficulties.

REFERENCES

Adams, K. M. (1980). In search of Luria's battery: A false start. *Journal of Consulting and Clinical Psychology, 48*, 511–516.

Adams, K. M. (1984). Luria left in the lurch: Unfulfilled promises are not valid tests. *Journal of Clinical Neuropsychology, 6*, 455–458.

Andreasen, N. C. (1988). Brain imaging: Applications in psychiatry. *Science, 239*, 1381–1388.

Asbury, A. K. (1986). Statistical issues concerning computerized analysis of brainwave topography: An editorial comment. *Annals of Neurology, 19*, 497.

Belliveau, J. W., Kennedy, D. N., McKinstry, R. C., Buchbinder, B. R., Weisskoff, R. M., Cohen, M. S., Vevea, J. M., Brady, T. J., & Rosen, B. R. (1991). Functional mapping of the human visual cortex by magnetic resonance imaging. *Science, 254*, 716–719.

Benton, A. L. (1992). Clinical neuropsychology: 1960–1990. *Journal of Clinical and Experimental Neuropsychology, 14*, 407–417.

Benton, A. L., Hamsher, K. deS., Varney, N. R., & Spreen, O. (1983). *Contributions to neuropsychological assessment.* New York: Oxford University Press.
Binder, L. M. (1993). Assessment of malingering after mild head trauma with the Portland Digit Recognition Test. *Journal of Clinical and Experimental Neuropsychology, 15,* 170–182.
Binder, L. M., & Willis, S. C. (1991). Assessment of motivation after financially compensable minor head trauma. *Psychological Assessment: A Journal of Consulting and Clinical Psychology, 3,* 175–181.
Bondi, M., & Kaszniak, A. W. (1991). Implicit and explicit memory in Alzheimer's disease and Parkinson's disease. *Journal of Clinical and Experimental Neuropsychology, 13,* 339–358.
Brandt, J., Corwin, J., & Krafft, L. (1992). Is verbal recognition memory really different in Huntington's and Alzheimer's disease? *Journal of Clinical and Experimental Neuropsychology, 14,* 773–784.
Cassens, G., Wolfe, L., & Zola, M. (1990). The neuropsychology of depressions. *Journal of Neuropsychiatry and Clinical Neurosciences, 2,* 202–213.
Christensen, A.-L. (1979). *Luria's neuropsychological investigation* (2nd ed.). Copenhagen: Munksgaard.
Coltheart, M. (1985). Cognitive neuropsychology and the study of reading. In M. Posner & O. S. M. Marin (Eds.), *Attention and performance XI* (pp. 3–37). Hillsdale, NJ: Lawrence Erlbaum.
Crease, R. P. (1993). Biomedicine in the age of imaging. *Science, 261,* 554–561.
Cummings, J. L. (Ed.). (1990). *Subcortical dementia.* New York: Oxford University Press.
Delis, D. C., & Kaplan, E. (1983). Hazards of a standardized neuropsychological test with low content validity: Comment on the Luria-Nebraska Neuropsychological Battery. *Journal of Consulting and Clinical Psychology, 51,* 396–398.
Duffy, F. H. (1986). *Topographic mapping of brain electrical activity.* Stoneham, MA: Butterworth.
Duffy, F. H., Bartels, P. H., & Neff, R. (1986). A response to Oken and Chiappa. *Annals of Neurology, 19,* 494–497.
Duncan, C. C. (1990). Current issues in the application of P300 to research in schizophrenia. In E. R. Straube & K. Hahlwag (Eds.), *Schizophrenia: Concepts, vulnerability, and intervention* (pp. 117–134). Berlin: Springer-Verlag.
Duncan-Johnson, C. (1981). P300 latency: A new metric of information processing. *Psychophysiology, 18,* 207–215.
Golden, C. J. (1980). In reply to Adam's: In search of Luria's battery: A false start. *Journal of Consulting and Clinical Psychology, 48,* 517–521.
Golden, C. J., Ariel, R. N., Moses, J. A., Wilkening, G. N., McKay, S. E., & MacInnes, W. D. (1982). Analytic techniques in the interpretation of the Luria-Nebraska Neuropsychological Battery. *Journal of Consulting and Clinical Psychology, 50,* 40–48.
Golden, C. J., Hammeke, T. A., Purisch, A. D., & Moses, J. A. (1984). *A manual for the administration and interpretation of the Luria-Nebraska Neuropsychological Battery.* Los Angeles: Western Psychological Services.
Golden, C. J., & Maruish, M. (1986). The Luria-Nebraska Neuropsychological Battery. In D. Wedding, A. M. Horton, & J. Webster (Eds.), *The neuropsychology handbook* (pp. 161–193). New York: Springer.
Goodglass, H. (1994). Diversity and unity in neuropsychology: A perspective on the discipline. *The Diplomate, 13*(2), 5–7.
Grant, I., & Heaton, R. K. (1990). Human immunodeficiency virus-type 1 (HIV-1) and the brain. *Journal of Consulting and Clinical Psychology, 58,* 22–30.
Halliday, R., Callaway, E., & Rosenthal, J. H. (1984). The visual ERP predicts clinical response to methylphenidate in hyperactive children. *Psychophysiology, 21,* 114–121.
Handelsman, L. Horvath, T., Aronson, M., Schroeder, M., Jacobson, J., Wiener, J., Peterson, A., Holloway, K., Ness, R., Herman, S., & Maurer, G. (1992). Auditory event-related potentials in HIV-1 infection: A study in the drug-user risk group. *Journal of Neuropsychiatry and Clinical Neurosciences, 4,* 294–302.
Harter, M. R., Diering, S., & Wood, F. B. (1988). I. Separate brain potential characteristics in children

with reading disability and attention-deficit disorder: Relevance-independent effects. *Brain and Cognition, 7*, 54–86.

Hartman, D. E. (1991). Reply to Reitan: Unexamined premises and the evolution of clinical neuropsychology. *Archives of Clinical Neuropsychology, 6*, 147–165.

Heaton, R. K., Nelson, L. M., Thompson, D. S., Burks, J. S., & Franklin, G. M. (1985). Neuropsychological findings in relapsing-remitting and chronic-progressive multiple sclerosis. *Journal of Consulting and Clinical Psychology, 53*, 103–110.

Hill, C. D., Stoudemire, A., Morris, R., Martino-Saltzman, D., Markwalter, H. R., & Lewison, B. J. (1992). Dysnomia in the differential diagnosis of major depression, depression-related cognitive dysfunction, and dementia. *Journal of Neuropsychiatry and Clinical Neurosciences, 4*, 64–69.

Huber, S. J., Bornstein, R. A., Rammohan, K. W., Christy, J. A., Chakeres, D. W., & McGhee, R. B. (1992). Magnetic resonance imaging correlates of neuropsychological impairment in multiple sclerosis. *Journal of Neuropsychiatry and Clinical Neurosciences, 4*, 152–158.

Hutchinson, G. L. (1984). The Luria-Nebraska Neuropsychological Battery controversy: A reply to Spiers. *Journal of Consulting and Clinical Psychology, 52*, 539–545.

John, E. R., Prichep, L. S., Fridman, J., & Easton, P. (1988). Neurometrics: Computer-assisted differential diagnosis of brain dysfunctions. *Science, 239*, 162–169.

Kaplan, E. (1988). A process approach to neuropsychological assessment. In T. Boll & B. K. Bryant (Eds.), *Clinical neuropsychology and brain function: Research, measurement, and practice* (pp. 129–167). Washington, DC: American Psychological Association.

Kaufman, A. S., & Kaufman, N. L. (1983). *Administration and scoring manual for the Kaufman Assessment Battery for Children*. Circle Pines, MN: American Guidance Service.

Kim, S.-G., Ashe, J., Hendrich, K., Ellermann, J. M., Merkle, H., Ugurbil, K., & Georgopoulos, A. P. (1993). Functional magnetic resonance imaging of motor cortex: Hemispheric asymmetry and handedness. *Science, 261*, 615–617.

Kolb, B., & Whishaw, I. Q. (1990). *Fundamentals of human neuropsychology* (3rd ed.). New York: W. H. Freeman.

Leonberger, F. T. (1989). The question of organicity: Is it still functional? *Professional Psychology: Research and Practice, 20*, 411–414.

Levin, H. S., Benton, A. L., & Grossman, R. G. (1982). *Neurobehavioral consequences of closed head injury*. New York: Oxford University Press.

Levin, H. S., Grafman, J., & Eisenberg, H. M. (Eds.). (1987). *Neurobehavioral recovery from head injury*. New York: Oxford University Press.

Lezak, M. D. (1982). The problem of assessing executive functions. *International Journal of Psychology, 17*, 281–297.

Lezak, M. D. (1983). *Neuropsychological assessment* (2nd ed.). New York: Oxford University Press.

Luria, A. R. (1980). *Higher cortical functions in man* (2nd ed.). New York: Basic Books.

Mapou, R. L. (1988a). An integrated approach to the neuropsychological assessment of cognitive function. In J. M. Williams & C. J. Long (Eds.), *Cognitive approaches to neuropsychology* (pp. 101–122). New York: Plenum Press.

Mapou, R. L. (1988b). Testing to detect brain damage: An alternative to what may no longer be useful. *Journal of Clinical and Experimental Neuropsychology, 10*, 271–278.

Mapou, R. L., & Law, W. A. (1994). Neurobehavioral aspects of HIV disease and AIDS: An update. *Professional Psychology: Research and Practice, 25*, 132–140.

Martin, A., Heyes, M. P., Salazar, A. M., Kampen, D. L., Williams, J., Law, W. A., Coats, M. E., & Markey, S. P. (1992). Progressive slowing of reaction time and increasing cerebrospinal fluid concentrations of quinolinic acid in HIV-infected individuals, *Journal of Neuropsychiatry and Clinical Neurosciences, 4*, 270–279.

Martin, A., Heyes, M. P., Salazar, A. M., Law, W. A., & Williams, J. (1993). Impaired motor-skill learning, slowed reaction time, and elevated cerebrospinal fluid quinolinic acid in a subgroup of HIV-infected individuals. *Neuropsychology, 7*, 149–157.

Massman, P. J., Delis, D. C., Butters, N., Dupont, R. M., & Gillin, J. C. (1992). The subcortical dysfunction hypothesis of memory deficits in depression: Neuropsychological validation in a subgroup of patients. *Journal of Clinical and Experimental Neuropsychology, 14*, 687–706.

Meier, M. J. (1992). Modern clinical neuropsychology in historical perspective. *American Psychologist, 47,* 550–558.

Mirsky, A. F. (1987). Behavioral and psychophysiological markers of disordered attention. *Environmental Health Perspectives, 74,* 191–199.

Mirsky, A. F., & Duncan, C. C. (1987). An introduction to modern techniques of clinical neuropsychology. *Advances in Psychosomatic Medicine, 17,* 167–184.

Monsch, A. U., Bondi, M. W., Butters, N., Paulsen, J. S., Salmon, D. P., Brugger, P., & Swensen, M. R. (1994). A comparison of category and letter fluency in Alzheimer's disease and Huntington's disease. *Neuropsychology, 8,* 25–30.

Oken, B. S., & Chiappa, K. H. (1986). Statistical issues concerning computerized analysis of brainwave topography. *Annals of Neurology, 19,* 493–494.

Ollo, C., Johnson, R., Jr., & Grafman, J. (1991). Signs of cognitive change in HIV disease: An event-related potential study. *Neurology, 41,* 209–215.

Randolph, C., Braun, A. R., Goldberg, T. E., & Chase, T. N. (1993). Semantic fluency in Alzheimer's, Parkinson's, and Huntington's disease: Dissociation of storage and retrieval failures. *Neuropsychology, 7,* 82–88.

Rao, S. M., Grafman, J., DiGiulio, D., Mittenberg, W., Bernardin, L., Leo, G. J., Luchetta, T., & Unverzagt, F. (1993). Memory dysfunction in multiple sclerosis: Its relation to working memory, semantic encoding, and implicit learning. *Neuropsychology, 7,* 364–374.

Reitan, R. M., & Davison, L. A. (Eds.). (1974). *Clinical neuropsychology: Current status and applications.* Washington, DC: Winston & Sons.

Reitan, R. M., & Wolfson, D. (1985). *The Halstead-Reitan Neuropsychological Test Battery: Theory and clinical interpretation.* Tucson, AZ: Neuropsychology Press.

Ryan, L., Clark, C. M., Klonoff, H., & Paty, D. (1993). Models of cognitive deficit and statistical hypotheses: Multiple sclerosis, an example. *Journal of Clinical and Experimental Neuropsychology, 15,* 563–577.

Sergent, J., Zuck, E., Terriah, S., & MacDonald, B. (1992). Distributed neural network underlying musical sight-reading and keyboard performance. *Science, 257,* 106–109.

Shallice, T., & Burgess, P. (1991). Deficits in strategy application following frontal lobe damage. *Brain, 114,* 727–741.

Spiers, P. A. (1984). Have they come to praise Luria or to bury him: The Luria-Nebraska Battery controversy. *Journal of Consulting and Clinical Psychology, 49,* 331–341.

Stambrook, M. (1983). The Luria-Nebraska Neuropsychological Battery: A promise that *may* be partly fulfilled. *Journal of Clinical Neuropsychology, 5,* 247–269.

Talbot, J. D., Marrett, S., Evans, A. C., Meyer, E., Bushnell, M. C., & Duncan, G. H. (1991). Multiple representations of pain in human cerebral cortex. *Science, 251,* 1355–1358.

Tröster, A. I., Butters, N., Salmon, D. P., Cullum, C. M., Jacobs, D., Brandt, J., & White, R. F. (1993). The diagnostic utility of savings scores: Differentiating Alzheimer's and Huntington's diseases with the Logical Memory and Visual Reproduction tests. *Journal of Clinical and Experimental Neuropsychology, 15,* 773–788.

Turkheimer, E., Yeo, R. A., Jones, C. L., & Bigler, E. D. (1990). Quantitative assessment of covariation between neuropsychological function and location of naturally occurring lesions in humans. *Journal of Clinical and Experimental Neuropsychology, 12,* 549–565.

Van Gorp, W. G., Hinkin, C., Satz, P. Miller, E. N., Weisman, J., Holston, S., Drebing, C., Marcotte, T. D., & Dixon, W. (1993). Subtypes of HIV-related neuropsychological functioning: A cluster analysis approach. *Neuropsychology, 7,* 62–72.

Walsh, K. (1987). *Neuropsychology: A clinical approach* (2nd ed.). Edinburgh: Churchill Livingstone.

Zatorre, R. J., Evans, A. C., Meyer, E., & Gjedde, A. (1992). Lateralization of phonetic and pitch discrimination in speech processing. *Science, 256,* 846–849.

I

Assessment of Specific Functions

2

Assessment of Attention across the Lifespan

ALLAN F. MIRSKY, BRYAN D. FANTIE, and JANET E. TATMAN

INTRODUCTION

Whenever the human central nervous system is compromised, whether as the result of disease, trauma, fatigue, or intoxication, the higher cognitive functions suffer. This cognitive machinery is typically described and conceptually divided by hypothetical constructs such as memory, language, and attention. These constructs are not unitary entities but, rather, constitute integrated medleys of more elemental processes.

Since the smooth operation of the cognitive ensemble is dependent on the integrity and harmony of its components, a failure anywhere in the system will likely result in diminished output. Although the precise details of what is going wrong can vary from case to case, depending on just what subsystem has faltered, the net result will be a reduced capacity in overall functioning. Thus, it is not surprising that memory problems, language difficulty (especially with word finding), and impaired concentration and attention are the most frequent complaints of patients, whatever the etiology of their individual problem.

In many clinical neuropsychological examinations, the assessment of the critical function of attention is conducted in a haphazard fashion. Despite the fact that no unambiguous assessment of memory can be made without a systematic evaluation of attentional functions, attention is often measured in an informal manner, if it is evaluated at all. What might at first appear to be deficits in learning and memory may actually be the secondary results of the patient's impaired ability to attend effectively

ALLAN F. MIRSKY • Laboratory of Psychology and Psychopathology, National Institute of Mental Health, Bethesda, Maryland 20892-1366. BRYAN D. FANTIE and JANET E. TATMAN • Human Neuropsychology Laboratory, The American University, Washington, DC 20016-8062.

Clinical Neuropsychological Assessment: A Cognitive Approach, edited by Robert L. Mapou and Jack Spector. Plenum Press, New York, 1995.

to the relevant stimuli. The inability to focus on the task at hand can produce misleading difficulties in any type of test.

All too often attention is conceptualized and, consequently, treated as a unitary entity. This follows the implicit assumption that attention is a basic cognitive skill underlying and supporting the "higher" cognitive functions. Attention, however, consists of a number of basic capacities. The ability to detect the nature and contents of the environment, through sensory receptors, is not sufficient for survival in a complex habitat.

When necessary, one must also be able to select the appropriate stimulus on which to act from all the information that bombards the sensorium. Having selected, one must then be able to maintain fixation on the target, thereby resisting the tendency to be attracted by competing, but irrelevant or redundant, stimuli. When required, one must be able to terminate one's fixation and switch one's focus to another target. Sometimes one must carry out two functions simultaneously, splitting one's attention between a main target while monitoring what is happening in the periphery. The specific dysfunction will determine the nature of the resulting behavioral deficit. The ubiquitous complaint "I have difficulty with concentration" can have many meanings.

Formal clinical examinations are frequently limited to one sensory modality. Emphasis is, almost exclusively, confined to the visual domain. It is quite clear, however, that specific deficits can occur within other modalities. For example, recent research has supported the conclusion that patients with absence epilepsy can be distinguished reliably from controls and patients with other types of epilepsy on their performance of an auditory task requiring sustained attention (Duncan, 1988; Mirsky, 1992). Patients with schizophrenia also show this enhanced auditory attention deficit (Mirsky et al., 1992).

Specific measures of attention are often derived from the examiner's preconception of the tests that best assess attention, which is, in turn, frequently an incidental function of the other tests employed to evaluate the patient. Thus, for example, if the Wechsler Adult Intelligence Scale-Revised (WAIS-R); Wechsler, 1981), the Wechsler Intelligence Scale for Children-Third Edition (WISC-III; Wechsler, 1991), or one of their predecessors, such as the WAIS (Wechsler, 1955) or WISC-R (Wechsler, 1974), is being used, then scores on the Digit Span and Digit Symbol (or Coding in the WISC-III) subtests and/or the Arithmetic subtest may be used to provide indices of attention. If the Halstead-Reitan Neuropsychological Battery (Reitan & Davidson, 1974; Reitan & Tarshes, 1959; Reitan & Wolfson, 1985) forms the basis of the assessment, then scores on the Trail Making Test or Seashore Rhythm Test might form the basis of an evaluation of attention or concentration.

We would consider these kinds of assessment methods (and the statements and judgments based on them) to be rather primitive. They are, however, clearly a cut above those evaluations in which the sole basis of the assessment is the examiner's clinical impression. The most preferred means of assessment, and the most defensible, involves the use of a test or, as will be seen, a group of tests, that has the following characteristics:

1. They measure different aspects or components of attention, thus recognizing that attentional functions are as highly articulated as mnemonic functions.

2. The reliability and validity of the measures have been established.
3. The independent factor structure of the tests is known.
4. Data exist for persons of different neurodiagnostic categories.
5. Normative data for the tests exist, preferably for groups of different ages and educational and socioeconomic (and/or cultural) backgrounds.

The last criterion is of particular importance if the tests are to be used cross-culturally or to evaluate the neuropsychological status of persons whose background is other than white, well educated, middle class, since one cannot conclude a priori that normative data from one group will necessarily apply to a group with different demographic characteristics (e.g., nonwhites, less well educated, working class). No group of tests satisfies all of these criteria. Nevertheless, we believe that we are able to present a reasonable proposal aimed at the development of competent assessment of attentional functions.

As we stated earlier, attention is multifaceted, and the quest to dissociate it into basic but still behaviorally meaningful components remains a challenge. Cognitive psychologists, in particular, have been quite fruitful in their exploration and discovery of a number of the more finely grained aspects of attention. These include arousal, effort, and intensity (e.g., Kahneman, 1973); degree of alertness, selection, and capacity (e.g., Craik & Byrd, 1982; Posner & Boies, 1971); focused and divided attention (e.g., McDowd & Craik, 1988; Somberg & Salthouse, 1982); and search and detection, automatization, consistency, and complex attentional processing (e.g., Schneider, Dumas, & Shiffrin, 1984; Schneider & Shiffrin, 1977; Shiffrin & Schneider, 1977). Cognitive neuroscientists interested in underlying physiological mechanisms have examined the attentional elements of anticipation, sensory analysis, the orienting response, and habituation (e.g., Campbell, Hayne, & Richardson, 1992; Posner & Petersen, 1990). Most, if not all, of this work focused on normal subjects.

Within the context of specifying the character of the attentional defect associated with schizophrenia, Zubin (1975) divided attention into three putatively more fundamental processes. These were designated as "selection," "maintenance," and "shift." Zubin concluded that, in schizophrenia, although selection and maintenance functions remain essentially normal, there is a deficit in shifting attentional focus. Subsequently, while also studying schizophrenics, Mirsky and several colleagues (Mirsky, 1988; Mirsky, Silberman, Latz, & Nagler, 1985; Nagler & Mirsky, 1985) organized a new battery specifically concerned with tests of attention based, in part, on Zubin's earlier work. A series of prior publications has described this factor analytically based model for the clinical neuropsychological assessment of attention, the Laboratory of Psychology and Psychopathology-National Institute of Mental Health (LPP-NIMH) Attention Battery (Mirsky, 1987, 1988, 1989; Mirsky, Anthony, Duncan, Ahearn, & Kellam, 1991). Since its inception, the LPP-NIMH Attention Battery has been administered to a spectrum of clinical populations (e.g., patients with petit mal and complex partial seizure disorders [Duncan, 1988; Mirsky, 1992], anorexia nervosa and bulimia nervosa [Jones, Duncan, Brouwers, & Mirsky, 1991], affective disorders, and closed head injuries) and to normal subjects, including a large sample of public school children (Mirsky et al., 1991).

THE LPP-NIMH ATTENTION BATTERY AND THE ELEMENTS OF ATTENTION

The Adult Sample

A summary description of the adult sample appears in Table 2.1. The table also contains the mean scores on the 13 attention test measures derived from the eight tests of the battery. As presently constituted, the adult version of the LPP-NIMH Attention Battery includes eight standard neuropsychological measures tapping different aspects or elements of attention identified by factor analysis (Mirsky, 1987, 1988, 1989; Mirsky et al., 1991). Principal components analyses revealed four factors (Table 2.2), three of which are comparable to Zubin's proposed elements of attention. These four factors explained 80% of the battery's variance in the scores of the group of adults (203 neuropsychiatric patients and normal control subjects) and 65% of its variance in 435 children attending public schools. The first factor comprises loadings from four tests of perceptual-motor speed or focusing, including Digit Symbol Substitution, Stroop, Letter Cancellation, and Trail Making, Parts A and B. The first factor would

TABLE 2.1. Descriptive Variables and Attention Test Battery Scores: Adult Sample ($N = 203$)

Measure	Mean	SD
Descriptive variables		
Age	28.4	8.9
Education level (years)	14.7	2.1
WAIS-R Full Scale IQ	109.6	14.6
WAIS-R Performance IQ	107.0	14.7
WAIS-R Verbal IQ	109.9	14.9
Attention test scores[a]		
WAIS-R Digit Span	11.3	2.7
WAIS-R Arithmetic	10.9	2.5
WAIS-R Digit Symbol Substitution	11.5	2.9
Stroop Test	48.6	8.4
Talland Letter Cancellation	73.4	15.6
Trail Making, Part A	31.2	18.6
Trail Making, Part B	61.7	38.2
CPT Correct Responses (%) (CPT Hits)[b]	94.0	10.6
CPT Commission Errors (%)	1.3	2.0
CPT Reaction Time (ms) (CPT RT)	447.7	69.9
Wisconsin Card Sorting Test (WCST) # of Categories	5.5	1.2
Wisconsin Card Sorting Test (WCST) % Correct	79.3	12.3
Wisconsin Card Sorting Test (WCST) Errors	21.1	17.9

[a]The scores on these tests were computed as described in Mirsky et al., 1991, and are the variables that were entered into the principal components (or factor) analysis.

[b]The decision to include correct responses (CPT Hits), commission errors (CPT Comm.) and reaction time (CPT RT) in this analysis and in those reported in other tables was made in order to describe the CPT (vigilance) performance more completely. This is supported by Parasuraman's (1986) statement, "Three main measures are required to evaluate vigilance performance: the target detection rate, false detection rate, and reaction time" (p. 43–33). From Mirsky et al. (1991). Analysis of the elements of attention: A neuropsychological approach. *Neuropsychology Review, 2*(2), 109–145.

TABLE 2.2. Rotated Factor (Component) Patterns: Adult Sample

	Factor 1	Factor 2	Factor 3	Factor 4
WAIS-R Digit Span	.22	.19	.02	*.80*
WAIS-R Arithmetic	.17	.13	.28	*.72*
WAIS-R Digit Symbol Substitution	*.82*[a]	.07	.12	.26
Stroop Test	*.69*	.24	.27	.29
Letter Cancellation	*.81*	.17	.22	.18
Trail Making, Part A	*.70*	.21	.43	−.06
Trail Making, Part B	*.63*	.34	.45	.14
CPT Hits	.32	.25	*.86*	.11
CPT Commission Errors	.33	.27	*.83*	.11
CPT Reaction Time	.18	−.10	*.81*	.16
WCST # of Categories	.22	*.89*	.16	.08
WCST % Correct	.17	*.94*	.09	.17
WCST Errors	.17	*.95*	.09	.18
Variance Explained	31.8	30.3	27.3	15.0
Proposed Identity of Factor	Perceptual-Motor Speed	Flexibility	Vigilance	Numerical-Mnemonic
Element of Attention	*Focus-Execute*	*Shift*	*Sustain*	*Encode*

[a]Italicized loadings are the highest within a column and were used in the interpretation of the identity of the factor. From Mirsky et al. (1991). Analysis of the elements of attention: A neuropsychological approach. *Neuropsychology Review*, 2(2), 109–145.

thus seem to be composed of two elements: a visual-perceptual ability to scan stimulus material for a preset target rapidly and efficiently and an ability to make either verbal (Stroop) or skilled manual responses (Digit Symbol Substitution, Letter Cancellation, Trail Making) quickly. Hence, the designation *focus-execute* for this factor is an effort to encompass both aspects of the performance required by these tasks.

The second factor to emerge ("flexibility") has loadings from the measures on a single test—the Wisconsin Card Sorting Test—and has been labeled *shift*. It appears to reflect the abstract capacity to shift from attending to one aspect or stimulus feature of the target objects to another aspect in an adaptive and flexible manner.

The third factor has very substantial loadings from the performance measures derived from the Continuous Performance Test (CPT). The CPT, like the Mackworth Clock (Mackworth, 1950), is designed to measure the capacity to sustain concentration (i.e., vigilance). The task requires sustained concentration for periods of 7 to 10 minutes and yields measures of correct responses (CPT hits), commission errors (CPT Comm.), and reaction time (CPT RT) (Table 2.1). The motor requirement of the CPT is not very demanding, since a response to the target within 700 milliseconds (ms) is scored as correct. Visual go/no-go responses, of which this is an example, usually occur in 500 ms or less (Parasuraman, 1986; Sperling & Dosher, 1986). The mean reaction time for our adult sample (Table 2.1)—X and AX tasks combined—is 447.7 ms. In addition to the very substantial loadings from the CPT on the third factor, there are modest loadings from Trail Making, Parts A and B, although not as high as on the first factor (*focus-execute*). It could therefore be argued that the capacity to sustain an attentive effort is also important to some extent in successful performance on the Trail Making Test.

The final factor, *encode,* arising from the Digit Span and Arithmetic subtests of the WAIS-R, is the least understood of the four factors in this model. A reasonable hypothesis is that *encode* embodies some sort of numerical-mnemonic quality of attention because both tasks require the serial incorporation, retention, cognitive manipulation, and ultimate recall of numeric information.

The Child Sample

In the course of a collaboration between the National Institute of Mental Health, Johns Hopkins University, and the Baltimore City Public School System, we have had the opportunity to measure the attention test performance of 435 Baltimore Public School children. In addition to contributing to the definition of attention, other goals included understanding the relation of attention to aspects of academic performance and measures of behavioral disturbance. Data that are relevant to the latter goals will be the subject of further communications. The tests of the attention battery applied to the child sample are equivalent to, or a modification of, the tests in the adult battery. They are listed in Table 2.3, along with the scores of the subjects and some descriptive measures. As in the case of the adult sample, these scores were subjected to a principal components analysis and varimax rotation, the results of which are reported in Table 2.4.

TABLE 2.3. Descriptive Variables and Attention Test Battery Scores: Child Sample (N = 435)

Measure	Mean	SD
Descriptive variables		
Age (months)[a]	95.3	5.4
Peabody Picture Vocabulary Test Revised[b]	87.4	16.7
Attention test scores		
WISC-R Digit Span	9.3	2.6
WISC-R Arithmetic	9.3	3.2
WISC-R Coding	10.9	3.3
Digit Cancellation Completion Time	72.8	18.8
Digit Cancellation Omissions	3.4	2.9
CPT Correct Responses (%) (CPT Hits)	80.3	14.4
CPT Commission Errors (%)	2.2	2.5
CPT Reaction Time (ms) (CPT RT)	610.6	55.3
Wisconsin Card Sorting Test (WCST) % Correct	48.9	14.6
Wisconsin Card Sorting Test (WCST) # of Categories	2.9	1.8

[a]Of the 435 children, 380 were in the second grade and 53 in the first grade at the time of testing. There were 217 males, mean age = 95.5 (SD = 6.0), and 218 females, mean age = 95.2 (SD = 5.2). The factor analysis in Table 2.4 is based on 427 subjects; the data on 8 subjects were incomplete.

[b]This test yields scores roughly equivalent to verbal IQ. The mean score for the males was 89.3 (SD = 17.2); for the females, it was 85.5 (SD = 16.1). These data are from Mirsky et al. (1991). Analysis of the elements of attention: A neuropsychological approach. *Neuropsychology Review, 2*(2), 109–145.

TABLE 2.4. Rotated Factor (Component) Patterns: Child Sample

	Factor 1	Factor 2	Factor 3	Factor 4
CPT Hits	−.03	−.19	*.85*	.01
CPT Commission Errors	.01	−.35	*.52*	−.13
CPT RT	−.14	.27	*.65*	.35
Digit Cancellation Completion Time	−.12	−.07	.14	*.80*
Digit Cancellation Omission Errors	−.27	−.16	.18	−*.57*
WISC-R Coding	.06	.38	−.11	−*.58*
WISC-R Arithmetic	.22	*.74*	−.16	.01
Digit Span	.03	*.75*	−.04	−.12
WCST % Correct	*.95*[a]	.10	−.03	−.01
WCST # of Categories	*.95*	.11	−.06	.01
Variance Explained (%)	19.7%	15.3%	15.1%	14.5%
Proposed Identity of Factor	Flexibility	Numerical-Mnemonic	Vigilance	Perceptual-Motor Speed
Element of Attention	*Shift*	*Encode*	*Sustain*	*Focus-Execute*

[a]Italicized values are the highest loadings within a column and were used in the interpretation of the identity of the factor.

The results of the principal components analysis of the data of the child sample yielded factors that appear to be quite similar to those seen in the adult sample (Table 2.4)—*focus-execute, shift, sustain,* and *encode*—and we have given them the same labels as those in the adult sample. The order in which the four components were extracted from the adult sample, however, was *focus-execute, shift, sustain,* and *encode;* whereas, for the child sample, it was *shift, encode, sustain,* and *focus-execute.* While there are a number of possible explanations for the difference in the rankings between the groups (including the relative immaturity of certain regions of the child's brain in comparison to that of the adult [Yakovlev & Lecours, 1967]), part of the difference may be due to the dissimilarities in administration and/or scoring of the tests for the adult and child samples. In any event, the data in Table 2.4 suggest that the pattern of component skills identified in the adult sample can also be identified in children, and support the view that these elements (Table 2.4) may reflect salient components of attentive behavior.

Description of Measures

The following provides a brief description of each of the measures included in the LPP-NIMH Attention Battery. The reader is referred to the appropriate references for more detailed information.

Digit Symbol Substitution Test (WAIS-R)/Coding (WISC-R)

The Digit Symbol subtest requires the examinee to match and transcribe the appropriate nonsense symbols that have been arbitrarily associated with the numerals 1 through 9. Coding is an equivalent task for children and adolescents. Normal performance is highly dependent on motor persistence, visuomotor coordination, response speed, and sustained attention (Lezak, 1983).

Digit Span (WAIS-R, WISC-R)

Digit Span tests the limits of the examinee's capacity for encoding and briefly retaining a series of numbers. There are two portions of this test, digits forward and digits backward. Although, in normal adults, performances on the two parts of Digit Span are highly correlated, digits forward relies less on a normally functioning memory than it does on attention (Spitz, 1972).

Arithmetic (WAIS-R, WISC-R)

Arithmetic assesses the examinee's capacity for attending to and processing basic arithmetic problems without the aid of pencil and paper.

Each of these subtests is administered as described in the WAIS-R or WISC-R (WISC-III) manual. Factor analysis repeatedly has linked the Digit Symbol Substitution, Digit Span, and Arithmetic tests from the WAIS-R (or the WISC-R, as appropriate) into what is often referred to as the Attentional Triad (Kaufman, 1975; Leckliter, Matarazzo, & Silverman, 1986; Parker, 1983). The general consensus is that these subtests represent an aspect of attention corresponding to "freedom from distractibility" (Kaufman, 1979). Customarily, neuropsychologists use poor performance on this group of tests (often also including the Information subtest) to serve as an indication of attentional dysfunction. The so-called ACID (Arithmetic-Coding-Information-Digit Span) profile is of particular relevance to diagnosing children with attention-deficit disorder (ADD) and/or learning disabilities (LD). Some controversy exists, however, over whether ADD children always do more poorly on these specific subtests (Greenblatt, Mattis, & Trad, 1991; Schwartz et al., 1989). Although usually indicative of attentional dysfunction, a deficit related to "freedom from distractibility" may not be the primary, identifying characteristic of ADD. In fact, the ACID profile is more often associated with developmental dyslexia (Kolb & Whishaw, 1990; Rugel, 1974; Whishaw & Kolb, 1984).

Talland Letter Cancellation Test

Talland (1965) originally described the Letter Cancellation task that has, since that time, given rise to many versions, including ones constructed from letters, digits, or symbols. The LPP-NIMH version includes three variations of the basic task. In each trial, the examinee scans rows of upper- and lowercase letters to find and cross out as many of an assigned target as possible in 60 seconds. Either single or double spaces separate the letters. On trials 1 and 2 (Capitals), subjects must draw a line through all capital letters. During trials 3 and 4 (Spaces), subjects draw a line through the letters immediately before and after each double space, ignoring the letter's case. On trials 5 and 6 (Both), subjects cross out both types of targets previously assigned (i.e., Capitals and Spaces). Scores include the mean number correctly crossed out for each of the three task types, the total number of commission errors, and the number of omissions.

Stroop Color-Word Interference Test

Like Letter Cancellation, there are many versions of the Stroop Test (Stroop, 1935). The LPP-NIMH battery uses stimuli and instructions described by Golden (1978), which include color-word reading, color naming, and an interference condition. In addition to assessing lexical response speed to printed words and color, the measure evaluates the ability to focus attention on one aspect of a stimulus, while inhibiting a normally, more automatic response.

Trail Making Test

The Trail Making Test (Reitan & Davidson, 1974; Reitan & Wolfson, 1985) requires motor speed and focused attention while assaying visuomotor coordination and speed of processing in the sequencing of both numbers and letters (Reitan & Tarshes, 1959). Standard instructions are used for administration (Reitan & Wolfson, 1985). Part A of the task calls simply for sequencing overlearned material, while Part B requires conceptual alternation and behavioral inhibition.

Continuous Performance Test (CPT)

Rosvold, Mirsky, Sarason, Bransome, and Beck (1956) devised the CPT as a measure of the capacity to sustain a focus of attention. Various versions of the CPT have been devised: the standard visually presented X and AX tasks of the CPT require the subject to press a response key for certain target stimuli ("press as quickly as possible whenever you see the letter X" or "press for the X only if it is preceded by the letter A," respectively). The current version used in the LPP-NIMH battery runs on software operated by a Toshiba T1000 laptop computer (or other compatible DOS-based computer, with an 80286 or higher microprocessor) that communicates with a separate Stimulus/Response Unit.

The X task reflects a highly automatic vigilance test that is dependent almost exclusively on sensory-perceptual processing, whereas the AX task has a clear memory component linked to the subject's distinguishing between target and nontarget Xs. Further, the latter assesses the subject's ability to inhibit the previously established task of pressing for each X.

There are several additional, different versions of the CPT that have not yet become regular parts of the LPP-NIMH Attention Battery but are presently being investigated. Two of these are the Degraded Visual-X task and the Auditory task. The Degraded Visual-X task is essentially the same as the standard X task described previously except that the stimuli are masked. Instead of clearly defined illuminated letters with sharp borders contrasting with the solid black background, the letters now appear as slightly more dense clusters of tiny dots against a background of similar dots. This task seems to require more perceptual effort on the part of subjects, because they must extract a meaningful gestalt from a nebulous display. During the Auditory task, the stimuli consist of three tones of distinctly different pitches. Participants must push the response button as quickly as possible whenever they hear the highest pitched tone.

Halperin and his colleagues (Halperin, 1991; Halperin, Newcorn, Sharma, Healey, Wolf, Pascualvaca, & Schwartz, 1990; Halperin, O'Brien, Newcorn, Healey, Pascualvaca, Wolf, & Young, 1990; Halperin, Wolf, Greenblatt, & Young, 1991; Halperin et al., 1988; O'Brien et al., 1988) have presented data suggesting that an analysis of the types of errors committed during the AX version of the CPT test might be useful in differentiating between various subtypes of cognitive and behavioral dysfunction in children. For example, they could distinguish children diagnosed as having attention-deficit/hyperactivity disorder (ADHD), according to DSM-III criteria (American Psychiatric Association, 1980), from those with conduct disorder (CD). Children with ADHD and ADHD + CD had significantly more omission errors than children diagnosed with CD alone. Similarly, the authors found that the correlation between teachers' ratings of a group of normal, nonreferred children on measures of inattention, from both the DSM-III and the Conners Teacher Questionnaire (Goyette, Conners, & Ulrich, 1978), and the number of omission errors on the CPT AX task was significant and selective. Measures of conduct problems, hyperactivity, and impulsivity correlated with the tendency to respond incorrectly to letters other than an X that followed an A (A-Not-X errors), although these errors did not correlate with inattention ratings. Incorrectly responding to an X that was not preceded by an A (X-only errors) correlated only with the inattention/passivity factor of the Conners Teacher Questionnaire.

Halperin has suggested that omission errors plus slow reaction time X-only errors can be used to generate a CPT-inattention score. Similarly, fast A-Not-X errors (incorrectly responding to any letter that follows an A other than an X) plus slow A-only errors (incorrectly responding to an A instead of an X) produce a CPT impulsivity score. The other types of errors, slow A-Not-X, fast X-only, fast A-only, and random errors, compose a CPT dyscontrol score distinct from both impulsivity and inattention. Using the IOWA Conners Teachers Rating Scale (Loney & Milich, 1982) and their interpretation of CPT errors, Halperin and his colleagues found that children who were rated as "pure hyperactives" were significantly more inattentive than all the other groups. The "mixed hyperactive/aggressive" group was the most impulsive. Notably, the "pure aggressive" group was indistinguishable from normal controls on all aspects of CPT performance. On the putative measure of dyscontrol, all groups performed equivalently.

Wisconsin Card Sorting Test (WCST)

Grant and Berg (1948) constructed the WCST to examine a subject's ability to attend to and make decisions based on simple percepts. More specifically, the task gauges the subject's ability to shift attention from one sorting criterion to another in response to minimally informative prompts. Successful performance requires discerning the sort criterion from the examiner's feedback alone. This criterion changes after a predetermined number of consecutive correct responses. The testee must be able to disengage from the previous response set and shift attention to finding and following the new criterion. The LPP-NIMH battery uses stimuli and instructions described by Heaton (1981) thus generating several scores, including the number of cards sorted correctly and incorrectly, category shifts achieved, and perseverative responses. Although impairment on the test is commonly associated with frontal lobe dysfunction (e.g., Milner, 1963), it is a particular characteristic pattern of perseverative errors, rather than poor performance on the instrument, per se, that appears to be indicative of frontal lobe dysfunction. The WCST, however, like all neuropsychological tests, assays behavioral function and not anatomy.

NEUROLOGICAL CORRELATES OF THE ATTENTION SYSTEM

There is evidence from neuroanatomical, clinical, and neuropsychological studies that an attention "system" can be described within the brain (Mirsky, 1987; Posner, Inhoff, Friedrich, & Cohen, 1987), and that different parts of it may have some degree of specialization for different functions. Figure 2.1 summarizes this conception. The structures included within this cerebral model are similar to those included within models proposed earlier by Heilman, Watson, Valenstein, and Damasio (1983) and by Mesulam (1987). Their models are based on anatomical data from human clinical cases in which neglect was a symptom, as well as on some animal lesion studies. Our model (Mirsky et al., 1991) is also based on human and animal data; however, it differs from previous models in that distinct functions have been proposed for specific cerebral regions. It is thus similar to the models proposed by Pribram and McGuinness (1975) and by Posner and Petersen (1990). The evidence of our model of attention is detailed in Mirsky et al. (1991).

The *Sustain* Element

The tectum and the mesopontine regions of the reticular formation and other structures of the brainstem are depicted in the lower right portion of Figure 2.1. The work of Moruzzi and Magoun (1949) and Lindsley, Bowden, and Magoun (1949) established these areas as essential to the maintenance of consciousness and to the regulation of levels of arousal. In our view, these structures make up the basic, fundamental, phylogenetically most primitive component of the attention system of the brain. We are strongly influenced in this assertion by the theorizing of MacLean (1990), who has pointed out that the brain of the reptile, although little more than a brainstem and a few ganglia, supports a complex series of behaviors, including many of the attention functions discussed in our model.

A number of other studies could be cited in support of the role of midbrain and brainstem structures in the maintenance of vigilance or sustained attention. Mirsky and Oshima (1973) provided evidence that subcortical aluminum cream lesions in the brainstem of the monkey impair sustained visual attention. Using another technique, Bakay Pragay, Mirsky, Fullerton, Oshima, and Arnold (1975) demonstrated that subcortical electrical stimulation of the brainstem reticular formation impairs sustained

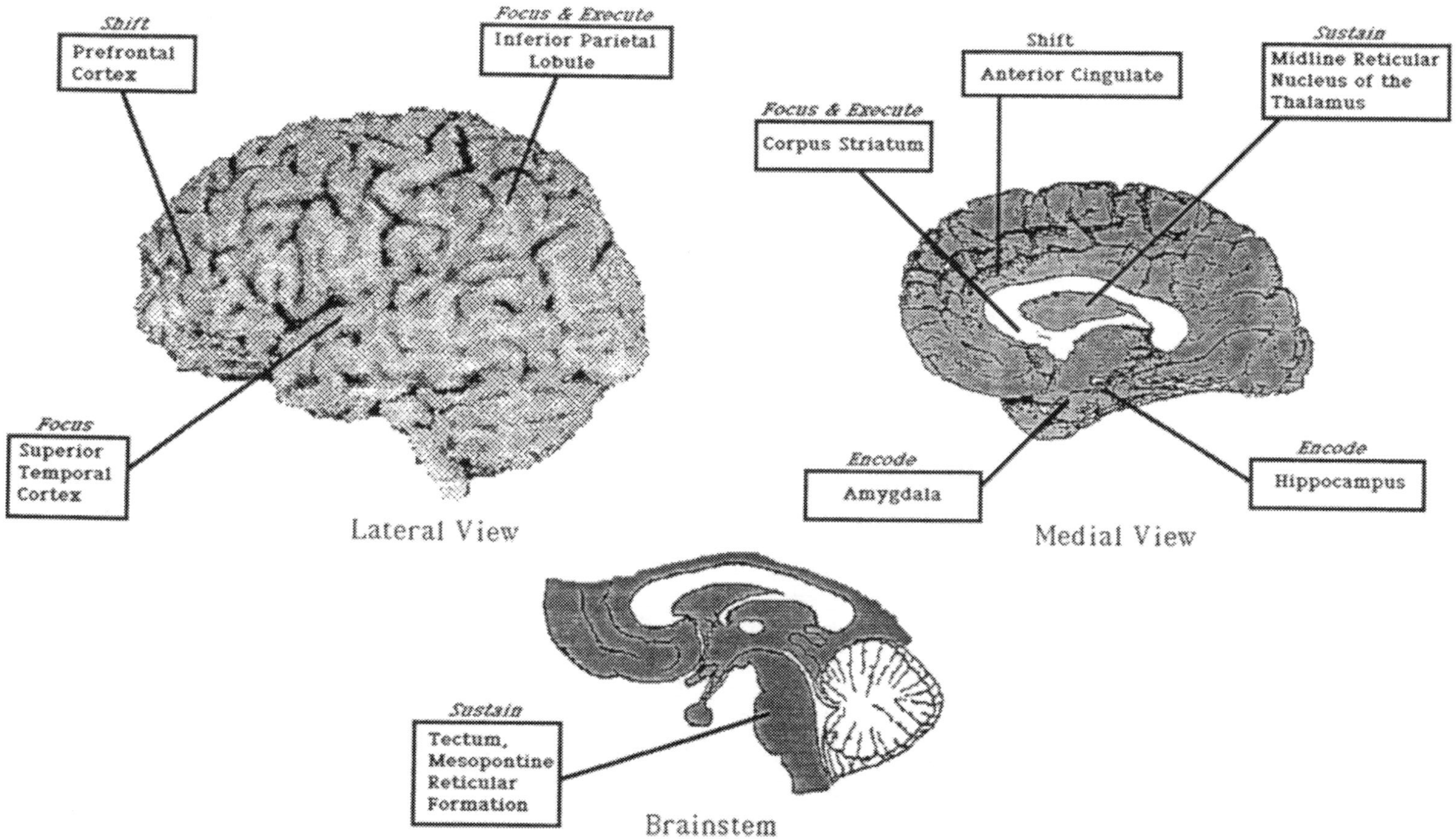

FIGURE 2.1. Anatomy of the attention system. Semischematic representation of brain regions involved in attention with tentative assignment of functional specializations to the regions. Adapted from Mirsky, A. F. (1987). Behavioral and psychophysiological markers of disorded attention. *Environmental Health Perspectives, 74*, 191–199.

visual attentive behavior in the monkey. Mirsky, Bakay Pragay, and Harris (1977) showed that electrical stimulation of the brain in regions that produce impairment of sustained attention also produce reduced visual evoked potentials. In all of these studies, a monkey version of the CPT was used so as to increase the likelihood that animal data could be generalized to human clinical data (e.g., Mirsky & Van Buren, 1965). Furthermore, in all of these studies, the findings support the view that mesencephalic brainstem structures are critical for the maintenance of sustained attention.

A somewhat modified version of this monkey CPT (i.e., a go/no-go visual attention task) was also used in the successful search for single neural units involved in attention (Bakay Pragay, Mirsky, Ray, Turner, & Mirsky, 1978). The following is a brief summary of that work. Basically, these experiments employed simultaneous measurement of behavior and neuronal firing in trained monkey subjects. Bakay Pragay and coworkers identified cells in the midline thalamus, deep layers of the superior colliculus, tectal and pretectal regions, and pontine and mesencephalic portions of the brainstem that apparently support attention (Bakay Pragay et al., 1978; Ray, Mirsky, & Bakay Pragay, 1982). These "Type II" cells increased their firing on both go and no-go trials of a go/no-go visual discrimination task designed to be analogous to the CPT (Rosvold et al., 1956). Type II cells ceased responding to the task stimuli when they were no longer associated with reinforcement. Moreover, in some instances, Type II cells began firing hundreds of milliseconds before the occurrence of task stimuli—as though in anticipation of the appearance of the reinforced stimuli in this repetitive, predictable task. The firing of these cells was unrelated to the occurrence of eye movements, supporting the view that they are not part of a visual orientation or signal detection system (Ray et al., 1982) of the type described by Posner and Petersen (1990).

Bakay Pragay, Mirsky, and Nakamura (1987) also found Type II cells in regions of the monkey prefrontal cortex extending from the midprincipal sulcus to the central sulcus, although the frequency with which they were encountered diminished in the more caudal (and thus more purely motor) locations. Type II cells were also identified in the medial prefrontal regions and in the cingulate gyrus. Moreover, Bakay Pragay, Mirsky, and Nakamura (1988) also found Type II cells in the inferior parietal lobule (Area 7) and the prestriate cortex (Area V4). Every region of the monkey brain that has been explored by Bakay Pragay and coworkers on the basis of a presumptive role in attention (i.e., mesopontine brainstem structures, medial thalamus, prefrontal and frontal association cortex, inferior parietal and prestriate cortex) has been found to contain attention-related Type II cells. There are no contradictions between their distribution and the schematic map of the human brain in Figure 2.1.

The emphasis in this section is on the neural substrate of the sustain element. Type II cells can sustain task-related firing over hundreds of trials and could thus qualify as the neural substrate of this element. The characteristics of some "asymmetric" Type II cells, however, could also be construed as essential to the function of focusing on some aspect of the environment: although both "go" and "no-go" stimuli elicit cell firing, the response to "go" stimuli is more vigorous (Bakay Pragay et al., 1987). Furthermore, as the task stimuli are dissociated from reinforcement, the cells almost immediately cease task-related firing; such a rapid disconnection would be part of the capacity necessary for rapid shifting to other aspects of the environment that may hold more promise as reinforcers.

The data are insufficient to conclude that Type II cells have distinct functions in different attention-related areas of the brain. The prefrontal cells in the study by Bakay Pragay et al. (1987) showed great sensitivity in response to changes in task parameters, thus supporting a role for these cells in the *shift* element of attention. Since these experimental maneuvers were not tried in most of the mesopontine cells (or cells in other locations), however, it is not clear whether this flexibility is unique to cells of the frontal cortex. Other characteristics by which Type II cells differ include the degree of symmetry in firing pattern between "go" and "no-go" trials, the latency at which the cell fires in "anticipation" of stimulus onset, and whether the cell increases or decreases firing in relation to the stimuli. The Type II cell may thus represent a kind of primordial attention cell that, depending on the network in which it is embedded, can support the several functions necessary for attention that are postulated here.

The medial view of the right hemisphere (Figure 2.1) depicts the midline thalamic region (and the reticular nuclei), for which a role in attention is supported by the anatomical and physiological studies of Ajmone Marsan (1965) and Jasper and co-workers (Jasper, 1958). The studies of Yingling and Skinner (1975), on the role of the reticular nucleus of the thalamus in modulating visual information, also support the role of thalamic structures in sustained attention. These authors demonstrated that stimulation of this thalamic nucleus could modify the influence of reticular formation effects on visual signals. We are proposing that these brainstem and thalamic structures are essential for the maintenance of vigilance, rather than simply to regulate levels of arousal (i.e., stages of sleep). This is an extension of the Moruzzi-Magoun-Lindsley concept (that dealt primarily with the role of the reticular formation in arousal) but is certainly compatible with it. The writings of Lindsley (e.g., Lindsley, 1960) are conducive to the view that, within the general state of wakefulness, there exist degrees of behavioral tuning. One of the ways in which this is expressed is in variations in the readiness to respond. Readiness to respond (as measured by reaction time and number of correct responses in a visual discrimination task) can be modified by low-intensity stimulation of the reticular formation (Fuster & Uyeda, 1962). Scheibel (1980) has speculated that the brainstem reticular formation and portions of the nonspecific or reticular thalamus act in concert with certain cortical regions to provide the "structuro-functional" basis of awareness.

Clearly, our argument that these reticular structures are specific substrates of the *sustain* element of attention would be stronger if we had more information than that provided by disruptions of performance on a monkey version of the CPT (and other similar data). Animal models of some of the tasks used in our attention battery are difficult or impossible to achieve; previously, however, one of us tried with some success (using drugs rather than lesions) to show differential effects of various classes of drugs on different cognitive-attentive tasks (i.e., match-to-sample versus CPT) in the monkey (Bakay Pragay, Mirsky, & Abplanalp, 1969). Greenblatt (1986) recently provided some reasonably direct evidence of the effects of brainstem pathology on the CPT. She found that posterior fossa tumors that compressed the brainstem (and impaired the function of the reticular formation) affected speed of response on a CPT-type task. A correlation of 0.82 was found between tumor size and reaction time on the CPT. We may add that the specificity of the localization of sustained attention in the brainstem and reticular thalamus is indirectly supported by human clinical studies showing the relative lack of effect of large temporal lobe resections on the CPT (e.g., Lansdell & Mirsky, 1964).

Nevertheless, despite the difficulties in reaching an unequivocal conclusion, we believe that the information presented here supports the view that the element of attention that we have labeled *sustain* is particularly dependent on the brainstem and thalamic portions of the attention system of Figure 2.1.

The *Encode* Element

The hippocampus and amygdala are presented in phantom on this brain view. The involvement of the hippocampus in attention is suggested by both behavioral and electrophysiological measures (e.g., Blakemore, Iversen, & Zangwill, 1972). The classical hippocampal theta rhythm, associated with heightened attention, has been amply characterized (Adey, 1969). We assume from other studies of the neuropsychological role of the hippocampus (Mishkin, 1978; Scoville & Milner, 1957) that it is involved primarily in the mnemonic (encode) aspects of attention, as defined by our model. Mishkin (1978) has provided animal data that the amygdala may also be involved in the support of memory functions.

The *Shift* Element

The localization of the capacity to shift in the prefrontal cortex is based primarily on the work of Milner (1963). Milner demonstrated that resections of the dorsolateral prefrontal cortex for relief of seizure disorders impair performance on the WCST. The resection of other cerebral areas (i.e., the anterior temporal lobe) fails to produce the deficit. This test has been used in conjunction with radioactive xenon-imaging of cerebral blood flow in schizophrenic patients (Weinberger, Berman, & Zec, 1986). The results have led to speculation that the prefrontal areas of patients with schizophrenia are relatively inactive.

We have taken the liberty of including the medial frontal cortex and the anterior cingulate gyrus in the focal representation of the *shift* element; this is primarily on the basis of our monkey data indicating that "attention" cells are equally well represented in the medial and dorsolateral prefontal regions of the cortex (Bakay Pragay et al., 1987). Obviously, more human lesion data would be necessary to establish whether this is a correct assignment of function.

Another issue concerns whether it is more useful to consider the *shift* element of the WCST as a component of an overarching classification of behaviors—that of executive function—rather than that of attention per se. The boundaries between "attention" and "executive function" are rather indistinct; therefore, the decision to consider shift behavior assessed by the WCST as attention appears reasonable. Other empirical (or theoretical) information may suggest the need to revise this view.

The *Focus-Execute* Element

When assessed with neuropsychological tests, impaired attention is often identified with poor performance on such measures as Digit Symbol Substitution, Letter Cancellation, Stroop and Trail Making; moreover, the loss of ability to focus on specific environmental cues and to respond appropriately to them would seem to constitute a reasonable working definition of neglect, at least in its milder form.

We could turn to the clinical literature on neglect to provide clues as to the location of the *focus-execute* elements in the attention system of the brain. Unfortunately, this does not lead to a specific localization of this element(s) of attention; Heilman et al. (1983) and Mesulam (1987), on the basis of their own observations and the reports of others, have concluded that neglect may follow damage to any of the cerebral structures shown in Figure 2.1. The possibility exists, therefore, that *focus-execute* functions are represented everywhere in the system delineated in Figure 2.1.

We would like to propose, however, that the inferior parietal, superior temporal, and striatal regions have a special role in the support of these functions. The first two are major multimodal sensory convergence areas of the brain. The posterior parietal cortex, in particular, has connections with sensory, limbic (i.e., cingulate cortex), thalamic, and brainstem reticular areas as well as motor regions of the brain (Mesulam, 1987). The multiplicity of these connections, as well as the many reports of neglect following parietal lesions (particularly on the right side) (Heilman et al., 1983), led to the selection of this brain area as the primary cerebral locus of the *focus-execute* element. The connection of the parietal cortex with the corpus striatum, as well as the important modulatory motor role of this nuclear complex, dictates its inclusion in the *focus-execute* (with special emhasis on the execute) cerebral support system. Of possible relevance, as well, is the role of the caudate nucleus (a component of the corpus striatum) in support of such behavioral tasks as delayed alternation and delayed response (Battig, Rosvold, & Mishkin, 1960).

The role of the superior temporal cortex, or, more accurately, the superior temporal sulcus, as a multimodal sensory convergence area with a role in focused attention is supported by the anatomical studies of Pandya and coworkers (e.g., Pandya & Yeterian, 1985). Recent studies of attention-related behavior in patients with complex partial seizures (with foci of abnormal tissue in the temporal lobe), some of whom have undergone anterior temporal lobectomy for relief of seizures, support the view that the anterior temporal lobe is part of the brain system involved in the *focus-execute* element of attention. Roth, Connell, Faught, and Adams (1988) reported that patients with left or right temporal epileptogenic foci have "mild" attentional deficits, as assessed by tests that included (among others) the Stroop, Trail Making, Digit Span, and Digit Symbol Substitution. Those with right-sided foci had significantly greater deficits on Trail Making, Part B, than the group with left-sided foci. Similarly, Hermann and Wyler (1988) reported that there was a decline in 40% of their measures of attention and concentration in a study of 38 patients who underwent anterior temporal lobectomy. Their attention measures included the Stroop and Trail Making tests. Also of interest in their study was the finding that indicated a sparing of performance on the WCST (the *shift* element) after anterior temporal lobe resections. Moreover, Lansdell and Mirsky (1964) had previously reported no impairment on the CPT (the *sustain* element) following temporal lobe resections.

The pattern of findings in these studies supports the view that performance on tests assessing what we have labeled the *focus-execute* element of attention (Stroop, Trail Making) is impaired with dysfunction or destruction of temporal lobe tissue. We have, however, insufficient data on these tests to claim that the superior temporal cortex has a different or unique role with respect to attention than the inferior parietal or striatal regions. Nevertheless, since the superior temporal sulcus is not clearly implicated in motor (i.e., *execute*) functions, we have not included the *execute* function in the temporal region in Figure 2.1.

Another complication in the interpretation of the data of Roth et al. (1988) and Hermann and Wyler (1988) is that patients with complex partial seizures may have, in addition to their temporal cortical abnormalities, abnormal tissue in the amygdala and anterior hippocampus (Penfield & Jasper, 1954). Concurrent involvement of the temporal cortex, hippocampus, and amygdala, according to our model, would suggest that two of the elements of attention (*focus-execute* and *encode*) would be impaired in such patients and that this impairment might increase with anterior temporal lobe resection.

There is little doubt that the brain structures presented in Figure 2.1 could be construed to form a system; anatomical connections among the various areas have been well described (e.g., Jones & Peters, 1986). Considerable evidence indicates that performance on tests of attention may be impaired selectively by different brain lesions. This implies that distinct elements of attention (*focus-execute, sustain, shift, encode*) are supported by distinct brain regions (Figure 2.1).

Please note, at the outset, that this effort of assigning functional specialization of components of attention to different brain regions is not meant to be absolute, and it is likely that some brain regions share more than one attentional function. Caveats aside, the model purposes the following:

1. Attention is a complex process or set of processes. It can be subdivided into a number of distinct functions, including *focus-execute, sustain, encode,* and *shift.*
2. These functions are supported by different brain regions, which have become specialized for this purpose but which nevertheless are organized into a system.
3. The function of focusing on environmental events is shared by superior temporal and inferior parietal cortices as well as by structures that make up the corpus striatum.
4. The execution of responses must depend heavily on the integrity of inferior parietal and corpus striatal regions. (See discussion in Mesulam, 1987.)
5. Sustaining a focus of attention on environmental events is the major responsibility of rostral midbrain structures, including the mesopontine reticular formation and midline and reticular thalamic nuclei. This is obviously a major component of this model; however, the evidence is largely inferential, indirect, or based on animal models.
6. Encoding of stimuli is dependent on the amygdala and hippocampus.

7. The capacity to shift from one salient aspect of the environment to another is supported by the prefrontal cortex (Milner, 1963).
8. Damage or dysfunction in one of these brain regions can lead to circumscribed or specific deficits in a particular attentional function.

PRACTICAL APPLICATIONS

Thus far, we have established our concept of attention as a multifaceted construct. In doing so, we have described the Laboratory of Psychology and Psychopathology's unique approach to assessing attention with an "attention battery." We have outlined the bases of our notion of the components of attention, what they are, how they can be measured, and their putative neurological substrata. We turn now to focus more fully on practical issues associated with assessing attention in the clinical setting.

Normative Data Stratified by Age

In Table 2.5, we present normative data from the performance on the LPP-NIMH Attention Battery of a group of 188 normal, healthy subjects. They ranged from 5 through 94 years of age and comprised two groups: 111 subjects recruited for this study who were tested at a variety of locations in the Washington, DC, area, including the campus of The American University (Tatman, 1992; Tatman, Fantie, & Mirsky, 1992), and 77 normal control subjects who were part of research protocols at the Intramural Program of the NIMH. We hope that these data help to promote the systematic evaluation of attentional capacities and the use of an attention battery as part of the neuropsychological examination.

A Model for the Development of Some Forms of Attention Deficit

These normative data (Table 2.5) may serve to remind us of the importance of intact attentional processes in achieving a successful adaptation to the school environment. Aside from, or in addition to, the children identified as having ADHD (discussed above in relation to error types on the CPT), there exist many children who are identified as making poor or marginal adjustments to the classroom; however, their initial distinguishing characteristics are not necessarily poor attention. Instead, they may be seen by their teachers as shy or aggressive (or as having both sets of characteristics). Many of these children are unable to achieve mastery of first- and second-grade work. Kellam attributed this early failure, manifest as shyness or aggressiveness, to impaired "concentration" (Kellam, Branch, Agrawal, & Emsminger, 1975). Thus, behaviors that are not immediately recognized as due to poor attention are, in fact, the sequelae of this deficit. These behaviors are associated with early school dropout and the later development of antisocial acts and other symptoms of disorder. Elsewhere (Mirsky & Siegel, 1994), we have speculated on the possible pathophysiological etiology of such outcomes in relation to our neuropsychological model of the localization of attention elements in the brain. This speculation is based, in part, on unpublished data from a cohort of 435 East Baltimore children, in which the attention factors of *encode* and *sustain* were found to be impaired in children manifesting a marked degree of shyness and/or aggressiveness. The model, expressed as a flow diagram, is summarized in Figure 2.2.

Some Observations on Cultural/Socioeconomic Factors

In the course of an investigation of the familial transmission of disordered attention, we recently studied attentional capacities in two predominantly non-American subject cohorts, one from Ireland and the other from Israel (Mirsky et al., 1992). For the Irish subjects, the cohort included a group of schizophrenic persons, their first-degree relatives, and matched controls. For the Israeli portion of the project, the cohort included Israeli first-degree relatives of schizophrenics and Israeli control subjects, but the schizophrenic subjects were actually inpatients at NIMH and were unrelated to the Israeli subjects.

There were striking differences in the level of performance on some of the attention tests between the Irish and the Israeli-NIMH cohorts. The raw scores indicate that a gradient of performance was observed across the groups within each population such that controls performed best, followed by first-degree relatives of schizophrenics, and finally by schizophrenic subjects, who performed most poorly. The data were interpreted to indicate that the attention deficit seen in the schizophrenic patients is also present in the first-degree relatives of schizophrenics, although in milder form. The absolute scores of the subjects in the two cohorts differed, however, in a striking and statistically significant manner. Two examples of this are seen in Figures 2.3 and 2.4, showing the range of mean scores on the Digit Symbol Substitution subtest and WCST for the groups in the Israeli-NIMH and Irish cohorts. The mean performance level of the Irish controls is about the same as that of the NIMH schizophrenic subjects.

The question arises as to how to interpret the low scores seen in the Irish sample, and in particular the schizophrenic subjects. The poor scores of the Irish schizophrenic subjects may be a reflection of the increased severity of the disorder in this population; another factor may be the age of the subjects (they were on the average 46 years of age as compared with a mean age of approximately 30 years for the Israeli-NIMH cohort). The Irish subjects also had a more limited educational background (i.e., a mean educational level of 10 years as compared to 14 years for the Israeli-NIMH group). In the schizophrenic subjects, age is, of course, confounded with years of identified illness; in the group of Irish schizophrenics this was in excess of 20 years. Age and educational level seem the likely explanation for the differences between the respective groups of relatives and controls. Age per se, however, probably does not account for the poor scores of the Irish groups, since there was an overall lack of correlation of test scores with age in both the probands and the nondisordered controls (these data are reported elsewhere). Duration of illness and its consequences (Chapman, Chapman, & Raulin, 1976) and the relatively modest education of this group of rural subjects (leading to unfamiliarity with cognitive tasks and assessment procedures)

TABLE 2.5. Normative Data Stratified by Age: LPP-NIMH Attention Battery

Age—years	5–15	16–24	25–34	35–44	45–54	55–64	65–74	75–84	85–94
N	8	32	48	23	11	17	27	16	6
Education (years)									
Mean	4.1	14.7	15.9	16.6	15.7	15.6	16.3	15.6	13.0
SD	*2.9*	*1.5*	*1.9*	*2.2*	*2.1*	*3.2*	*3.2*	*3.9*	*4.6*
WAIS-R Full Scale IQ									
Mean	127.1	116.5	114.7	121.4	117.2	121.3	122.1	118.4	101.8
SD	*14.9*	*12.5*	*10.4*	*10.7*	*14.0*	*15.9*	*13.7*	*15.0*	*12.5*
WAIS-R Digit Symbol									
Mean	12.6	12.7	12.5	12.3	12.3	12.4	13.1	10.5	9.2
SD	*3.7*	*2.3*	*2.6*	*2.2*	*2.9*	*2.7*	*3.1*	*1.9*	*1.7*
Trails A									
Mean	42.2	24.2	27.3	26.8	28.0	31.3	42.7	46.1	62.2
SD	*19.9*	*7.5*	*11.4*	*5.7*	*8.5*	*19.4*	*23.1*	*16.7*	*17.5*
Trails B									
Mean	115.5	48.9	53.6	54.3	61.3	74.2	114.9	120.4	168.8
SD	*65.9*	*14.7*	*19.0*	*15.5*	*21.0*	*46.9*	*107.6*	*63.5*	*60.8*
Letter Cancellation									
Mean	37.3	81.3	80.0	72.8	69.6	62.1	54.9	42.7	32.2
SD	*17.9*	*11.5*	*11.0*	*11.2*	*11.9*	*17.6*	*11.4*	*11.6*	*5.1*
Stroop									
Mean	47.9	52.3	50.7	47.9	51.1	50.8	51.3	43.5	39.3
SD	*7.7*	*6.3*	*7.4*	*7.2*	*5.9*	*6.4*	*8.0*	*7.5*	*5.1*
CPT X Hits									
Mean	81.1	98.9	99.1	99.8	97.8	98.7	96.6	96.2	92.8
SD	*25.3*	*1.3*	*1.6*	*0.4*	*3.0*	*2.8*	*6.1*	*4.5*	*8.4*
CPT AX Hits									
Mean	80.3	95.0	95.6	97.3	91.6	94.9	94.2	90.3	83.2
SD	*18.3*	*5.8*	*4.7*	*4.1*	*17.9*	*6.1*	*6.8*	*9.3*	*14.0*

CPT X % Commission Errors									
Mean	0.54	0.37	0.36	0.20	0.24	0.29	0.26	0.26	0.44
SD	*0.39*	*0.36*	*0.51*	*0.25*	*0.32*	*0.49*	*0.40*	*0.34*	*0.34*
CPT AX % Commission Errors									
Mean	1.30	1.05	0.81	0.37	0.17	0.26	0.46	0.49	1.11
SD	*0.82*	*1.14*	*1.15*	*0.60*	*0.31*	*0.37*	*0.59*	*0.41*	*0.76*
CPT X Reaction Time									
Mean	476.2	426.3	428.6	386.3	450.0	390.8	420.7	440.0	453.3
SD	*105.1*	*51.9*	*53.3*	*31.4*	*62.3*	*43.3*	*43.9*	*62.2*	*48.9*
CPT AX Reaction Time									
Mean	352.9	404.2	431.0	377.0	443.3	386.2	400.9	416.7	410.0
SD	*107.5*	*80.1*	*64.9*	*51.8*	*85.8*	*65.0*	*47.9*	*55.8*	*79.4*
Wisconsin Card Sorting Task (Categories)									
Mean	5.6	5.6	5.9	5.6	5.8	5.1	5.0	4.3	3.2
SD	*0.5*	*1.0*	*0.5*	*1.3*	*0.6*	*1.6*	*1.5*	*1.7*	*3.0*
Wisconsin Card Sorting Task (Number Correct)									
Mean	73.8	67.3	69.0	67.0	68.4	71.6	73.1	74.8	63.0
SD	*10.2*	*6.8*	*7.4*	*9.3*	*2.8*	*11.1*	*10.4*	*9.8*	*23.4*
Wisconsin Card Sorting Task (Errors)									
Mean	27.0	18.4	14.8	19.3	19.5	32.7	31.7	40.6	59.0
SD	*5.5*	*18.3*	*10.4*	*15.8*	*16.7*	*24.7*	*20.7*	*18.0*	*28.8*
WAIS-R Digit Span									
Mean	11.6	12.2	11.8	12.0	12.3	12.6	11.8	12.0	9.0
SD	*3.6*	*2.4*	*2.5*	*1.8*	*3.4*	*3.6*	*2.6*	*3.2*	*2.2*
WAIS-R Arithmetic									
Mean	14.4	12.5	11.3	13.1	12.3	11.4	11.5	10.9	10.0
SD	*3.1*	*2.7*	*2.0*	*2.3*	*1.4*	*3.7*	*2.9*	*2.8*	*2.1*

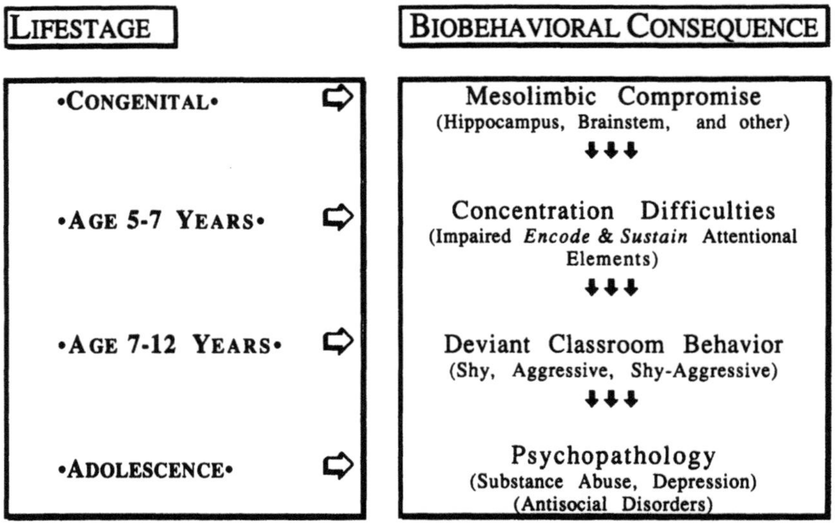

FIGURE 2.2. Lifestage model of attentional pathology.

cannot be ruled out as contributing to the low scores obtained by the Irish schizophrenics in this study. The Israeli subjects, in contrast, were more likely to have been exposed to assessment procedures in school or while serving in the Israeli Defense Force. Education and related socioeconomic factors are thus probably responsible for the lower performance of the nonpatient Irish groups.

Results such as these temper the interpretation of the absolute scores of these tests and encourage us to bear in mind the socio-cultural-educational milieu from which test subjects are derived. The low scores of these rural Irish subjects on the WCST are of

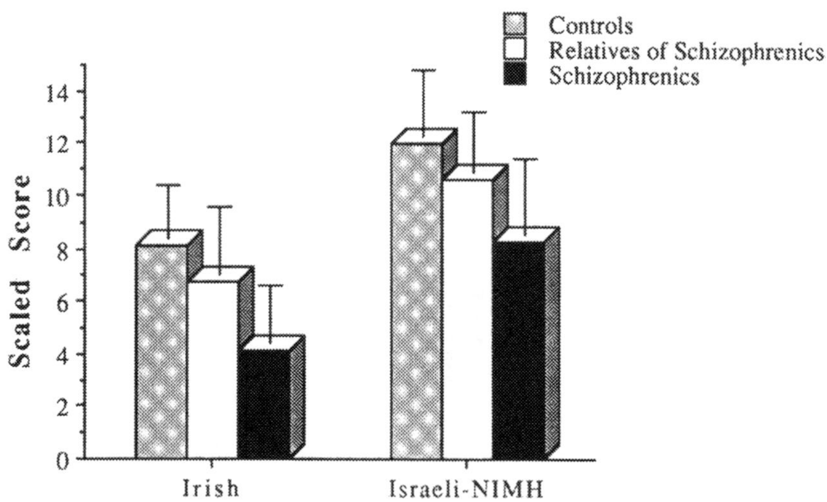

FIGURE 2.3. Digit Symbol Substitution Test: Israeli-NIMH versus Irish samples. The mean scores on the Digit Symbol Substitution Test for the groups in the Israeli-NIMH and Irish samples.

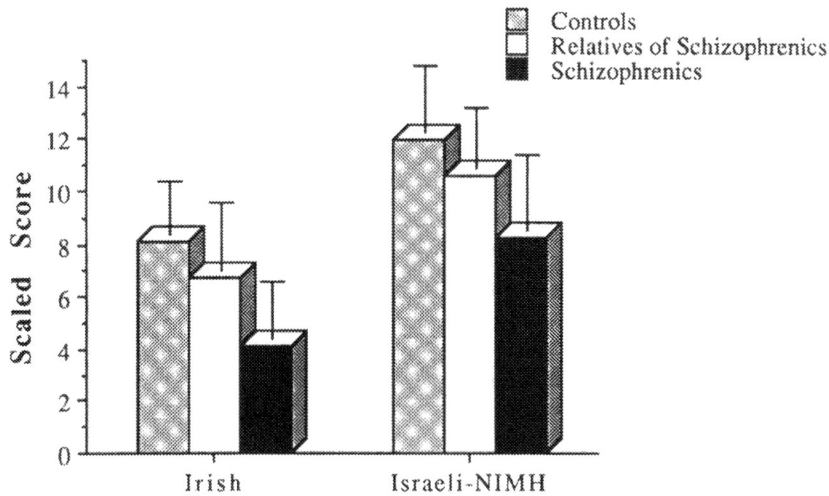

FIGURE 2.4. Wisconsin Card Sorting Test: Israeli-NIMH versus Irish samples. The mean scores on the Wisconsin Card Sorting Test for the groups in the Israeli-NIMH and Irish samples.

particular interest, in view of the fact that several studies have shown that by age 10, the majority of a group of U.S. school children are able to achieve six categories on this test (Chelune & Baer, 1986; Fey, 1951). Moreover, in the data reported in the present chapter, the subjects between the ages of 5 and 15 years (with an average of only 4.1 years of education) performed as well as the adult Irish controls on the WCST.

In contrast, the scores on the CPT tended to be very similar for comparable subjects for the two cohorts (Figure 2.5): the control subjects, the relatives, and the schizophrenic subjects are more similar between cohorts than they are within cohorts. This result suggests that tests such as the CPT may be more useful (or more robust) in cross-national or cross-socioeconomic investigations of schizophrenia (and possibly, other neuropsychiatric disorders) than measures that appear to be strongly influenced by the education, background, and/or cultural milieu of the subjects.

CASE EXAMPLES

The Case of Mrs. L.L.

The following narrative is presented as an example of the use of the Laboratory of Psychology (LPP)-NIMH Attention Battery in a case of closed head injury in which one of the presenting symptoms was difficulty with short-term memory. The results of the testing indicated that the patient was experiencing pervasive problems with attention that may have been sufficient to account for her impaired memory.

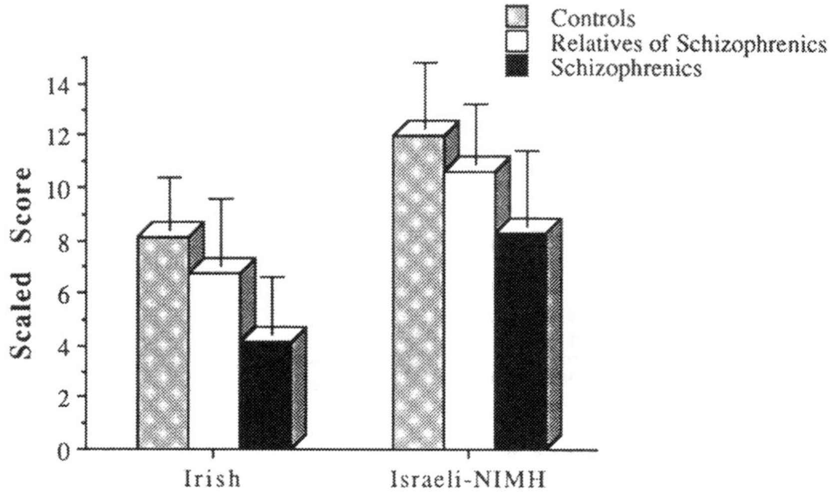

FIGURE 2.5. CPT: Israeli-NIMH versus Irish samples. The mean scores on the CPT for the groups in the Israeli-NIMH and Irish samples.

Mrs. L.L., a 34-year-old mother of five children, had been in a motor vehicle accident approximately 14 months prior to her neuropsychological evaluation. In the accident, she struck the left side of her body and was rendered unconscious for several hours. Since the accident, she had suffered from pain related to injuries to her neck, shoulder, left arm, and hand. She had been referred for neuropsychological testing by her neurologist because, in addition to these symptoms, she had complaints of headache, occasional dizziness, word-finding problems, visual-spatial confusion, and problems with short-term memory. Mrs. L.L.'s education had included 3 years of college, and she taught school for a number of years while raising her family of five. Her youngest child was 2 when Mrs. L.L. was seen. She had not taught school for 6 years prior to the evaluation.

She was dressed casually but carefully at the time of the examination, and conversed freely and in a relaxed manner with the examiner. At times she seemed concerned about her performance, but persevered in all the tests and appeared to be performing up to the limits of her abilities. While she was right-handed, she was noticeably impaired in the use of her left hand and arm, and occasionally this caused some delay in her ability to manipulate test materials. Nevertheless, it did not appear that any of the scores obtained had been affected substantially by that disability.

The tests administered included the LPP-NIMH Attention Battery and the following measures of memory: the Wechsler Memory Scale, Form I; the Rey-Osterrieth Complex Figure Test; and the California Discourse Memory Test.

Mrs. L.L.'s performance was evaluated by observing the way in which she coped with the demands of the various asessment procedures and by comparing her scores with those of a group of 20 normal control subjects whose ages ranged from 20 to 49, and whose educational background (approximately 3 years of college) was similar to hers.

The results indicated that there was a pervasive pattern of deficit in most of the tests of the LPP-NIMH Attention Battery. This was evident in the *encode* (Arithmetic, Digit Span), *focus-execute* (Digit Symbol Substitution, Stroop, Trail Making, Talland Letter Cancellation), and *sustain* (CPT) attention elements. The *encode* tests were perhaps the least impaired, with scores falling approximately two standard deviations below those of the comparison groups. The most severe impairment was seen in the tests measuring *focus-execute* and *sustain* attentional capacities, where the scores ranged from two to seven standard deviations below the norms (*focus-execute*) to between 10 and 20 standard deviations below expectation (*sustain*). The poorest *focus-execute* performance was seen on the Trail Making Test, Part B. Mrs. L.L.'s execution here was slow, halting, and confused. On *sustain* tests (various versions of the CPT, both visual and auditory), Mrs. L.L. scored as poorly as persons with severe absence epilepsy or untreated ADHD.

On both the *focus-execute* and *sustain* tests, Mrs. L.L. was penalized for her inability to perform skilled motor acts in rapid fashion. But her deficit was clearly not due merely to lack of speed; she made many errors of omission as well (seen on the visual and auditory subtasks of the CPT and in the Talland Letter Cancellation task). Her performance on the CPT tasks was also marked by numerous impulsive errors, in which she responded to nontarget stimuli.

In contrast to these performances, Mrs. L.L. achieved relatively normal scores on the test of the capacity to shift from one stimulus concept to another, the WCST.

On the Wechsler Memory Scale, Mrs. L.L. achieved a Memory Quotient of 93. In comparison with an assumed premorbid IQ of 110–115, this score suggested a moderate impairment of her overall memory. The subtests that she performed most poorly tended to be those requiring memory for verbal material. Impairment in the recall of prose was also seen in the California Discourse Memory Test, where Mrs. L.L.'s success in the immediate recall of short narratives fluctuated from normal to impaired, and in which her delayed recall was in the range seen in cases of closed head injury. The memory loss was clearly not restricted to verbal material, however. In the Rey-Osterrieth Test (recall of a complex visual figure), her scores were in the impaired range, and similar to those reported by Taylor (cases seen at the Montreal Neurological Institute) following right temporal lobe resections. The copies of the figure were clearly reminiscent of the productions of brain-injured persons and showed perseverative repetition of some of the figure elements.

Thus, Mrs. L.L. showed a clear pattern of impairment in tests of memory and attention that was rather pervasive and not confined to a single mode of functioning or to a particular aspect of attention. Her scores were in the impaired range in the tasks measuring the ability to *encode*, *focus-execute*, and *sustain* attention. The only aspect of these performances that appeared to be relatively intact was the capacity to shift attention from one stimulus aspect to another.

Her presenting complaint of short-term memory problems was substantiated: her memory was clearly defective in both the verbal and visual-spatial spheres. Although the memory impairment was indisputable, it appeared to have been secondary to the deficits seen in the several elements of attention described above. This interpretation is supported to some extent by the fact that the moderate memory impairment was fairly diffuse and widespread and did not worsen appreciably in the delayed (in contrast to the immediate) recall tests. This suggests that she was able to retain material, to a reasonable degree, to which she had been able to attend.

The area of injury to Mrs. L.L.'s brain would be difficult to specify on the basis of these test results. The substantial impairment seen in the tests of sustained visual and auditory attention, however, pointed to some dysfunction in subcortical structures or in the connections between these structures and their cortical targets.

The pattern of attention and memory deficits seen on these tests was without doubt the result of the head injury, since it was not credible that Mrs. L.L. could have achieved a career as a teacher (and 3 years of college education) with attention (and memory) performances this poor.

Some of the impairment seen in these tests may be expected to dissipate with time. The improvement would not be expected to be substantial or dramatic, however, in view of the fact that 15 months had already elasped since the accident. The recommendations that were made included treatment with stimulant medication (which can improve attention in ADHD), cognitive (including attention) retraining, and possible membership in a head-injury support group. Unfortunately, the patient was lost to follow-up so that the long-term outcome is not known.

The Case of E.T.

The report that follows highlights the use of LPP-NIMH Attention Battery in evaluating the efficacy of the drug methylphenidate (Ritalin) in an adolescent boy hospitalized for severe anxiety and depression, with a prior history of treatment for ADHD. The results encouraged the continued use of the drug, since it seemed to produce beneficial effects on his capacity to sustain attention.

E.T., a 16-year-old in the 11th grade, had been hospitalized for depression and anxiety that had increased in severity to the point where it could not be managed on an outpatient basis. E.T. had a long-standing history of learning disability and ADHD (diagnosed by one of the world's leading experts in the field) and was attending special education classes for all of his academic subjects. Prior to his hospitalization, he had experienced the loss of two close friends in an automobile accident and the termination of a relationship by his girlfriend. His parents described him as having difficulties in behavioral, psychosocial, and cognitive spheres.

The question that led to his neuropsychological evaluation had two facets; the first concerned whether his cognitive problems could be contributing to his adjustment difficulties. The second had to do with the development of an overall treatment strategy for the patient. As a second grader, E.T. had been placed on methylphenidate to control his ADHD. At age 15, he had terminated the medication but had recently reinstated it because he thought it might help with some of his symptoms. To determine whether, at this stage, the drug was in fact producing a beneficial effect on his cognitive abilities (via the amelioration of attention), he was tested on the LPP-NIMH Attention Battery both on and off methylphenidate. Eighteen days separated the two examinations, and when he was tested the second time (off medication), he had been free of the drug for 3 days.

E.T. was friendly, cooperative, and hard working during his evaluations, both on and off the drug, suggesting that he was working to the best of his ability on both occasions. He complained of being tired on the second evaluation, despite the fact that he was sleeping 8 to 10 hours per night. While he seemed noticeably more fidgety and restless during the no-drug than the drug evaluation, this impression may have been confounded by the examiner's knowledge of the medication status of the patient.

With respect to the first issue, namely, whether there had been a contribution to his adjustment problems stemming from his cognitive difficulties, the test results supported this inference. The data suggested that he had marked difficulty in processing verbal information. New learning in the verbal modality, in particular, was seen as subject to the strong interfering effects of distraction. This disability had in all likelihood contributed to the development of a maladaptive mode of coping characterized by impulsive acting-out, incessant arguing, manipulativeness, and denial.

With respect to the second issue, the comparison of his performance on the LPP-NIMH Attention Battery on the two occasions was revealing. On neither test was there any evidence of impairment in the *encode, focus-execute,* or *shift* elements of the battery. Scores were within normal limits for his age group both times. In contrast, measures of sustained attention showed a marked drop when E.T. was off medication; his scores fell from the normal range when on methylphenidate to four to five standard deviations below expectation when off the drug. Moreover, the decrement in performance increased directly with task complexity and was also accompanied by a substantial increase in reaction time.

The results of the testing were seen as consistent with research demonstrating that the primary impairment in children with ADHD is in sustained attention. In view of the substantial improvement in this capacity with methylphenidate, it was recommended that the drug be continued, since it could play a significant role in a comprehensive treatment regimen.

CONCLUSIONS

We have presented arguments for the careful evaluation of attention during neuropsychological assessment. In fact, we suggest that the accurate examination of other cognitive systems, like language or memory, is dependent on the prior establishment of intact attentional processes. Although attention is a complex multipartite hypothetical construct, its elements or, at the very least, more stochastic subdivisions are dissociable in a meaningful way. We have reviewed the factor analytically derived four elements of attention and described briefly a likely neuroanatomical substrate for the attention system.

We have presented normative data for the LPP-NIMH Attention Battery that extends across most of the lifespan, and we have discussed some of the possible problems that may arise because of the influence of socioeconomic and cultural factors, particularly in non-U.S. populations. We have introduced some of the possible manifestations of disordered attention and presented a sampling of illustrative case reports.

Recent evidence (Streissguth et al., 1994) suggests that parts of the LPP-NIMH Attention Battery (especially the CPT and Letter Cancellation Task) are particularly sensitive to the effects of maternal alcohol ingestion during pregnancy. These findings encourage the assessment of attention in clinical projects concerned with the effects of environmental toxic agents. We have found that the WCST may be sensitive to an attentional deficit associated with HIV seropositivity in individuals who, otherwise, appear asymptomatic (Fantie, Mirsky, & Bowes, 1990). Clinicians who overlook or undervalue the importance of assessing attention properly do so at their own peril; a greater risk, however, is borne by their patients.

REFERENCES

Adey, W. R. (1969). Spectral analysis of EEG data from animals and man during alerting, orienting and discriminative responses. In C. R. Evans & T. B. Mulholland (Eds.), *Attention and neurophysiology: An international conference* (pp. 194–229). London: Butterworths.

Ajmone Marsan, C. (1965). The thalamus: Data on its functional anatomy and on some aspects of the thalamo-cortical integration. *Archives Italiennes de Biologie, 103*, 847–882.

American Psychiatric Association. (1980). *Diagnostic and statistical manual of mental disorders* (3rd ed.). Washington, DC: Author.

Bakay Pragay, E. (1982). Functional analysis of attention-related unit activity in the reticular formation of the monkey. *Experimental Neurology, 77*, 544–562.

Bakay Pragay, E., Mirsky, A. F., & Abplanalp, J. M. (1969). The effects of chlorpromazine and secobarbital on matching from sample and discrimination tasks in monkeys. *Psychopharmacologia, 7*, 128–138.

Bakay Pragay, E., Mirsky, A. F., Fullerton, B. C., Oshima, H. I., & Arnold, S. W. (1975). Effect of electrical stimulation of the brain on visually controlled (attentive) behavior in the *Macaca mulatta*. *Experimental Neurology, 49*, 203–220.

Bakay Pragay, E., Mirsky, A. F., & Nakamura, F. K. (1987). Attention-related activity in the frontal association cortex during a go/no-go visual discrimination task. *Experimental Neurology, 96*, 481–500.

Bakay Pragay, E., Mirsky, A. F., & Nakamura, F. K. (1988). *Attention-related activity in the inferior-parietal and prestriate cortex of the monkey during a go/no-go visual discrimination task*. Unpublished manuscript.

Bakay Pragay, E., Mirsky, A. F., Ray, C. L., Turner, D. F., & Mirsky, C. V. (1978). Neuronal activity in the brain stem reticular formation during performance of a "go-no go" visual attention task in the monkey. *Experimental Neurology, 60*, 83–95.

Battig, K., Rosvold, H. E., & Mishkin, M. (1960). Comparison of the effects of frontal and caudate lesions on delayed response and alternation in monkeys. *Journal of Comparative and Physiological Psychology, 53*, 400–404.

Blakemore, C., Iversen, S. D., & Zangwill, O. L. (1972). Brain functions. *Annual Review of Psychology, 23*, 413–456.

Campbell, B. A., Hayne, H., & Richardson, R. (1992). *Attention and information processing in infants and adults: Perspectives from human and animal research*. Hillsdale, NJ: Lawrence Erlbaum.

Chapman, L. J., Chapman, J. P., & Raulin, M. L. (1976). Scales for physical and social anhedonia. *Journal of Abnormal Psychology, 85*(4), 374–382.

Chelune, G. J., & Baer, R. A. (1986). Developmental norms for the Wisconsin Card Sorting Test. *Journal of Clinical and Experimental Neuropsychology, 8*, 219–228.

Craik, F. I. M., & Byrd, M. (1982). Aging and cognitive deficits: The role of attentional resources. In F. I. M. Craik & S. Trehub (Eds.), *Aging and cognitive processes* (pp. 191–211). New York: Plenum Press.

Duncan, C. C. (1988). Application of event-related brain potentials to the analysis of interictal attention in absence epilepsy. In M. S. Myslobodsky & A. F. Mirsky (Eds.), *Elements of petit mal epilepsy* (pp. 341–364). New York: Peter Lang.

Fantie, B. D., Mirsky, A. F., & Bowes, R. T. (1990). A cognitive-behavioural deficit associated with HIV-seropositivity. *Society for Neuroscience Abstracts, 16*(2), 1240.

Fey, E. T. (1951). The performance of young schizophrenics and young normals on the Wisconsin Card Sorting Test. *Journal of Consulting Psychology, 15*, 311–319.

Fuster, J. M., & Uyeda, A. (1962). Facilitation of tachistoscopic performance by stimulation of midbrain tegmental points in the monkey. *Experimental Neurology, 6*, 384–406.

Golden, C. J. (1978). Stroop Color and Word Test (Cat. No. 30150M). *A manual for clinical and experimental uses*. Chicago: Stoelting.

Goyette, C. H., Conners, C. K., & Ulrich, R. F. (1978). Normative data on revised Connors parent and teacher rating scales. *Journal of Abnormal Child Psychology, 6*, 221–236.

Grant, D. A., & Berg, E. A. (1948). A behavioral analysis of degree of reinforcement and ease of shifting to new responses in a Weigl-type card-sorting problem. *Journal of Experimental Psychology, 38*, 404–411.

Greenblatt, E., Mattis, S., & Trad, P. V. (1991). The ACID pattern and the freedom from distractibility factor in a child psychiatric population. *Developmental Neuropsychology, 7*, 121–130.

Greenblatt, R. M. (1986). The effects of brain stem compression on attention and memory (Doctoral dissertation, The City University of New York, 1986). *Dissertation Abstracts International, 47*, 1301B.

Halperin, J. M. (1991). The clinical assessment of attention. *International Journal of Neuroscience, 58*, 171–182.

Halperin, J. M., Newcorn, J. H., Sharma, V., Healey, J. M., Wolf, L. E., Pascualvaca, D. M., & Schwartz, S. (1990). Inattentive and non-inattentive ADHD children: Do they constitute a unitary group? *Journal of Abnormal Child Psychology, 18*, 437–449.

Halperin, J. M., O'Brien, J. D., Newcorn, J. H., Healey, J. M., Pascualvaca, D. M., Wolf, L. E., & Young, J. G. (1990). Validation of hyperactive, aggressive, and mixed hyperactive/aggressive disorders in children: A research note. *Journal of Child Psychology and Psychiatry and Allied Disciplines, 31*, 455–459.

Halperin, J. M., Wolf, L. E., Greenblatt, E. R., & Young, J. G. (1991). Subtype analysis of commission errors on the continuous performance test in children. *Developmental Neuropsychology, 7*, 207–217.

Halperin, J. M., Wolf, L. E., Pascualvaca, D. M., Newcorn, J. H., Healey, J. M., O'Brien, J. D., Morganstein, A., & Young, J. G. (1988). Differential assessment of attention and impulsivity in children. *Journal of the American Academy of Child and Adolescent Psychiatry, 27*, 326–329.

Heaton, R. K. (1981). *The Wisconsin Card Sorting Test manual*. Odessa, FL: Psychological Assessment Resources.

Heilman, K. M., Watson, R. T., Valenstein, E., & Damasio, A. R. (1983). Localization of lesions in neglect. In A. Kertesz (Ed.), *Localization in neuropsychology* (pp. 471–492). New York: Academic Press.

Hermann, B. P., & Wyler, A. R. (1988). Neuropsychological outcome of anterior temporal lobectomy. *Journal of Epilepsy, 1*, 135–145.

Jasper, H. H. (1958). Recent advances in our understanding of ascending activities of the reticular system. In H. H. Jasper (Ed.), *Reticular formation of the brain* (pp. 319–331). Boston: Little, Brown.

Jones, B. P., Duncan, C. C., Brouwers, P., & Mirsky, A. F. (1991). Cognition in eating disorders. *Journal of Clinical and Experimental Neuropsychology, 13*(5), 711–728.

Jones, E. G., & Peters, A. (Eds.). (1986). *Cerebral cortex: Sensory-motor areas and aspects of cortical connectivity*. New York: Plenum Press.

Kahneman, D. (1973). *Attention and effort*. Englewood Cliffs, NJ: Prentice-Hall.

Kaufman, A. S. (1975). Factor analysis of the WISC-R at 11 age levels between 6½ and 16½ years. *Journal of Consulting and Clinical Psychology, 43,* 135–147.

Kaufman, A. S. (1979). *Intelligence testing with the WISC-R.* New York: Wiley & Sons.

Kellam, S. G., Branch, J. D., Agrawal, K. C., & Emsminger, M. E. (1975). *Mental health and going to school.* Chicago: University of Chicago Press.

Kolb, B., & Whishaw, I. Q. (1990). *Fundamentals of human neuropsychology* (3rd ed.). New York: W. H. Freeman.

Lansdell, H., & Mirsky, A. F. (1964). Attention in focal and centrencephalic epilepsy. *Experimental Neurology, 9,* 463–469.

Leckliter, I. N., Matarazzo, J. D., & Silverman, A. B. (1986). A literature review of factor analytic studies of the WAIS-R. *Journal of Clinical Psychology, 42,* 332–342.

Lezak, M. D. (1983). *Neuropsychological assessment* (2nd ed.). New York: Oxford University Press.

Lindsley, D. B. (1960). Attention, consciousness, sleep and wakefulness. In J. Field, H. W. Magoun, & V. E. Hall (Eds.l), *Handbook of physiology* (pp. 1553–1593). Washington, DC: American Physiological Society.

Lindsley, D. B., Bowden, J. W., & Magoun, H. W. (1949). Effect upon the EEG of acute injury to the brain stem activating system. *Electroencephalography and Clinical Neurophysiology, 1,* 475–486.

Loney, J., & Milich, R. (1982). Hyperactivity, inattention, and aggression in clinical practice. *Advances in Developmental and Behavioral Pediatrics, 3,* 113–147.

Mackworth, N. H. (1950). Researches on the measurement of human performance. *Medical Research Council Special Report* (No. 268). London: HMSO.

MacLean, P. D. (1990). *The triune brain in evolution: Role in paleocerebral functions.* New York: Plenum Press.

McDowd, J. M., & Craik, F. I. M. (1988). Effects of aging and task difficulty on divided attention performance. *Journal of Experimental Psychology: Human Perception and Performance, 14,* 267–280.

Mesulam, M.-M. (1987). Attention, confusional states and neglect. In M.-M. Mesulam (Ed.), *Principles of behavioral neurology* (pp. 125–168). Philadelphia: F. A. Davis.

Milner, B. (1963). Effects of different brain lesions on card sorting. *Archives of Neurology, 9,* 90–100.

Mirsky, A. F. (1987). Behavioral and psychophysiological markers of disordered attention. *Environmental Health Perspectives, 74,* 191–199.

Mirsky, A. F. (1988). Research on schizophrenia in the NIMH Laboratory of Psychology and Psychopathology, 1954–1987. *Schizophrenia Bulletin, 14,* 151–156.

Mirsky, A. F. (1989). The neuropsychology of attention: Elements of a complex behavior. In E. Perecman (Ed.), *Integrating theory and practice in clinical neuropsychology* (pp. 75–91). Hillsdale, NJ: Lawrence Erlbaum.

Mirsky, A. F. (1992). Neuropsychological assessment of epilepsy. *New Issues in Neurosciences, 4*(1), 25–39.

Mirsky, A. F., Anthony, B. J., Duncan, C. C., Ahearn, M. B., & Kellam, S. G. (1991). Analysis of the elements of attention: A neuropsychological approach. *Neuropsychology Review, 2*(2), 109–145.

Mirsky, A. F., Bakay Pragay, E., & Harris, S. (1977). Evoked potential correlates of stimulation-induced impairment of attention in *Macaca mulatta. Experimental Neurology, 57,* 242–256.

Mirsky, A. F., Lochhead, S. J., Jones, B. P., Kugelmass, S., Walsh, D., & Kendler, K. S. (1992). On familial factors in the attentional deficit in schizophrenia. A review and report of two new subject samples. *Journal of Psychiatric Research, 26*(4), 383–403.

Mirsky, A. F., & Oshima, H. I. (1973). Effect of subcortical aluminum cream lesions on attentive behavior and the electroencephalogram in monkeys. *Experimental Neurology, 39,* 1–18.

Mirsky, A. F., & Siegel, A. (1994). The neurobiology of violence and aggression. In A. J. Reiss, K. A. Miczek, & J. A. Roth (Eds.), *Understanding and preventing violence, Volume 2: Biobehavioral influences* (pp. 59–172). Washington, DC: National Academy Press.

Mirsky, A. F., Silberman, E. K., Latz, A., & Nagler, S. (1985). Adult outcomes of high-risk children: Differential effects of town and kibbutz rearing. *Schizophrenia Bulletin, 11,* 150–154.

Mirsky, A. F., & Van Buren, J. M. (1965). On the nature of the "absence" in centrencephalic epilepsy:

A study of some behavioral, electroencephalographic and autonomic factors. *Electroencephalography and Clinical Neurophysiology, 18,* 334–348.
Mishkin, M. (1978). Memory in monkeys severely impaired by combined but not separate removal of amygdala and hippocampus. *Nature, 273,* 297–298.
Moruzzi, G., & Magoun, H. W. (1949). Brain stem reticular formation and activation of the EEG. *Electroencephalography and Clinical Neurophysiology, 1,* 455–473.
Nagler, S., & Mirsky, A. F. (1985). Introduction: The Israeli high-risk study. *Schizophrenia Bulletin, 11,* 19–29.
O'Brien, J., Morganstein, A., Newcorn, J., Sharma, V., Wolf, L., & Halperin, J. M. (1988). Psychometric and neuropsychological differentiation of conduct disorder and attention deficit disorder. *Scientific Proceedings of the Annual Meeting of the American Academy of Child and Adolescent Psychiatry, 4,* 67.
Pandya, D. N., & Yeterian, E. H. (1985). Architecture and connection of cortical association areas. In A. Peters & E. G. Jones (Eds.), *Cerebral cortex: Association and auditory cortices* (pp. 3–61). New York: Plenum Press.
Parasuraman, R. (1986). Vigilance, monitoring and search. In K. R. Boff, L. Kaufman, & J. P. Thomas (Eds), *Handbook of perception and human performance* (pp. 43.1–43.39). New York: Wiley.
Parker, K. (1983). Factor analysis of the WAIS-R at nine age levels between 16 and 74 years. *Journal of Consulting and Clinical Psychology, 51,* 302–308.
Penfield, W., & Jasper, H. (Eds.). (1954). *Epilepsy and the functional anatomy of the human brain.* Boston: Little, Brown.
Posner, M. I., & Boies, S. J. (1971). Components of attention. *Psychological Review, 78,* 391–408.
Posner, M. I., Inhoff, A., Friedrich, F. J., & Cohen, A. (1987). Isolating attentional systems: A cognitive-anatomical analysis. *Psychobiology, 15*(2), 107–121.
Posner, M. I., & Petersen, S. E. (1990). The attention system of the human brain. *Annual Review of Neuroscience, 13,* 25–42.
Pribram, K. H., & McGuinness, D. (1975). Arousal, activation, and effort in the control of attention. *Psychological Review, 82,* 116–149.
Ray, C. L., Mirsky, A. F., & Bakay Pragay, E. (1982). Functional analysis of attention-related activity in the reticular formation of the monkey. *Experimental Neurology, 77,* 544–562.
Reitan, R. M., & Davidson, L. A. (Eds.). (1974). *Clinical neuropsychology: Current status and applications.* Washington, DC: Winston & Sons.
Reitan, R. M., & Tarshes, E. L. (1959). Differential effects of lateralized brain lesions on the Trail Making Test. *Journal of Nervous and Mental Disease, 129,* 257–262.
Reitan, R. M., & Wolfson, D. (1985). *The Halstead-Reitan Neuropsychological Test Battery.* Tucson, AZ: Clinical Neuropsychology Press.
Rosvold, H. E., Mirsky, A. F., Sarason, I., Bransome, E. D., Jr., & Beck, L. H. (1956). A continuous performance test of brain damage. *Journal of Consulting Psychology, 20,* 343–350.
Roth, B. E., Connell, R. E., Faught, R. E., & Adams, B. (1988). Attention deficits in patients with complex partial seizures. *Epilepsia, 29,* 693.
Rugel, R. P. (1974). WISC subtest scores of disabled readers: A review with respect to Bannatyne's recategorization. *Journal of Learning Disability, 17,* 48–55.
Scheibel, A. B. (1980). Anatomical and physiological substrates of arousal: A view from the bridge. In J. A. Hobson & M. A. B. Brazier (Eds.), *The reticular formation revisited* (pp. 55–60). New York: Raven Press.
Schneider, W., Dumas, S. T., & Shiffrin, R. M. (1984). Automatic and control processing and attention. In R. Parasuraman & D. R. Davies (Eds.), *Varieties of attention* (pp. 1–27). Orlando, FL: Academic Press.
Schneider, W., & Shiffrin, R. M. (1977). Controlled and automatic human information processing: 1. Detection, search, and attention. *Psychological Review, 84,* 1–66.
Schwartz, S. T., Healey, J. M., Halperin, J. H. Wolf, L. E., Pascualvaca, D. M., Newcorn, J., & Sharma, V. (1989). Is the "Attentional Triad" of the WISC-R related to attention? *Journal of Clinical and Experimental Neuropsychology, 11,* 27.

Scoville, W. B., & Milner, B. (1957). Loss of recent memory after bilateral hippocampal lesions. *Journal of Neurology, Neurosurgery, and Psychiatry, 20,* 11–21.

Shiffrin, R. M., & Schneider, W. (1977). Controlled and automatic human information processing: 2. Perceptual learning, automatic attending, and a general theory. *Psychological Review, 84,* 127–190.

Somberg, B. L., & Salthouse, T. A. (1982). Divided attention abilities in young and old adults. *Journal of Experimental Psychology: Human Perception and Performance, 8,* 651–663.

Sperling, G., & Dosher, B. A. (1986). Handbook of perception and human performance. In K. R. Boff, L. Kaufman, & J. P. Thomas (Eds.), *Strategy and optimization in human information processing* (pp. 2.1–2.65). New York: Wiley.

Spitz, H. H. (1972). Note on immediate memory for digits: Invariance over the years. *Psychological Bulletin, 78,* 183–185.

Streissguth, A. P., Sampson, P. D., Carmichael Olson, H., Bookstein, F. L., Barr, H. M., Scott, M., Feldman, J., & Mirsky, A. F. (1994). Maternal drinking during pregnancy: Attention and short-term memory performance in 14-year-old offspring: A longitudinal prospective study. *Alcoholism: Clinical & Experimental Research, 18,* 202–218.

Stroop, J. R. (1935). Studies of interference in serial verbal reactions. *Journal of Experimental Psychology, 18,* 643–662.

Talland, G. A. (1965). *Deranged memory.* New York: Academic Press.

Tatman, J. E. (1992). *Elements of attention and concentration in normal aging adults: Focus on decline.* Unpublished master's thesis, The American University, Washington, DC.

Tatman, J. E., Fantie, B. D., and Mirsky, A. F. (1992). Elements of attention: Performance of healthy adults and neuropsychiatric patients on the NIMH-LPP Attention Battery. *Society for Neuroscience Abstracts, 17*(2), 1208.

Wechsler, D. (1955). *Manual for the Wechsler Adult Intelligence Scale.* New York: Psychological Corporation.

Wechsler, D. (1974). *Wechsler Intelligence Scale for Children* (rev. ed). New York: Psychological Corporation.

Wechsler, D. (1981). *Wechsler Adult Intelligence Scale* (rev. ed.). New York: Psychological Corporation.

Wechsler, D. (1991). *Wechsler Intelligence Scale for Children* (3rd ed.). San Antonio: Psychological Corporation.

Weinberger, D. R., Berman, K. F., & Zec, R. F. (1986). Physiological dysfunction of dorsolateral prefrontal cortex in schizophrenia. 1. Regional cerebral blood flow (rCBF) evidence. *Archives of General Psychiatry, 43,* 114–125.

Whishaw, I. Q., & Kolb, B. (1984). Neuropsychological assessment of children and adults with developmental dyslexia. In R. N. Malatesha & H. A. Whitaker (Eds.), *Dyslexia: A global issue* (pp. 375–404). The Hague: Martinus Nijhoff.

Yakovlev, P. I., & Lecours, A.-R. (1967). The myelogenetic cycles of regional maturation of the brain. In A. Minkowski (Ed.), *Regional development of the brain in early life* (pp. 3–70). Oxford: Blackwell.

Yingling, C. D., & Skinner, J. E. (1975). Regulation of unit activity in nucleus reticularis thalami by the mesencephalic reticular formation and the frontal granular cortex. *Electroencephalography and Clinical Neurophysiology, 39,* 635–642.

Zubin, J. (1975). Problem of attention in schizophrenia. In M. L. Kietzman, S. Sutton, & J. Zubin (Eds.), *Experimental approaches to psychopathology* (pp. 139–166). New York: Academic Press.

3

Assessment of Problem Solving and Executive Functions

FELICIA C. GOLDSTEIN and ROBERT C. GREEN

The assessment of problem solving and executive functions is one of the most challenging tasks facing clinicians involved in the evaluation of behavior. Although there are numerous neuropsychological measures to examine these abilities, no single test captures their full complexity. The skills necessary for performing behaviors such as planning, hypothesis testing, and self-monitoring are interrelated and often subtle. Successful performance depends not only on the integrity of these specific skills, but on other domains such as language, attention, and memory. The ability to use feedback, for example, may be disrupted because the patient has forgotten a previous response rather than being insensitive to environmental contingencies. Motivational level also influences whether the patient is willing to formulate strategies and to select behaviors necessary to achieve goals. Assessment requires a comprehensive approach that employs an array of methods and includes careful analysis of the underpinnings of impairments.

In this chapter, we present assessment techniques for evaluating disorders of problem solving and executive functions. First, the critical elements of these abilities will be described. Neuropsychological tests will then be covered, and general guidelines for assessment will be considered. Finally, illustrative case examples will be provided in order to demonstrate application of these principles.

FELICIA C. GOLDSTEIN and ROBERT C. GREEN • Neurobehavioral Program, Department of Neurology, Emory University School of Medicine and Wesley Woods Center, Atlanta, Georgia 30329.

Clinical Neuropsychological Assessment: A Cognitive Approach, edited by Robert L. Mapou and Jack Spector. Plenum Press, New York, 1995.

CONCEPTUAL FRAMEWORKS

Problem solving and *executive functions* are terms that have been used to describe the most complex of all human cognitive skills. Descriptions of the problem-solving process abound in early theoretical discussions (e.g., Lhermitte et al., 1972, cited in Jouandet & Gazzaniga, 1979; Luria, 1963, 1966, 1973), whereas *executive functions* is a relatively newer term (e.g., Lezak, 1983; Stuss & Benson, 1986). *Problem solving* refers to specific behaviors, such as concept formation and the ability to shift mental sets, that affect the quality with which a task is performed. *Executive functions* is a broader term that encompasses processes including anticipation, goal selection, and planning/organization. These two nomenclatures are often used collectively to describe the process of perceiving the relevant parameters of a situation, calling on stores of experience, and planning novel sequences of behavior. Frameworks for conceptualizing problem solving and executive functions emphasize motivation, selection and implementation of a plan, and self-evaluation of final performance. These behaviors are presented in Table 3.1 and are also elaborated below.

Motivation

Motivation is a common theme within almost any conceptual framework that addresses problem solving and executive functions. According to Luria (1973), thinking "arises only when the subject has an appropriate motive which makes the task urgent and its solution essential" (p. 327). Similarly, for Lezak (1983), the correlates of goal formation, that is, determining what one needs and wants, involve both motivation and self-awareness. Individuals with deficits of executive function may maintain established responses to familiar situations, but when confronted with novelty, they may fail to formulate new behaviors to achieve a goal. In other descriptions, initiation of executive functions depends on "drive" and motivation (Stuss & Benson, 1986). Drive refers to physiological states such as hunger, whereas motivation "reflects a greater degree of intellectual control" (p. 243). Motivational disturbances are difficult to disentangle from other aspects of activation and initiation, but often appear to be particularly impaired in patients who exhibit symptoms of depression. Depression is a common concomitant of head injury that is associated with diminished motivation

TABLE 3.1. Similarities among Behaviors Involved in Problem Solving and Executive Functioning as Delineated in Various Frameworks

Luria (1973)	Lezak (1983)	Stuss and Benson (1986)
I. Motivation	Goal formulation	Anticipation Motivation Self-awareness
II. Task analysis Selection of plan Selection of behaviors	Planning	Goal selection
III. Implementation	Carrying out activities	Preplanning
IV. Evaluation	Effective performance	Monitoring

(Levin, 1987; Prigatano, 1987). Reduced motivation can also be seen in conditions where affect is absent, or in cases of anosognosia or denial of illness where a failure to appreciate deficits may produce impaired capacity for formulating goals and realistic plans (Prigatano, 1991). In these conditions, altered mediation of motivation is presumed to influence whether problem solving is attempted and the manner in which the patient approaches a task.

Planning

The next stage of problem solving and executive functions involves analyzing the task and considering solutions prior to engaging in any overt action. Luria (1973) identifies components including (1) restraining impulsivity, investigating the conditions of the problem, and recognizing the critical components and their relations; (2) selecting one alternative and devising a strategy; and (3) choosing the tactics essential to the strategy. Impulsivity, the failure to analyze a task before responding, leads to erroneous answers caused by focusing only on superficial qualities. For example, in solving the problem "Jack has four apples, and Jill has two apples more. How many apples had they together?" patients may respond "six" without performing the intermediate step required by the word *more* (Luria, 1973).

Lezak's (1983) *planning* stage of the executive functions consists of determining and arranging the integral elements to achieve a particular goal. For Lezak, the necessary prerequisites for successful completion include anticipation of the future in relation to the present circumstances, conceptualization and weighing of alternatives, and evolution of a framework. The importance of anticipation, goal selection, and preplanning (establishment of means–end relationships) is also highlighted by Stuss and Benson (1986).

Execution

Following a description of the strategy and tactics needed to achieve a goal, the next emphasis in several frameworks is on the execution of the necessary behaviors to accomplish the goal. Lezak (1983) refers to this stage as "carrying out activities." Successful completion of a task "requires the actor to initiate, maintain, switch, and stop sequences of complex behavior in an orderly and integrated manner" (p. 512). Two types of behavior frequently interfere with the implementation of strategies and tactics. One deficit is *perseveration,* which refers to the continuation of a response that is no longer relevant. Sandson and Albert (1987) have identified three subtypes of perseveration including recurrent (repeating a previous response to a new stimulus), stuck-in-set (incorrectly maintaining the same category of response), and continuous (abnormally prolonging a behavior without stopping). *Impersistence,* or difficulty in maintaining a voluntary response over time, is another deficit that may interfere with performance. Luria accounts for these impairments by hypothesizing that the patient's speech or self-verbalizations no longer serve to maintain or to modify their responses. He states, "If a verbal program involves the arrest of a former action or an association, it loses its controlling function, and the action turns into an unselective, impulsive 'field reaction' or 'perseveration'" (Luria & Homskaya, 1964, p. 360). Stuss, Delgado, and Guzman (1987), however, reported that verbalizations were helpful in restoring control over motor behavior in two patients with right frontal lobe dysfunction. These patients were unable to continue keeping their eyelids closed but could so when they repeated the command out loud during performance of the activity. Stuss et al. (1987) suggested that Luria's hypothesis referred specifically to left frontal lobe damage. They proposed that patients with right frontal lobe deficits could be taught self-talk techniques as a rehabilitation intervention.

Evaluation of Performance

A final stage in the completion of a task concerns evaluation of one's performance. For Luria (1973), the solution of a problem entails subsequent "comparison of the results obtained with the original conditions of the task" (p. 329). The process ends only if the solution matches the original goal. If not, then the search for strategies and facts continues. Lezak (1983) describes the critical behaviors in this stage as the ability to self-monitor and self-correct. She notes that patients may fail a task either because they do not perceive their errors or because they know they are occurring but do not correct them.

Thus, there are multiple skills that contribute to problem solving and executive functions. Our approach in this chapter is to elaborate and describe the methodology for clinical neuropsychological assessment of these abilities. In the following section, we describe procedures including measures of hypothesis generation and shifting of response sets, divergent thinking, reasoning, and planning and organization. These areas are by no means exhaustive but have been chosen because they are the best developed in terms of available neuropsychological procedures.

ASSESSMENT TECHNIQUES

Our discussion of neuropsychological procedures is organized by the primary behavioral domains they assess. It should be highlighted, however, that these tests do not fall into discrete categories but span a number of abilities. Inclusion in a particular section is based on a test's most salient qualities. Pure deficits in any one area are exceptional, and a skillful and experienced practitioner may be needed to describe and differentiate deficits that are both complementary and additive. Moreover, some of these tests do not have normative data for older patients. Results must be interpreted cautiously with an elderly patient, since studies of nonneurological populations have reported a decline in abstraction and problem solving with advancing age (e.g., Albert, Wolfe, & Lafleche, 1990; Haaland, Vranes, Goodwin, & Garry, 1987; Salthouse & Prill, 1987). Finally, the impact of the patient's educational level and estimated premorbid abilities needs to be considered when interpreting performance. For example, one may miss an impairment in a highly educated individual who can compensate for the task demands. In contrast, individuals from other cultural backgrounds may perform less well on some measures, despite an absence of brain pathology (see, for example, Mirsky, Fantie, & Tatman, this volume). Thus, the pattern of performance on a number of tests, observations of behavior during the session, and family reports of functioning outside the examination should all contribute to clinical decision making.

Generation of Hypotheses and Shifting of Response Sets

Cognitive flexibility or the capacity to exhibit a "win–stay, lose–shift" strategy is an important component of problem solving. Tests of sorting are used to examine hypothesis generation and the patient's ability to shift concepts. The patient must develop a hypothesis and engage in a particular response type based on environmental contingencies. Successful performance requires an evaluation of one's behavior by comparing it with the initial task requirements. Neurologically impaired individuals may exhibit deficits in benefiting from feedback, modifying their behavior in response to current task demands, and shifting response sets.

The Category Test (Halstead, 1947) examines the patient's ability to infer similarities and differences, to form grouping principles, and to make novel responses based on previous experiences. The original test uses 208 items that are projected on a screen, although a booklet form exists that allows bedside administration and ease of transportation (DeFilippis & McCampbell, 1987). The Category Test includes sets of items that are organized by different principles. For example, in one set, the Roman numerals I through IV appear on the screen, and the patient must learn to match a particular numeral to the Arabic number (e.g., match II to 2) on the response lever. In another set, four figures appear, and the patient must press the lever corresponding to the item that is most different from the others. The patient receives auditory feedback on whether a response is correct or incorrect, and thus learns the correct principle from the pattern of successes and failures. The score consists of the total number of errors.

The Wisconsin Card Sorting Test (WCST; Grant & Berg, 1948; Heaton, 1981; Heaton, Chelune, Talley, Kay, & Curtiss, 1993) is another frequently employed measure of hypothesis generation and response shifting. As shown in Figure 3.1, the WCST uses cards that vary along the dimensions of color, form, and number. The patient is shown four key cards, and places cards from a deck below the key cards he or she thinks they match. The patient must determine the correct sorting rule (i.e., whether the sort is right or wrong) based on feedback from the examiner following each trial. After 10 correct consecutive sorts based on the concept "color," the principle changes without warning to "form," and the patient finds that previously correct responses are now incorrect. Following 10 more consecutive correct trials, the rule becomes "number." The Modified Card Sorting Test (MCST) was developed by Nelson (1976) as a simplified version of the WCST. The MCST takes less time to administer (using 48 instead of 128 trials and requiring only six correct sorting trials before the concept shifts), the sequence of the principles is determined by the patient rather than being set by the examiner, and the key cards share only one attribute with the cards in the deck. On the WCST, a stimulus card can match a key card in more than one way such as both color and form, thus making the examiner's feedback ambiguous. The most striking difference between the measures, however, is that on the

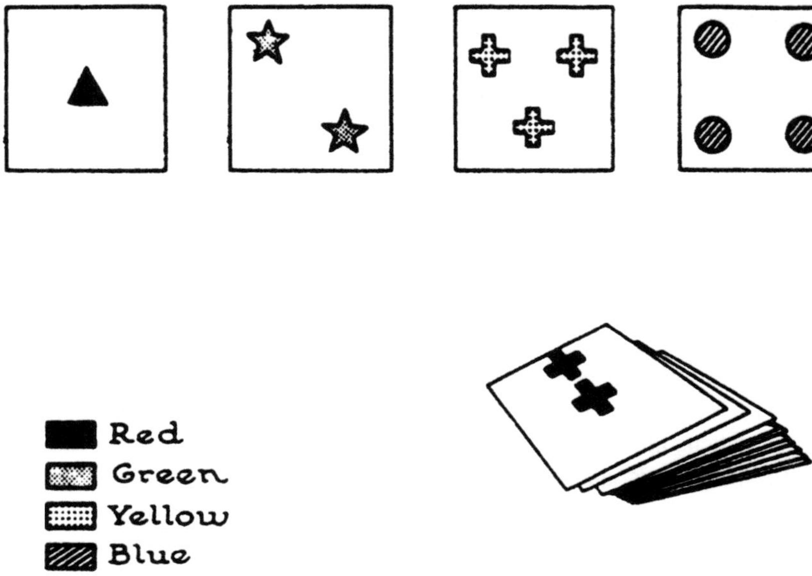

FIGURE 3.1. Wisconsin Card Sorting Test stimulus materials. From Milner, B. (1963). Effects of different brain lesions on card sorting. *Archives of Neurology, 9,* 90–100. Reproduced with permission of the author.

MCST, the examiner *tells* the patient that the rule has now changed and that he or she must figure out a different way to match the cards. On the WCST, no warning is given, and the patient must infer this switch based on being told that he or she is no longer correct. Nelson (1976) found that the warning to shift sets on the MCST reduced the distress level of subjects because they were not given unexpected negative feedback.

The WCST and the MCST yield a number of indices for isolating the features of an executive processing deficit. *Perseveration* consists of staying with an incorrect rule despite being continuously told after each trial that the sorting principle is wrong. Nelson (1976) observed that telling patients that the rule changed did not reduce their tendency to engage in this behavior. Our own experience with patients who have a variety of neurobehavioral problems also indicates that the MCST is remarkably sensitive to problems in set shifting. Perseveration on the WCST and MCST has been associated with frontal lobe pathology (Drewe, 1974; Milner, 1963; Nelson, 1976; Robinson, Heaton, Lehman, & Stilson, 1980). It is important to realize, however, that perseveration also occurs in association with lesions outside the frontal lobes (Allison, 1966; Helmick & Berg, 1976; Sandson & Albert, 1987). Further, a recent study using magnetic resonance imaging found no significant differences in WCST performance between patients with and without frontal lobe damage (Anderson, Damasio, Jones, & Tranel, 1991).

Other performance indices on the card sorting tasks include *failure to maintain set,* which occurs whenever the patient switches to a new rule after at least five consecutive trials of using a correct sorting strategy. This behavior may indicate an attentional problem as opposed to an executive processing deficit. *Number of categories achieved* provides information about the patient's ability to recognize the sorting principles. For patients who achieve fewer than three correct sorts, we have found that it is useful to ask about their understanding of the test requirements and what concepts were involved. This can help determine whether poor performance was caused by confusion about instructions or an inability to hypothesize. *Nonperseverative errors* involve sorting to the wrong principle and may indicate guessing, forgetting the principle, or developing an elaborate hypothesis that is not part of the test (Lezak, 1983). Heaton (1981) observed that normal controls greater than 59 years of age achieved fewer categories and made more total errors and perseverative errors/responses than younger subjects. More recently, Axelrod and Henry (1992) reported a similar age-associated decrement in WCST performance in their comparison of normal subjects ranging from their fifties through their eighties. With increased age, individuals made more total errors and perseverative errors/responses.

Both the WCST and the MCST are sensitive to problems in the ability to reason and to shift response sets. The choice between these two measures is best guided by the ability level of the patient. Examiners working with premorbidly high-functioning individuals or those who exhibit only mild levels of cognitive deterioration may prefer the WCST because it is more challenging. Unlike the WCST, there are no norms available for the MCST, but as noted by Lezak, "[I]n clinical practice norms are rarely needed for determining whether or how a performance is unsatisfactory" (1983, p. 492).

Delayed alternation tasks provide another means of examining the patient's capacity to form rules and to shift mental sets (Freedman & Oscar-Berman, 1986a; Oscar-Berman, McNamara, & Freedman, 1991). In the delayed alternation (DA) procedure, the patient must learn to alternate responding from the left to the right sides on subsequent trials. On trial 1, a reward such as a coin is placed behind a screen to the patient's right side. Following a brief delay of a few seconds, the screen is lifted, and the patient chooses the side where he or she thinks the coin is hidden. If the patient is correct, the examiner now places the coin on the left side (hidden by the screen), and after another brief interval, the patient again chooses. If the response is again correct, the coin shifts to the right side until the patient can demonstrate on a series of consecutive trials that he or she has learned the rule to switch responding. If responding is incorrect (i.e., the patient chooses the side where the coin is not hidden), the coin remains in the same place until that side is eventually chosen. The delayed alternation procedure provides information about the patient's ability to use feedback to modify responses. Memory and attentional demands come into play as well, since successful performance depends on the patient attending to and remembering the placement of the reward on the previous trial. Oscar-Berman and colleagues (Freedman & Oscar-Berman, 1986a, b; Oscar-Berman et al., 1991) have demonstrated DA deficits in numerous patient populations including Alzheimer's disease (AD), Parkinson's disease (PD), and Korsakoff's syndrome. Errors on this task have been correlated with bilateral frontal lobe lesions (Freedman & Oscar-Berman, 1986a). However, as seen with the WCST, even patients without frontal lobe pathology can perform poorly (Chorover & Cole, 1966).

The Visual-Verbal Test (Feldman & Drasgow, 1951) also evaluates the capacity for mental flexibility. This test requires the individual to form a rule for unifying items such as their color, shape, size, position, or structure and then to switch to another principle. The patient is shown a total of 42 cards that each depict four objects. The task is to determine how three of the four objects on a card are alike and then decide another way in which three objects are similar. Albert and colleagues (1990) examined the performance of healthy subjects aged 30–79 years. They found that individuals 70 years and older obtained fewer correct responses and had difficulty establishing and switching mental sets compared to younger subjects 30–39 and 50–59 years of age.

The Twenty Questions procedure (Mosher & Hornsby, 1966) is another technique that can be used to examine problem-solving abilities and response shifting (Goldstein & Levin, 1991; Laine & Butters, 1982). For example, Goldstein and Levin (1991) evaluated survivors of severe closed head injury with this task by showing them an array of pictures that belonged to different categories such as animals and foods. The items were randomly arranged so that the shared conceptual features were not obvious. Patients were told to guess the item the examiner had in mind in the fewest number of trials by asking questions that could be answered "yes" or "no." This procedure was repeated for three items. Questions were scored for strategies including hypotheses (asking about a specific item: Is it the shoe?), pseudoconstraints (asking about a specific item in an indirect fashion: Does it have shoelaces?), and constraints (asking about a category that referred to two or more pictures and thus narrowed down the alternatives: Is it an article of clothing?). Compared to age and education matched controls, the patients required more trials to guess the items. As depicted in Figure 3.2, patients asked about a specific item (pseudoconstraint) rather than simultaneously eliminating several items from one category by referring to their shared conceptual features (constraint). The patients' poorer performance was not due to forgetting their questions, since they did not provide more repetitions than controls, and they understood the conceptual nature of the task, since they could group the pictures into categories. Rather, they lacked the capacity to formulate sophisticated questions and to use the examiner's feedback to narrow the alternatives.

In the motor domain, mental flexibility can be examined by having the patient perform copying tasks that require sequencing and response shifting. For example, the patient can be asked to copy alternating cursive letters (e.g., *m n m n,* etc.) or a ramparts figure (e.g., a square connected to a triangle connected to another square, etc.). Motor perserveration is the inability to inhibit continuous reproduction of one of the figures. Procedures that require the patient to make responses opposite to those of the examiner (Luria, 1966; Luria & Homskaya, 1964) are sensitive to difficulties in motor regulation. For example, if the examiner taps the table twice, the patient must tap once, and, conversely, if the examiner taps once, the patient must tap twice. Go/no-go tasks, in which the patient must inhibit responding, also can detect motor regulation problems. Thus, if the examiner taps twice, the patient must lift a finger, but if the examiner taps once, the patient must do nothing. Patients with self-regulation deficits may mimic the examiner's response rather than producing the correct, alternate response (Lezak, 1983).

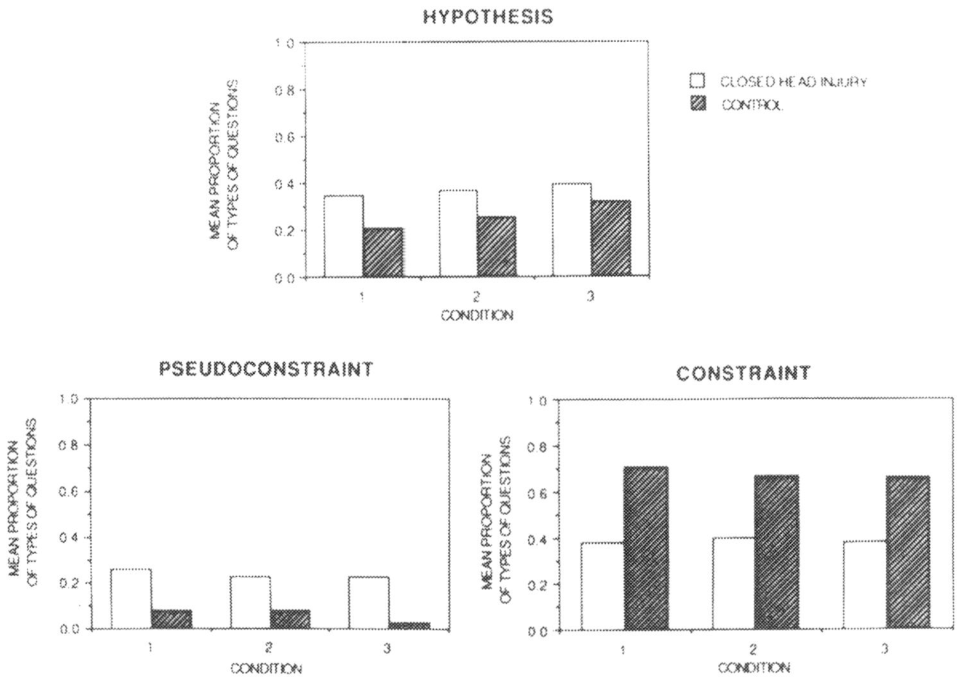

FIGURE 3.2. Mean proportion of types of questions asked for the three conditions of the Twenty Questions procedure. From Goldstein, F. C., & Levin, H. S. (1991). Question-asking strategies after severe closed head injury. *Brain and Cognition, 17*, 23–30. Reproduced with permission of the publisher.

Divergent Thinking

The neuropsychological evaluation commonly stresses convergent thinking, in which there is only one answer to a problem or one means of accomplishing a goal. Divergent thinking, or the ability to produce alternative approaches, however, is also critical to successful problem solving.

Fluency tasks are useful in examining divergent thinking. On a verbal fluency measure such as the Controlled Oral Word Association Test (COWAT; Benton & Hamsher, 1989), patients are instructed to say as many words in 1 minute that begin with a specific letter. They are warned against using the same word or a similar variant (e.g., saying both *cough* and *coughing*) and also against providing proper nouns such as names of people or places. Performance is scored for the number of correct responses, perseverative errors such as repeating a word, and nonperseverative errors such as providing a proper noun or a word beginning with a different letter. Reduced verbal fluency is a feature of left frontal injury even in nonaphasic patients (Benton, 1968). Table 3.2 displays word generation to the letters *F, A,* and *S* by a 61-year-old, right-handed man with a college degree, evaluated through the Emory Neurobehavioral Program. The patient underwent resections of bifrontal lobe meningiomas. His verbal fluency on this task was severely diminished, and he exhibited both perseverative and

TABLE 3.2. Controlled Oral Word Association in a Patient with Bifrontal Lobe Meningiomas

Letters

F	A	S
full	able	such
fanny	at last (NP)	simple
fantastic	at	soothe
frugal	around	simple (P)
fun loving (NP)[a]	asinine	shirt
full (P)	articulate	
funky		
funny		

Categories

Animals		Fruits/vegetables	
zebra	chicken	apple	lettuce
lion	goat	peach	peach (P)
tiger	sheep	orange	pear
wild beast (NP)	zebra	tangerine	apple (P)
elephant	giraffe	kumquat	grapes
cow	rhinoceros	cauliflower	cherries
bull	hippopotamus	broccoli	
pig			

[a]NP, nonperseverative error; P, perseverative error.

nonperseverative errors. In contrast, his verbal output improved when he was asked to say words that belong to categories. We have found that the inclusion of a category fluency measure to compare with word fluency provides useful clinical information about the nature of the underlying disturbance. Patients who exhibit impaired divergent thinking frequently show a facilitation when given the structure of categories, since this task provides external guidance. The failure to significantly increase output when given categories is observed in AD. Monsch et al. (1992) found that category fluency discriminated between patients with AD versus normal controls, a finding they attributed to impaired semantic knowledge and search in AD.

Jones-Gotman and Milner (1977) developed a nonverbal analog of verbal fluency. On the design fluency test, patients are told to generate as many designs as they can within a specified time period. In the Free Condition, patients have 5 minutes to make different drawings that cannot be named (i.e., that do not depict real objects) and to avoid scribbles. In the Fixed Condition, patients are given 4 minutes to make drawings that have exactly four lines. Definitions of lines include angular and curved shapes as well as circles. Again, patients are instructed to make designs that cannot be named and that differ from each other. They are given only one warning whenever they break a particular rule. Jones-Gotman and Milner studied epileptic patients with unilateral surgical excisions and normal controls. They found that patients with right-hemisphere lesions tended to have lower productivity scores. In addition, patients with right frontal and right fronto-central lesions displayed a higher incidence of perseveration.

Reasoning

Reasoning entails the capacity for understanding relations, identifying essential components, synthesizing them, and deriving a common theme. Impairments can occur anywhere in the process of formulating a strategy for problem solution. Patients may focus on only one aspect of a problem and thus fail to appreciate the overall implications. Kurt Goldstein (Goldstein, 1942; Goldstein & Scheerer, 1941) distinguished between a concrete and an abstract attitude. The former involved the tendency to be bound by the stimulus properties of a task, whereas the latter entailed the ability to go beyond the present, to simultaneously consider several aspects of a problem, and to think symbolically.

The Similarities subtest of the Wechsler Adult Intelligence Scale-Revised (WAIS-R; Wechsler, 1981) is frequently used to evaluate reasoning. This test requires the patient to infer the shared conceptual features between items such as an orange and banana, and to state the way in which they are the same or alike. The WAIS-R manual includes scoring criteria that award points depending on the level of abstraction (e.g., one point for "you eat them" and two points for "fruit"). A common response of brain-injured patients with impaired verbal reasoning is to say that items are not the same or to provide answers that emphasize differences, such as responding that an eye is for seeing and an ear is for hearing. Age-related decrements also may be observed. Axelrod and Henry (1992) found a significant age-related decline on the Similarities subtest, with healthy community-residing adults greater than 70 years manifesting abstraction difficulties relative to those in their fifties and sixties. The Dementia Rating Scale (Mattis, 1988) provides choices for patients who perform poorly when asked to spontaneously generate similarities. For example, they are given three possible answers (e.g., coat-shirt: *clothing*, wool, fruit) and are asked to select the best response. Patients are also told to select an item that does not belong with the others (e.g., boy, *door,* man). Clinically, we find these techniques useful for circumventing problems, such as dysnomia, that may interfere with the patient's ability to state relationships. A similar format is provided in the WAIS-R as a Neuropsychological Instrument (Kaplan, Fein, Morris, & Delis, 1991).

Reasoning skills are also evaluated through the use of proverb interpretation and verbal absurdity tasks. The former measure examines the patient's ability to go beyond the concrete meaning of a statement to a more abstract generalization. One widely used measure is the Proverb Interpretation Task (Gorham, 1956). In the free condition, the patient is given 12 proverbs and is instructed to explain the meaning of each one. The patient is told to say what the proverb means, as opposed to providing a literal interpretation. Scoring occurs on a three-point system whereby abstract responses receive the most points. In the recognition form of the test, the patient is given 40 items, each having four possible answers, and is told to choose the best abstract meaning. Albert and colleagues (1990) reported a decrement in proverb interpretation with age, such that persons 70 years and older were more likely to provide concrete explanations. Sophisticated proverb interpretation is related to higher levels of education and vocabulary skills on the WAIS-R. Therefore, patients who lack formal education or have low premorbid intellectual abilities may perform at an impoverished level. The patient's ability to infer meaning from a statement and to determine whether the information is logical is another important component of assessment. On the Verbal Absurdities subtest of the Stanford-Binet (Terman & Merrill, 1973; Thorndike, Hagen, & Sattler, 1986), the patient is presented with vignettes and has to determine what is foolish or wrong with each story. For example, he or she may be told about a man who got the flu and died, but the second time he got the flu, he quickly recovered.

Estimation tasks are useful for examining reasoning skills because of their open-ended nature, the lack of an obvious strategy, and the fact that there are a range of probable responses. The patient must use general knowledge and apply a series of logical steps before producing a response. For example, in answering the question "What is the length of the average man's spine?" the patient could first think about the average man's height, then take into consideration the beginning and end points of the spine, and finally subtract the length of the head/neck and legs. Other solution paths, however, are also possible.

Impaired cognitive estimation has been associated with frontal lobe dysfunction (Shallice & Evans, 1978; Smith & Milner, 1984). Shallice and Evans (1978) designed a cognitive estimation questionnaire for patients with frontal or nonfrontal brain lesions. Twelve questions were quantitative (e.g., "How many slices in a sliced loaf?"), and three were qualitative (e.g., "What is the largest object normally found in a house?"). In comparison to the answers provided by normal controls, patients with frontal lobe lesions offered more bizarre estimates than those with lesions outside the frontal lobes. Shallice and Evans noted that this effect was not mediated by differences between the groups in the size of lesions or in general intellectual functioning and mathematical ability. Goldstein and colleagues (Goldstein et al., 1992) administered the cognitive estimation procedure to patients with AD or PD who had achieved comparable scores on the Dementia Rating Scale (Mattis, 1988). The answers of demographically matched normal elderly controls were used to judge the extremeness of the patients' responses. AD patients (Figure 3.3) provided significantly more unusual responses than PD patients when they had to spontaneously generate answers. Because of the word-finding demands of this task, which may have placed the AD patients at a disadvantage, we devised another procedure requiring subjects to select from a list of choices the best response to each question. Both patient groups choose bizarre answers relative to normal elderly controls. The researchers hypothesized that AD and PD patients had frontal lobe dysfunction that interfered with their estimations of real-world events.

We have thus far largely focused on verbal reasoning skills. Tests exist as well for measuring the patient's capacity to analyze and to derive logical relations from visual material. One such task is Picture Completion on the WAIS-R, which requires the patient to detect missing details. The missing elements become less obvious as the difficulty level increases. For example, an easy item requires detecting that the nose-piece is missing in a pair of eyeglassses, whereas a more abstract item requires realizing that a mirror does not show a woman's complete reflection. One can also examine concrete and abstract responses to the same card. Patients bound by the obvious may respond that in a scene of a man and a dog walking on a beach, the dog is missing a leash rather than the fact the man has left footprints in the sand, but the dog has not.

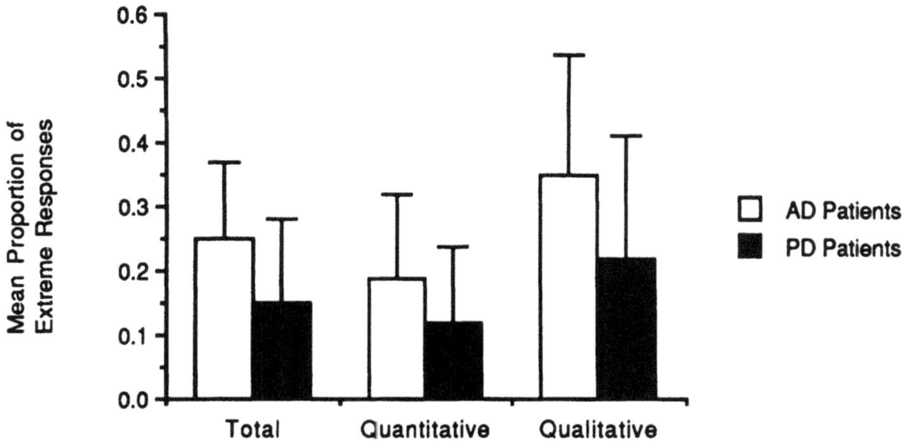

FIGURE 3.3. Mean proportion of extreme responses given by patients with Alzheimer's or Parkinson's disease cn the cognitive estimation procedure.

Picture Arrangement, also on the WAIS-R, examines the patient's capacity to sequence material. The patient is given cards in a mixed-up order and has to arrange them logically so that they "tell a story that makes sense." The Raven's Standard Progressive Matrices (Raven, 1960) was developed as a measure of nonverbal analogical reasoning and is useful to administer to patients with expressive language problems, since the test does not require a verbal response. As shown in Figure 3.4, the patient views a pattern and must choose the figure from a set of alternatives that best completes the sequence. The test is untimed and consists of 60 problems, which become increasingly difficult within each set of 12 patterns. The Raven's Coloured Progressive Matrices

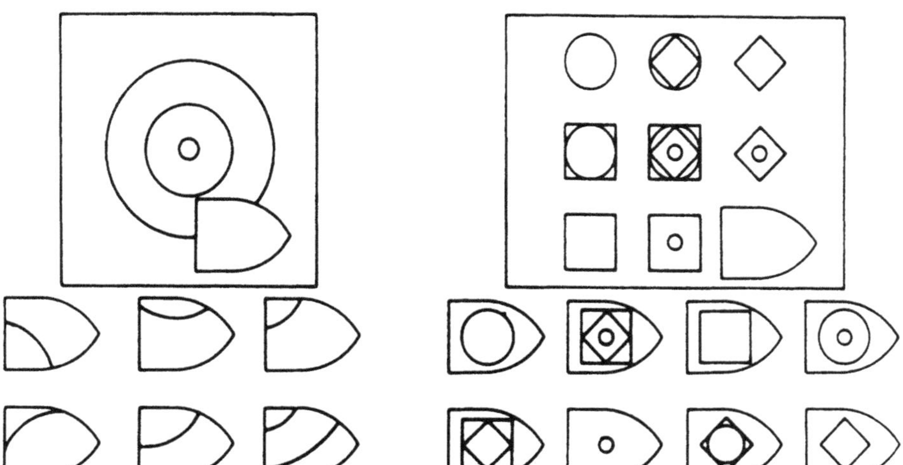

FIGURE 3.4. Examples of two Progressive Matrices-type items. From Lezak, M. D. (1983). *Neuropsychological assessment* (2nd ed.). New York: Oxford University Press. Reproduced with permission of the author and publisher.

(Raven, 1965) is an easier version that can be used with children, adults older than age 65 years, aphasics, and adults suspected of mental deficiency.

Planning and Organization

This category of neuropsychological tests examines the patient's ability to inhibit impulsive tendencies and to consider the future consequences of his or her behavior toward the achievement of a goal. The Porteus Maze Test (Porteus, 1965) is widely used to evaluate these abilities. The patient is given a maze with a marked starting point and is instructed to use a pencil to trace his or her way out of the maze without going into a "blind alley" (Figure 3.5). Doing so is a "fatal error," which results in termination of the trial and repetition of the same maze, up to a specific criterion. The patient also is warned not to cross a solid line but to go through an opening in order to get into the next lane, although doing so is not a "fatal error" and results only in a warning. Successful completion of the mazes involves taking the time to scan the

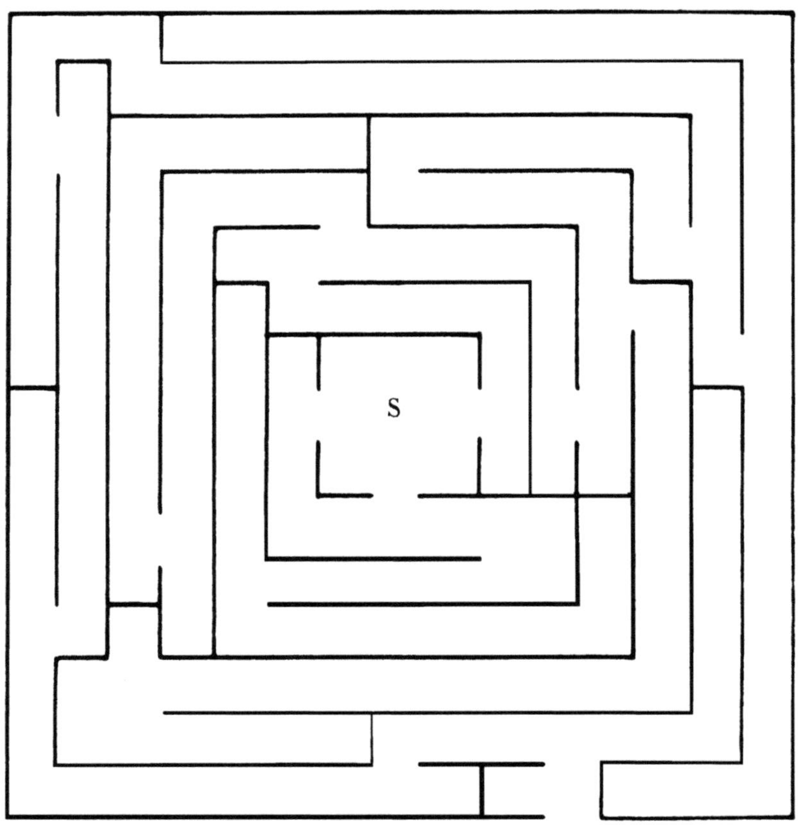

FIGURE 3.5. Sample item (Adult 1) from the Porteus Maze Test. From Porteus, S. D. (1965). *Porteus Maze Test: Fifty years' application*. New York: Psychological Corporation. Reproduced with permission of the publisher.

pattern and to think about the next move at a particular junction before responding. The number of trials required to complete a given maze provides a measure of the ability to benefit from feedback and to learn from errors. The number of seconds to complete each maze can be used as an indicator of cognitive efficiency, as well as a marker of impulsivity, since time is wasted on rapid but incorrect decisions. The difficulty level of the mazes increases from preschool to adult ages. A maze task is also included as a supplementary subtest on the Wechsler Intelligence Scale for Children (WISC-III; Wechsler, 1991). Lezak (1983) recommends this shorter version as a sensitive measure of planning, although it provides less information about the ability to learn from errors, since entering a blind alley does not result in repetition of the maze.

The Tower of London Test, designed by Shallice (1982), also evaluates the patient's capacity to "look ahead" and to think through a number of response alternatives. The patient is presented with three different colored beads that are displayed on a block having three pegs and is instructed to use the fewest number of moves to arrange the beads to look like a model. He or she is told to move only one bead at a time and that the beads must always rest on a peg (e.g., not the table). As shown in Figure 3.6, the number of moves needed to match a model ranges from two to five. Impulsivity is gauged by the time the patient takes before making an initial move, whereas general efficiency is measured by the number of moves needed to solve each problem. Shallice (1982) reported that patients with left anterior (frontal lobe) lesions solved significantly fewer problems on the first attempt than patients with right anterior and left or right posterior lesions.

Levin and colleagues (Levin, Goldstein, Williams, & Eisenberg, 1991) used both the Porteus Mazes and the Tower of London tasks with long-term survivors of severe closed head injury who were enrolled in a rehabilitation facility. Patients were classified as having frontal ($N = 7$) or nonfrontal ($N = 6$) lobe pathology based on lesions visualized by magnetic resonance imaging. Compared to the nonfrontal patients or demographically matched controls, those with frontal lobe lesions were slower to solve the Porteus Mazes. Other differences between frontal and nonfrontal lobe patients on these tasks did not reach significance. However, there were a small number of patients in these groups, and differentiation according to side of lesion could not be performed.

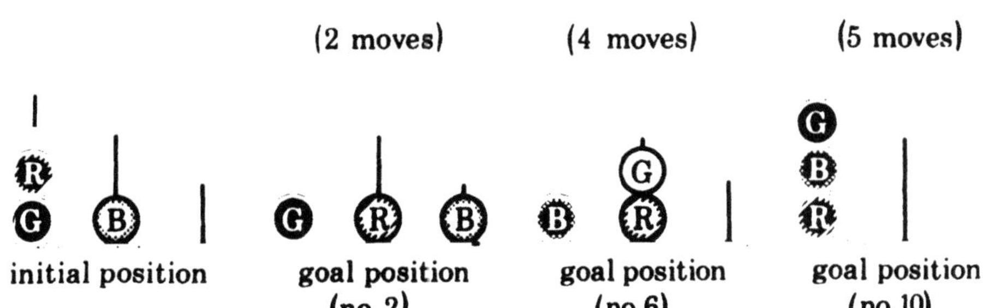

FIGURE 3.6. Three problems of the Tower of London Test. The initial position is the same for all. From Shallice, T. (1982). Specific impairments of planning. *Philosophical Transactions of the Royal Society of London, 298,* 199–209. Reprinted with permission of the author and publisher.

The Rey-Osterrieth Complex Figure Test (Osterrieth, 1944), originally designed as a measure of visual memory, can also offer a way to assess organizational strategies. The patient is shown a complex line drawing and is asked to copy the figure on a blank sheet of paper. Colored pencils may be handed sequentially to the patient at various points during execution, so that the examiner can monitor the order of completing the design. Alternatively, as discussed by Lezak (1983), the examiner can simultaneously reproduce on another sheet of paper the patient's drawing and number each element. Patients who are disorganized are more likely to jump randomly from one section to another rather than thoughtfully approaching the test. Apart from gauging planning ability, however, the patient's drawing can be impaired because of a host of other factors including visual neglect and motor problems. Therefore, it is important to rule out these alternative explanations by analyzing whether a visuomotor disturbance was observed on other measures such as a simple copying task.

As can be seen from our review of neuropsychological measures, there are a variety of procedures designed to evaluate these abilities. In the following section, we discuss some issues related to test selection and interpretation of findings.

ADDITIONAL CONSIDERATIONS FOR ASSESSMENT

The assessment of problem solving and executive functions offers several challenges. One is to select tools and environments that are sensitive to impairments. A second challenge is to separate the causes for difficulties that are revealed through these tests. An impaired score on an executive processing task does not always stem from an executive processing deficit. For example, another cognitive skill such as memory may be primarily involved. Finally, while the frontal lobes are associated with disorders of reasoning and problem solving, scores on neuropsychological tests can be "normal," even in patients with known frontal lobe damage, or quite abnormal with lesions in other brain regions (see Levin, Eisenberg, & Benton, 1991; Stuss & Benson, 1986, for reviews). In the following section, we consider these issues and highlight their implications for assessment.

Types of Procedures and Settings Sensitive to Impairments

It has been noted that the assessment environment is poorly designed to evaluate difficulties in problem solving and executive functions. Testing is typically structured by the examiner and conducted in a distraction-free room, measures are administered one at a time for short trials that last a few minutes, and there is frequently only one correct answer per problem (Lezak, 1983; Shallice & Burgess, 1991a). These circumstances lessen the need for the patient to plan and initiate independently.

Shallice presents an information-processing model that is useful for predicting the types of procedures and environments most likely to capture impairments (Norman & Shallice, 1986; Shallice & Burgess, 1991a, b). Shallice distinguishes between two levels of action and thought. At the first level, the individual is confronted with a setting for which established routines for carrying out a task already exist. A second level of processing occurs whenever routine operations cannot successfully achieve a goal. At this stage, the Supervisory System is called into play. This Supervisory System controls processes such as goal articulation, plan formulation, and creation and triggering of "markers." Markers are defined as messages that some future behavior needs to be evaluated before it is undertaken. An example of the processes performed by the Supervisory System is shown in Table 3.3. The scenario is one in which an individual must respond to an urgent letter. The first two steps require that the individual articulate a goal and develop a plan. Next, markers are created to remind the person at some future point to stop at the post office to buy stamps, to write a letter at work, and then to mail it. Each of these markers, in turn, is triggered by an environmental cue such as leaving the train station, arriving at work, and taking a break for lunch. New markers are created whenever the plan requires modification, such as finding that one cannot write the letter at work.

One implication of Shallice's model is that processes under the domain of the Supervisory System will be tapped whenever neuropsychological tasks introduce novelty and do not depend on routine methods or knowledge for solution. Stuss and Benson (1986) similarly emphasize the importance of novelty. They observe that activation of the frontal lobes, the presumed seat of the executive functions, occurs "at the time a new activity is being learned and active control is required." They go on to note, "After the activity has become routine, however, these activities can be handled by other brain areas, and frontal participation is no longer demanded" (p. 245). It is not surprising that many patients with frontal lobe compromise score normally on standardized tests of intelligence, since these measures examine "crystallized" knowledge but fail to examine "fluid" capacity to solve new problems (Newcombe, 1982). Thus, open-ended measures using divergent reasoning are more likely to elicit deficits than are rote procedures. An example of this approach is the previously described estimation procedure, which requires an individual to perform a number of intermediate steps in order to arrive at an answer. As shown in Table 3.4, a patient with resection of the

TABLE 3.3. Simple Scenario to Illustrate Component Processes in Practical Problem Solution

7:45 a.m.	Situation: receive urgent letter.
7:50 a.m.	Goal articulation: to reply as soon as possible (no stamp available).
8:00 a.m.	Plan formulation: decide to buy stamps at post office on way to work, write letter immediately on arrival and post it at lunchtime.
	Marker creation 1—When leaving underground—Go to post office.
	Marker creation 2—When arrive at work, write brief letter (if not possible on arrival, then carry out plan modification).
	Marker creation 3—When go to lunch, post letter.
9:00 a.m.	(Leave underground) Marker trigger 1—Go to post office.
9:15 a.m.	(Arrival work) Marker trigger 2—Write letter.[a]
12:30 p.m.	(Go lunch) Marker trigger 3—Post letter.

[a]If not possible to write letter at that time, plan modification occurs and new markers are set up.

Note. From T. Shallice, & P. W. Burgess. (1991). Deficits in strategy application following frontal lobe damage in man. *Brain, 114*, 727–741. Reprinted with permission of the author and publisher.

TABLE 3.4. Performance of Patient with Resection of Right Frontal Lobe

Q.	What is the length of one quarter of the Eiffel Tower?
A.	(After long hesitation, he said he did not know.)
Q.	What is the height of the Eiffel Tower?
A.	300 meters.
Q.	What is half of 300?
A.	150
Q.	What is half of 150?
A.	75
Q.	What is the length of one quarter of the Eiffel Tower, which measures 300 meters?
A.	(After long cogitation) . . . 300 meters (and despite many attempts, he failed each time).

Note. From J. Barbizet (1970). *Human memory and its pathology*. San Francisco: W. H. Freeman. Reprinted with permission of the author and publisher.

right frontal lobe is unable to calculate one-fourth the length of the Eiffel Tower despite knowledge of the overall length and the necessary arithmetic abilities to perform the task (Barbizet, 1970). To elicit impairments, Lezak (1983) recommends unstructured tasks such as having the patient put Tinkertoy pieces together to form a construction of his or her own choosing rather than being told what to build. The final product can be scored for qualities including the number of pieces used and the presence of moving parts. Lezak found that patients who were classified as dependent (relied on others to perform daily routines or to assist with transportation) used fewer pieces and constructed less complex objects than patients who were independent.

A second implication of Shallice's framework is that impairments will be seen whenever tasks require that behavior be organized over longer periods of time than traditionally used in the assessment setting. One can evaluate whether individuals are able to modify their plans in response to changes in environmental contingencies. Tasks that require the weighing of priorities and time sharing are most effective at detecting impairments in the Supervisory System. To illustrate this approach, Shallice and Burgess (1991a) required patients with prefrontal damage to quickly perform open-ended tasks in a way that maximized their overall score. The tasks included dictating a route, solving arithmetic problems, and writing the names of 100 pictured objects. These activities could not be completed in the time frame, and the investigators were interested in the extent to which each patient exhibited planning and time sharing. Relative to controls, patients attempted fewer tasks and spent more time on one particular task.

Many components of problem solving and executive functions, such as motivation and self-awareness, do not have formal assessment techniques but depend on careful observations of the patient's behaviors during the session. The manner in which the patient accepts new challenges, his or her level and maintenance of effort throughout the assessment process, and his or her frustration tolerance and perseverance when tasks become difficult provide insight toward whether and under what conditions a motivational disturbance exists. Evaluation of patients' and families' agreement concerning the presence and severity of deficits can help determine whether the patient has realistic self-appraisal.

Separation of Primary versus Secondary Impairments

Another guideline for assessment involves the need to conduct a detailed analysis of the mechanisms responsible for a breakdown in performance. Stuss and Benson (1986) conceptualize a lower tier of abilities, such as attention, memory, and language, and a higher level of behaviors such as goal selection, planning, and monitoring. Disorders can represent a direct deficit (e.g., a breakdown in planning) or an indirect deficit due to a disruption in lower level functions (e.g., memory). A breakdown in an area such as memory may be caused by damage to a structure such as the temporal lobes responsible for the basic ability or may represent frontal lobe damage that, in turn, modulates the efficiency of the mnestic process.

One issue that must be addressed during testing concerns the reasons why a patient fails a particular task. Is the impaired performance due to an executive processing deficit or to a disruption at a lower level? Such distinctions are eloquently described by Luria (1973). For example, he contrasts the performance of two groups of patients attempting to arrange blocks to form spatial designs. Both groups fail the task but for different reasons. Patients with parietal–occipital lesions "turn the Koh's blocks over helplessly without knowing how to fit them together, or in what position to put the diagonal so that it will match the outlines of the design" (p. 332). Patients with frontal lobe lesions, in contrast, "have no difficulty in finding the necessary spatial relationships. . . . The patients do not analyze the diagram, they make no attempt to convert the 'units of impression' into 'units of construction,' and they manipulate the cubes impulsively" (p. 333). During assessment, separation of higher order deficits from disruptions of lower level abilities can be determined in several ways. First, as emphasized by Luria's "syndrome analysis" approach, structured tasks should be given to see if they facilitate performance. If there is a disruption of higher order processes, tasks that remove the need for behaviors such as anticipation and planning should ameliorate the deficit. Thus, a patient with an apparent visuomotor impairment on a spontaneous clock drawing task may perform quite well when copying a clock from a model, implicating a disturbance in purposeful activity rather than a visual synthesis problem. A patient who cannot recall more than five words of a list over repeated trials may exhibit normal memory when given category cues, thus suggesting difficulty with active retrieval. Observations of behaviors can also help determine the underlying cause of the impairment. In learning a list of words that belong to categories, does the patient cluster them at recall, or is retrieval haphazard? The latter approach may implicate an organizational deficit interfering with memory. On a card sorting task, can the patient verbalize the correct strategy despite the inability to change to a new concept? If so, then the problem may not be due to a failure to recall the correct hypothesis but rather to an inability to modify behaviors. Qualitative observations are also critical to establishing the nature of the underlying deficit. Lezak (1983) recommends noting features of performance such as carelessness (e.g., skipping problems on a paper-and-pencil-type measure), poor planning (e.g., inadequate spacing of drawings), and failures to self-correct even when errors are acknowledged.

Inferences Concerning Frontal Lobe Dysfunction

Another consideration during assessment concerns inferences regarding cerebral localization. Should impairments in problem solving and executive functions be taken as evidence that the frontal lobes are involved? As shown in Figure 3.7, the frontal lobes have extensive connections with brain regions including the parietal, temporal, and occipital lobes, the telencephalic limbic system, and subcortical areas including the hypothalamus and the dorsal medial nucleus of the thalamus (see Damasio, 1991; Stuss & Benson, 1986, for reviews). Stuss and Gow (1992), in the context of closed head injury, note that "frontal dysfunction" may stem not only from focal damage but from secondary mechanisms. For example, diffuse axonal injury may result in attentional deficits that resemble those seen in focal frontal lobe injury. Shearing may cause a disconnection of the frontal lobes from other areas including limbic and association regions that, in turn, are known to produce impairments in attention and personality. Finally, postinjury consequences such as pain and depression may lead to impaired reasoning and inefficiency of cognitive processing.

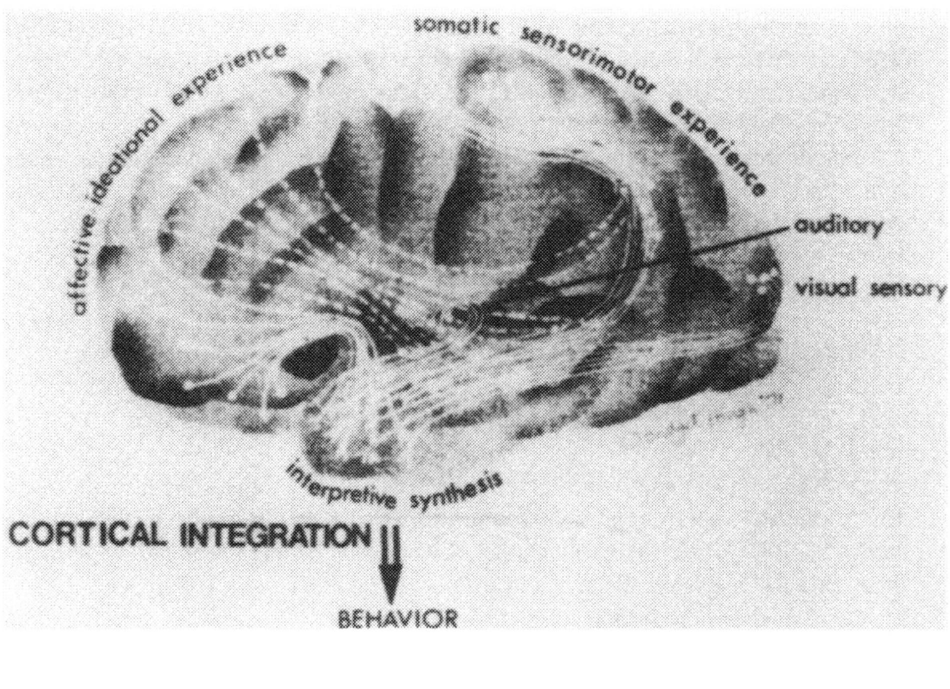

FIGURE 3.7. Convergence of sensory information onto the convexity of the anterior frontal lobe. Adapted from Powell, T. P. S. (1972). Sensory convergence in the cerebral cortex. In L. V. Laitinen & K. E. Livingston (Eds.), *Surgical approaches in psychiatry. Proceedings of the Third International Congress of Psychosurgery*. University Park, Baltimore, MD. Reproduced with permission of the author and publisher.

The complexities of attempts to localize brain functions are demonstrated whenever patients perform normally on tests sensitive to frontal lobe functioning, and yet have documented focal damage. It has been reported, for example, that a patient with extensive bilateral orbitofrontal and dorsolateral atrophy scored normally on the WCST, a measure widely viewed as sensitive to frontal lobe damage (Heck & Bryer, 1986). The converse of this exception is demonstrated whenever patients with lesions outside the frontal lobes perform as poorly as those with known dysfunction.

These previous issues raise several important caveats. First, as recommended by Stuss and Gow (1992), it may be more prudent to use the term "executive control" as opposed to "frontal lobe function" in discussing abilities such as anticipation, planning, and goal selection, and when communicating neuropsychological findings. Second, as noted by Heck and Bryer (1986), "Absence of evidence is not evidence for absence." A negative finding is not proof that the ability is normal. The assessment setting sometimes provides so much structure that patients do not need to exhibit executive abilities. In addition, premorbid functioning can determine the challenge level of any test. A particularly bright individual may not find the processing demands of a test to be "executive" at all. Finally, neuropsychological tests should be used in conjunction with the results of neurological and neuroimaging evaluations, functional history, and reports of family members and friends. Patients may score normally in the testing session and yet have gross disturbances in organizing their daily activities.

Below, we present the neuropsychological findings of two patients referred to the Emory Neurobehavioral Program. These cases highlight issues we have raised concerning the types of tasks likely to elicit deficits, the importance of qualitatively analyzing test performance, and the fact that scores can be within normal limits even though a patient has definite frontal lobe pathology.

CLINICAL CASES

Case 1: J.H.

J.H., a 52-year-old, left-handed male with 4 years of college education, was referred for an evaluation of memory and personality changes. One year prior to referral, J.H. began exhibiting impaired judgment, such as driving a lawn mower down the street to a repair shop. He also lost his family savings in a jewelry investment deal conducted over the telephone, resulting in his filing for bankruptcy. J.H. displayed increased irritability, social withdrawal, and lack of interest in hobbies. His wife stated that she had noticed "subtle changes" for the previous 3 to 4 years; these were initially attributed to depression. J.H. underwent psychiatric evaluation and was subsequently referred for a neurological evaluation, which was normal. A computed tomography (CT) scan revealed generalized cortical atrophy that was substantially greater in the frontoparietal region. Previous medical history was significant for an automobile accident 10 years prior, which had resulted in a severed aorta that required surgery. At the time of this accident, J.H. had sustained brief loss of consciousness but had been able to resume work without obvious neurobehavioral deficits.

Behavioral Observations

J.H. was a neatly dressed gentleman. When asked if he was having any problems, he responded, "None that I can think of." He denied changes in his personality or his cognitive functioning such as memory ("as good as it ever was"). Later in the interview, J.H. remarked that he was not as "outgoing" as he had been. He denied depression, although he did acknowledge that he was "concerned" about finances. The most striking feature of the interview was J.H.'s lack of insight concerning any difficulties or reasons for seeking medical consultation. He said that he was referred to the neurologist for a "check-up," and he could not elaborate when pressed for more details.

During testing, J.H. was pleasant but did not establish rapport. He displayed a flat affect. There was no frustration or defensiveness evident in his performance of the neuropsychological procedures. Even when he was repeatedly told that he was incorrectly matching the cards on the WCST, J.H. never became frustrated. He thought that he did well on every measure, irrespective of his actual functioning. J.H. frequently digressed into long-winded stories when answering questions and had to be redirected to the task at hand. Impulsivity was observed on verbal recall and picture arrangement measures. On this latter task, he quickly sequenced the pictures and then realized that they were in the wrong order.

Test Results

Scores on the neuropsychological procedures are summarized in Table 3.5.

J.H.'s performance improved whenever he was provided with structure, suggesting problems with planning and initiation as opposed to a primary disturbance of language, visuospatial processing, or memory. For example, J.H. produced low output on the COWAT, requiring him to generate words beginning with the letters *F, A*, and *S*. However, as seen in Table 3.5, there was a noticeable improvement when he was asked to say words belonging to categories such as Animals or Fruits/Vegetables. Improvement with structure was also observed on visuospatial measures. J.H. exhibited an apparent disturbance on the Block Design subtest of the WAIS-R. He could configure the easiest designs using four blocks, but his functioning deteriorated when using nine blocks. In contrast, J.H. was able to judge the angular orientation of designs (Judgment of Line Orientation; Benton, Hamsher, Varney, & Spreen, 1983), indicating that his visuospatial abilities were actually intact. This latter test simply required J.H. to point to lines that were oriented in the same direction as a model, and therefore did not require him to organize his responses. J.H. showed impaired verbal recall when he recalled words the examiner read to him on the California Verbal Learning Test (CVLT; Delis, Kramer, Kaplan, & Ober, 1987), and his ability to reproduce designs he had just seen (Visual Reproduction of the Wechsler Memory Scale-Revised [WMS-R]; Wechsler, 1987) was also impaired. However, when given a recognition format, his memory for recurring pictures on the Continuous Recognition Memory Test (Hannay & Levin, 1988) or for words on the CVLT was normal. For example, although he recalled only 6 of 16 words after 20 minutes, he recognized all 16 words

TABLE 3.5. Neuropsychological Test Scores for J.H.

Measure	Score	Norms[a]
Controlled Oral Word Association		
Total correct for three letters	21 words	$z = -1.80$
Total correct for three categories	36 words	
WAIS-R Block Design (Age-Scaled Score)	7	$z = -1.00$
Judgment of Line Orientation, total correct (30 max.)	28	$M = 24.3$ (no SD provided)
California Verbal Learning Test—Free and Cued Recall		
List A: Total trials 1–5 (80 max.)	41	$T = 34$
List B: (16 possible)	5	$z = -1$
List A: Short recall (16 max.)	7	$z = -2$
List A: Cued recall (16 max.)	9	$z = -1$
List A: Long delay free recall	6	$z = -2$
List A: Long delay cued recall	7	$z = -2$
WMS-R Visual Reproduction		
Immediate recall	30	Percentile = 41
Delayed recall	24	Percentile = 27
Continuous Recognition Memory		
Correct responses (100 max.)	90	$z = 0.60$
California Verbal Learning Test—Recognition		
Long delay recognition	16	$z = 1.00$
False positives	2	$z = 0.00$
Design Fluency (Fixed Condition)		
Total output	80 designs	
Number correct	21 designs	$M = 19.7$ (no SD provided)
Percent perseverative errors	74%	$M = 15\%$ (no SD provided)
Percent nonperseverative errors	0%	
Wisconsin Card Sorting Test		
Number of categories (6 max.)	2	$z = -3.27$
Percent perseverative errors	39%	$z = -6.04$
Percent nonperseverative errors	0%	$z = 1.55$
WAIS-R Similarities Scaled Score (Age-Scaled Score)	7	$z = -1.00$
Other WAIS-R Subtests (Age-Scaled Scores)		
Information	10	$z = 1.00$
Digit Span	10	$z = 1.00$
Vocabulary	8	$z = -0.67$
Arithmetic	11	$z = 0.33$
Picture Completion	10	$z = 1.00$
Picture Arrangement	8	$z = -0.67$
Digit Symbol	8	$z = -0.67$
Verbal IQ	96	$z = -0.27$
Performance IQ	88	$z = -0.80$
Full Scale IQ	93	$z = -0.47$
Boston Naming Test, number correct (60 max.)	56	$z = .07$

[a]Norms are based on published values and are provided when available.

(two false-alarm errors) with choices. This finding indicated that J.H.'s difficulty involved actively searching and retrieving material rather than a storage deficit, per se.

Other indications for an executive processing deficit were J.H.'s failures to display a learning curve and to organize material semantically on free recall. On the CVLT, J.H. showed an initial improvement from trial 1 (5 words) to trial 2 (10 words), but he did not exhibit a further improvement (trial 3 = 8 words, trial 4 = 9 words, trial 5 = 10 words). J.H. rapidly recalled these words and then abruptly ended each trial by commenting, "That's it, I guess." His pattern was reminiscent of Luria's (1973) observations regarding the impact of frontal lobe lesions on memory performance. Luria noted that subjects with brain lesions outside the frontal lobes improved their recall over repeated trials, but their performance fell off after capacity was reached or fatigue set in. Subjects with frontal lobe lesions, in contrast, retained two to five words on every trial, with no attempt to retrieve additional words from memory. J.H. also did not take advantage of the semantic structure of the word list. The CVLT includes words from the categories of clothing, tools, spices/herbs, and fruits. J.H.'s recall was unorganized, and he randomly jumped from one category to the next rather than clustering the words. For example, J.H.'s recall on trial 5 was "Drill, plums, slacks, pliers, sweater, apricots, nutmeg, parsley, grapes, slacks (perseveration), wrench." This lack of clustering may be clinically relevant, since some investigators have suggested that the frontal lobes are involved in semantic processing (Moscovitch, 1982; Squire, 1982; Zatorre & McEntee, 1983). For example, patients with Korsakoff's syndrome do not exhibit a normal facilitation in recall when they are switched from learning one group of conceptually related words to a new category. This finding has been interpreted to indicate that these patients do not process material semantically as a result of underlying frontal lobe involvement.

The inability to use feedback to monitor performance, another characteristic of an executive processing disorder, was observed on the Design Fluency task (Jones-Gotman & Milner, 1977) in which J.H. was given 4 minutes to generate nonsense drawings that had four lines. As shown in Figure 3.8, his drawings were highly perseverative. Poor performance was not due to a failure to comprehend or to remember the task demands. In fact, J.H. was given several warnings that his designs needed to be different from each other. J.H. always stated that he understood this rule, and then he proceeded to make another perseverative drawing.

Impaired reasoning was also characteristic of J.H.'s performance. He quickly achieved two correct sorts in 28 trials on the WCST and then could not obtain the third concept of "number." He was repeatedly told for the next 36 trials that his sorting was incorrect, but he continued to make perseverative responses. Impaired reasoning was further observed on the Similarities subtest of the WAIS-R. J.H. could not think of shared relationships between items such as table and chair ("need a chair to sit at a table"), poem and statue ("not alike"), and work and play ("first you work and then you play").

Other features of J.H.'s performance are shown in Table 3.5. His general intellectual functioning was in the low average to average range, certainly below expectation for estimated premorbid functioning. Digit Span and Arithmetic, measures of attention and mental control, were relative strengths. Language was well preserved.

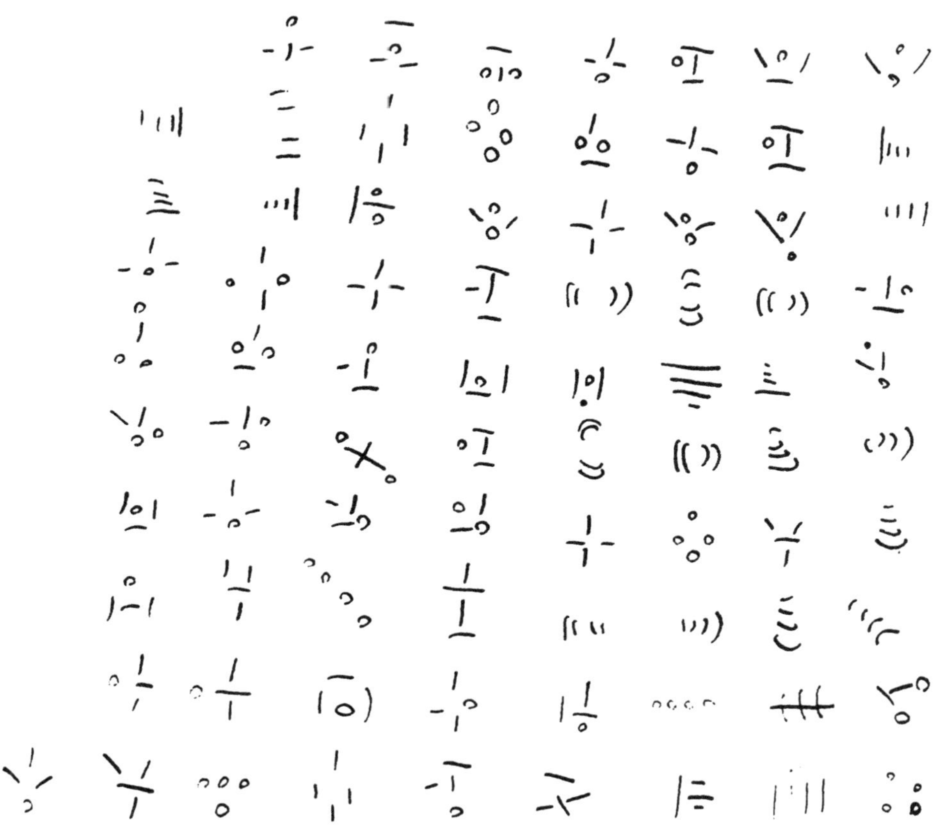

FIGURE 3.8. Design Fluency performance (fixed condition) of patient J.H.

Naming of pictured items (Boston Naming Test; Kaplan, Goodglass, & Weintraub, 1983) was normal, as was comprehension of task instructions and questions.

Synthesis

Several features of J.H.'s performance were consistent with an executive processing disturbance. He benefited whenever tests provided structure, he exhibited problems with divergent thinking and the ability to use feedback, and his reasoning was impaired. In contrast, attention, naming, and visuospatial abilities were relatively preserved.

J.H.'s history and pattern of results suggest a dementia of the frontal lobe type (Gustafson, Brun, & Risberg, 1990; Miller et al., 1991; Neary, Snowden, Northen, & Goulding, 1988; see also Walsh, this volume). Behavioral and personality changes such as social withdrawal, unconcern, and disinhibition are prominent early features of frontal lobe dementia, whereas cognitive deficits occur later. Neuropsychological testing reveals impairments of executive processing and memory with relative preservation of attention, language, and visuospatial skills (Miller et al., 1991). Single photon emission computerized tomography, not performed on J.H., indicates hypoperfusion in the frontal and temporal regions, and on autopsy, these patients may exhibit Pick bodies or only gliosis and neuronal loss.

Case 2: H.B.

The second patient, H.B., a 44-year-old, right-handed, former medical technician with a college degree, was referred for neuropsychological evaluation of sequelae related to a left frontal lobe cyst. Four months prior to referral, H.B. experienced sudden onset of vomiting, headache, and aphasia. A CT scan revealed a 7-cm left frontal cyst, and she underwent a craniotomy for subtotal resection. H.B. developed a secondary seizure disorder that was well controlled with phenobarbital and valproic acid at the time of testing. Her previous medical history included poliomyelitis as a child with consequent muscle stiffness. She also had had a hysterectomy, a tonsillectomy, an appendectomy, and a motor vehicle accident over 20 years earlier, which resulted in a concussion.

Neuropsychological testing was requested to monitor any cognitive changes caused by her cyst and/or subsequent surgery. A magnetic resonance imaging scan on the same day as the evaluation indicated a large area of encephalomalacia in the left frontal lobe, with focal round areas of intra-axial fluid thought to be encephalomalacia change. There was no evidence of mass effect, midline shift, or hydrocephalus.

Behavioral Observations

H.B. was neatly dressed and groomed. She presented as an anxious individual and, in contrast to J.H. who denied any problems, H.B. reported numerous changes in her cognitive status. She described difficulty with her memory for everyday events, poor concentration, and impaired mathematical abilities. She noted that mood was "fluctuating" and stated that she felt nervous and experienced heart palpitations. H.B. denied a premorbid history of psychiatric treatment and drug/alcohol abuse. At the time of neuropsychological testing, she was also undergoing a psychiatric evaluation for depression.

During testing, H.B. put forth good effort. Her speech was rapid (reported as a premorbid characteristic), and she had difficulty concentrating. She frequently requested short breaks so that she could gather her thoughts before proceeding.

Test Results

H.B.'s neuropsychological test scores are shown in Table 3.6.

Like J.H., H.B. exhibited difficulties with hypothesis testing. On the WCST, she generated only three correct sorts after 64 trials. In contrast to J.H., however, she understood that the cards could be classified according to color, form, and number, and her performance was not perseverative. Instead, she made the task unnecessarily complicated and devised elaborate strategies. For example, she stated, "Different

TABLE 3.6. Neuropsychological Test Scores for H.B.

Measure	Score	Norms[a]
Wisconsin Card Sorting Test		
Number of categories (6 max.)	3	$z = -1.00$
Percent perseverative errors	19%	$z = -0.50$
Percent nonperseverative errors	5%	$z = 0.67$
Design Fluency (Fixed Condition)		
Total output	23	
Number correct	18	$M = 19.7$ (no SD provided)
Percent perseverative errors	13%	$M = 15\%$ (no SD provided)
Percent nonperseverative errors	9%	
Controlled Oral Word Association		
Total correct for three letters	48	$z = -0.34$
Total correct for three categories	58	
WAIS-R Similarities (Age-Scaled Score)	13	$z = 1.00$
Other WAIS-R Subtests (Age-Scaled Scores)		
Information	13	$z = 1.00$
Digit Span	8	$z = -0.67$
Vocabulary	16	$z = 2.00$
Arithmetic	9	$z = -0.33$
Picture Completion	11	$z = 0.33$
Picture Arrangement	11	$z = 0.33$
Block Design	12	$z = 0.67$
Digit Symbol	7	$z = -1.00$
Verbal IQ	111	$z = 0.73$
Performance IQ	102	$z = 0.13$
Full Scale IQ	107	$z = 0.47$
Wide Range Achievement Test-Revised (Standard Score)		
Arithmetic	105	$M = 100$, SD = 15
Reading	120	$M = 100$, SD = 15
WMS-R Mental Control: Errors (Seconds)		
Months forward	0 (6)	
Alphabet recitation	0 (5)	
Serial 3's (1 to 40)	0 (31)	
Months backward	1 (19)	
WMS-R Logical Memory		
Immediate recall	24	Percentile = 43
Delayed recall	22	Percentile = 51
WMS-R Visual Reproduction		
Immediate recall	34	Percentile = 59
Delayed recall	28	Percentile = 33

[a]Norms are based on published values and are provided when available.

colors and shapes and numbers have a pecking order. I can't figure it out. I think it's blue, red, green, yellow, and that star is over the circle, triangle, and cross."

Apart from her difficulties with the WCST, H.B. did not exhibit other executive processing deficits. Her ability to generate nonsense designs was within normal limits. However, in contrast to predictions based on her left frontal lobe lesion, H.B. also performed normally on the verbal fluency measure. She generated a large number of acceptable responses for both individual letters and categories, and she did not perseverate. Moreover, on a cognitive estimation procedure, H.B.'s responses were not extreme in comparison to controls (see Table 3.7). Finally, inferring relationships between concepts on the WAIS-R Similarities subtest was in the high average range and within expectation.

As she herself had noted, H.B. was found to have difficulty concentrating. The WAIS-R subtests of Digit Span, Arithmetic, and Digit Symbol Substitution were below expectation. H.B. could repeat five digits forward but reversed only three. Mental arithmetic was below estimated premorbid functioning, and her difficulty was due to forgetting the questions rather than to an inability to perform the calculations. When given written arithmetic problems (Wide Range Achievement Test-Revised [WRAT-R]; Jastak & Wilkinson, 1984), H.B. performed in the average range. Although abilities such as saying the months and the alphabet were fast and errorless, H.B. was slow in counting by 3's, and she made an error in reversing the order of the months.

Language skills including naming (Boston Naming Test), reading (WRAT-R), and vocabulary (WAIS-R) were normal. In addition, visuospatial functions as assessed by Block Design (WAIS-R) were intact. H.B.'s recall of stories and designs (WMS-R) was also within average limits.

TABLE 3.7. Responses to Cognitive Estimation Questionnaire for H.B.

		Norms[a]	
Question	Response	Mean	Range
On average, how many TV programs are there on one TV channel between 6:00 p.m. and 11:00 p.m.?	5	6.5	4–12
What is the age of the oldest person in America today?	105 years	108.7	100–115
What is the length of the average man's spine?	48 inches	30.3	20–36
How many slices are there in a loaf of sandwich bread?	32	27.1	15–47
How tall is the average American woman?	66 inches	65.6	62–70
What is the weight of the average American male?	190 pounds	174.5	150–205
What is the length of a dollar bill?	4 inches	6.0	4–10
How fast do race horses run?	30 mph	35.6	10–50
What is the seating capacity of a city bus?	50	46.4	22–103
How much does a full can of Coca-Cola weigh?	12 ounces	11.3	4–16

[a]Norms are based on control subjects 18–32 years old with high school and college educations.

Synthesis

H.B. did not exhibit striking evidence of executive processing deficits, particularly those attributable to left frontal lobe dysfunction. In this case, it is unclear when H.B. developed her left frontal cyst. If it developed in childhood, it is possible that her brain underwent some functional reorganization, as is known to occur when primary language areas are damaged in young children (Smith, 1984). Thus, this case illustrates the caveat that human brains may be organized differently from one another, as a result of genetically determined developmental variation or early neurological injury. Even in cases where brain organization is presumably "normal," neuropsychological tests can be within normal limits despite known frontal lobe involvement. In the case of H.B., for example, it is possible that more open-ended and time-sharing tasks of the type advocated by Shallice and Burgess (Shallice & Burgess, 1991a, b) would pick up deficits missed in the present exam. Moreover, although H.B. performed relatively well in the neuropsychological setting, she was having a great deal of difficulty managing at home. Her marriage was disintegrating, and she was unable to resume gainful employment. Thus, while deficits were not observed during the structured evaluation, the impact of executive processing impairments on daily functioning was likely considerable.

CONCLUSIONS

This chapter has reviewed neurocognitive models of problem solving and executive functions and has described the major neuropsychological tools that exist to evaluate deficits in these abilities. A number of limitations inherent to such evaluations have emerged that can be summarized as follows:

1. Deficits in problem solving and executive function are difficult to characterize unless more elemental cognitive abilities (attention, language, memory) are relatively intact. The clinician should always interpret executive impairments in light of other cognitive abilities.
2. The ability of a patient to "self-structure" is an important component of executive function, and the structure provided by conventional neuropsychological testing may actually mask the expression of deficits in this area. Therefore, in this arena, more than in any other, the clinician must elicit history of, and even observe, the patient's competency in the natural environment.
3. Deficits in problem solving and executive function are frequently associated with frontal lobe injury, but are not "localized" to the frontal lobes in the same way that we conceptualize sensorimotor or language localization. The clinician should not be wedded to the concept of finding evidence for or against frontal lobe damage, but should evaluate the competency of functional abilities in and of themselves.

Just as the astute clinician listens with his or her own linguistic cortex for subtle language deficits in a patient, so must clinicians use their own executive abilities in full measure as they evaluate their patients. Subtle failures in reasoning or roundabout ways of problem solving may signal impairments, even if the scores on neuropsychological tests are "normal." Neuropsychological testing is meaningful only when the examiner is respectful of these limitations and sensitive to the complexities of the "highest" of the higher cortical functions.

ACKNOWLEDGMENTS

Preparation of this chapter was supported in part by NIA grant P30AG10130 and NIDRR grant H133G30051.

REFERENCES

Albert, M. S., Wolfe, J., & Lafleche, G. (1990). Differences in abstraction ability with age. *Psychology and Aging, 5,* 94–100.

Allison, R. S. (1966). Perseveration as a sign of diffuse and focal brain damage. *British Medical Journal, 2,* 1095–1101.

Anderson, S. W., Damasio, H., Jones, R. D., & Tranel, D. (1991). Wisconsin Card Sorting Test performance as a measure of frontal lobe damage. *Journal of Clinical and Experimental Neuropsychology, 13,* 909–922.

Axelrod, B. N., & Henry, R. R. (1992). Age-related performance on the Wisconsin Card Sorting, Similarities, and Controlled Oral Word Association tests. *The Clinical Neuropsychologist, 6,* 16–26.

Barbizet, J. (1970). *Human memory and its pathology.* San Francisco: W. H. Freeman.

Benton, A. L. (1968). Differential behavioral effects in frontal lobe disease. *Neuropsychologia, 12,* 557–563.

Benton, A. L., & Hamsher, K. deS. (1989). *Multilingual aphasia examination* (2nd ed.). Iowa City: AJA Associates.

Benton, A. L., Hamsher, K. deS., Varney, N. R., & Spreen, O. (1983). *Contributions to neuropsychological assessment: A clinical manual.* New York: Oxford University Press.

Chorover, S. L., & Cole, M. (1966). Delayed alternation performance in patients with cerebral lesions. *Neuropsychologia, 4,* 1–7.

Damasio, H. C. (1991). Neuroanatomy of frontal lobe in vivo: A comment on methodology. In H. S. Levin, H. M. Eisenberg, & A. L. Benton (Eds.), *Frontal lobe function and dysfunction* (pp. 92–121). New York: Oxford University Press.

DeFilippis, N. A., & McCampbell, E. (1987). *Booklet Category Test.* Odessa, FL: Psychological Assessment Resources.

Delis, D. C., Kramer, J. H., Kaplan, E., & Ober, B. A. (1987). *California Verbal Learning Test: Research edition.* San Antonio: Psychological Corporation.

Drewe, E. A. (1974). The effect of type and area of brain lesion on Wisconsin Card Sorting Test performance. *Cortex, 10,* 159–170.

Feldman, M. J., & Drasgow, J. A. (1951). A visual–verbal test for schizophrenia. *Psychiatric Quarterly, 25,* 55–64.

Freedman, M., & Oscar-Berman, M. (1986a). Bilateral frontal lobe disease and selective delayed-response deficits in humans. *Behavioral Neuroscience, 100,* 337–342.

Freedman, M., & Oscar-Berman, M. (1986b). Selective delayed response deficits in Parkinson's and Alzheimer's disease. *Archives of Neurology, 43,* 886–890.

Goldstein, F. C., & Levin, H. S. (1991). Question-asking strategies after severe closed head injury. *Brain and Cognition, 17,* 23–30.

Goldstein, F., Presley, R., O'Jile, J., Freeman, A., Watts, R., & Green, R. (1992). Cognitive estimation in Alzheimer's and Parkinson's disease. *Journal of Clinical and Experimental Neuropsychology, 14,* 82.

Goldstein, K. (1942). *Aftereffects of brain injuries in war.* New York: Grune & Stratton.

Goldstein, K., & Scheerer, M. (1941). Abstract and concrete behavior: An experimental study with special tests. *Psychological Monographs, 53,* 1–151.

Gorham, D. R. (1956). A proverbs test for clinical and experimental use. *Psychological Reports, 1,* 1–12.

Grant, D. A., & Berg, E. A. (1948). A behavioral analysis of degree of reinforcement and ease of shifting to new responses in a Weigl-type card-sorting problem. *Journal of Experimental Psychology, 38,* 404–411.

Gustafson, L., Brun, A., & Risberg, J. (1990). Frontal lobe dementia of non-Alzheimer type. In R. J. Wurtman, S. Corkin, J. Growdon, & E. Ritter-Walker (Eds.), *Advances in neurology, Vol. 51: Alzheimer's disease* (pp. 65–71). New York: Raven Press.

Haaland, K. Y., Vranes, L. F., Goodwin, J. S., & Garry, P. J. (1987). Wisconsin Card Sort Test performance in a healthy elderly population. *Journal of Gerontology, 42,* 345–346.

Halstead, W. C. (1947). *Brain and intelligence.* Chicago: University of Chicago Press.

Hannay, H., & Levin, H. (1988). *The Continuous Recognition Memory Test.* Houston: Neuropsychological Resources.

Heaton, R. K. (1981). *The Wisconsin Card Sorting Test.* Odessa, FL: Psychological Assessment Resources.

Heaton, R. K., Chelune, G. J., Talley, J. L., Kay, G. G., & Curtiss, G. (1993). *Wisconsin Card Sorting Test (WCST)-Revised and expanded.* Odessa, FL: Psychological Assessment Resources.

Heck, E. T., & Bryer, J. B. (1986). Superior sorting and categorizing ability in a case of bilateral frontal atrophy: An exception to the rule. *Journal of Clinical and Experimental Neuropsychology, 8,* 313–316.

Helmick, J. W., & Berg, C. B. (1976). Perseveration in brain-injured adults. *Journal of Communication Disorders, 9,* 143–156.

Jastak, S., & Wilkinson, G. S. (1984). *The Wide Range Achievement Test-Revised administration manual.* Wilmington, DE: Jastak Associates.

Jones-Gotman, M., & Milner, B. (1977). Design fluency: The invention of nonsense drawings after focal cortical lesions. *Neuropsychologia, 15,* 653–674.

Jouandet, M., & Gazzaniga, M. S. (1979) The frontal lobes. In M. S. Gazzaniga (Ed.), *Handbook of behavioral neurobiology, Vol. 2: Neuropsychology* (pp. 25–59). New York: Plenum Press.

Kaplan, E., Fein, D., Morris, R., & Delis, D. C. (1991). *WAIS-R as a neuropsychological instrument.* San Antonio: Psychological Corporation.

Kaplan, E. F., Goodglass, H., & Weintraub, S. (1983). *The Boston Naming Test* (2nd ed.). Philadelphia: Lea & Febiger.

Laine, M., & Butters, N. (1982). A preliminary study of the problem solving strategies of detoxified long-term alcoholics. *Drug and Alcohol Dependency, 10,* 235–242.

Levin, H. (1987). Neurobehavioral sequelae of head injury. In P. Cooper (Ed.), *Head injury* (pp. 442–463). Baltimore: Williams & Wilkins.

Levin, H. S., Eisenberg, H. M., & Benton, A. L. (Eds.). (1991). *Frontal lobe function and dysfunction.* New York: Oxford University Press.

Levin, H. S., Goldstein, F. C., Williams, D. H., & Eisenberg, H. M. (1991). The contribution of frontal lobe lesions to the neurobehavioral outcome of closed head injury. In H. S. Levin, H. M. Eisenberg, & A. L. Benton (Eds.), *Frontal lobe function and dysfunction* (pp. 318–338). New York: Oxford University Press.

Lezak, M. D. (1983). *Neuropsychological assessment* (2nd ed.). New York: Oxford University Press.

Luria, A. R. (1963). *Restoration of function after brain injury.* New York: Pergamon Press.

Luria, A. R. (1966). *Higher cortical functions in man.* New York: Basic Books.

Luria, A. R. (1973). *The working brain.* New York: Basic Books.

Luria, A. R., & Homskaya, E. D. (1964). Disturbances in the regulative role of speech with frontal lobe lesions. In J. M. Warren & K. A. Albert (Eds.), *The frontal granular cortex and behavior* (pp. 353–371). New York: McGraw-Hill.

Mattis, S. (1988). *Dementia rating scale*. Odessa, FL: Psychological Assessment Resources.

Miller, B., Cummings, J. L., Villanueva-Meyer, J., Boone, K., Mehringer, C. M., Lesser, I. M., & Mena, I. (1991). Frontal lobe degeneration: Clinical, neuropsychological, and SPECT characteristics. *Neurology, 41*, 1374–1382.

Milner, B. (1963). Effects of different brain lesions on card sorting. *Archives of Neurology, 9*, 100–110.

Monsch, A. U., Bondi, M. W., Butters, N., Salmon, D. P., Katzman, R., & Thal, L. J. (1992). Comparisons of verbal fluency tasks in the detection of dementia of the Alzheimer's type. *Archives of Neurology, 49*, 1253–1258.

Moscovitch, M. (1982). Multiple dissociations of function in the amnesic syndrome. In L. S. Cermak (Eds.), *Human memory and amnesia* (pp. 337–370). Hillsdale, NJ: Lawrence Erlbaum.

Mosher, F. A., & Hornsby, J. R. (Eds.). (1966). *On asking questions*. In J. S. Brunen, R. R. Olver, & P. Greenfield (Eds.), *Studies in cognitive growth* (pp. 86–102). New York: Wiley.

Neary, D., Snowden, J. S., Northen, B., & Gouldin, P. (1988). Dementia of frontal lobe type. *Journal of Neurology, Neurosurgery, and Psychiatry, 51*, 353–361.

Nelson, H. E. (1976). A modified card sorting test sensitive to frontal lobe defects. *Cortex, 12*, 313–324.

Newcombe, F. (1982). The psychological consequences of closed head injury: Assessment and rehabilitation. *Injury: The British Journal of Accident Surgery, 14*, 111–136.

Norman, D. A., & Shallice, T. (1986). Attention to action: Willed and automatic control of behavior. In R. J. Davidson, G. E. Schwartz, & D. Shapiro (Eds.), *Consciousness and self-regulation: Advances in research and theory* (pp. 1–18). New York: Plenum Press.

Oscar-Berman, M., McNamara, P., & Freedman, M. (1991). Delayed-response tasks: Parallels between experimental ablation studies and findings in patients with frontal lesions. In H. S. Levin, H. M. Eisenberg, & A. L. Benton (Eds.), *Frontal lobe function and dysfunction* (pp. 230–255). New York: Oxford University Press.

Osterrieth, P. (1944). Le test de copie d'une figure complexe. *Archives de Psychologie, 30*, 206–356.

Porteus, S. D. (1965). *Porteus Maze Test: Fifty years' application*. New York: Psychological Corporation.

Prigatano, G. P. (1987). Personality and psychosocial consequences after brain injury. In M. Meier, A. L. Benton, & L. Diller (Eds.), *Neuropsychological rehabilitation* (pp. 355–378). New York: Guilford.

Prigatano, G. P. (1991). The relationship of frontal lobe damage to diminished awareness: Studies in rehabilitation. In H. S. Levin, H. M. Eisenberg, & A. L. Benton (Eds.), *Frontal lobe function and dysfunction* (pp. 381–397). New York: Oxford University Press.

Raven, J. C. (1960). *Guide to the Standard Progressive Matrices*. London: H. K. Lewis.

Raven, J. C. (1965). *Guide to using the Coloured Progressive Matrices*. London: H. K. Lewis.

Robinson, A. L., Heaton, R. K., Lehman, R. A. W., & Stilson, D. W. (1980). The utility of the Wisconsin Card Sorting Test in detecting and localizing frontal lobe lesions. *Journal of Consulting and Clinical Psychology, 48*, 605–614.

Salthouse, T. A., & Prill, K. (1987). Inferences about age impairments in inferential reasoning. *Psychology and Aging, 2*, 43–51.

Sandson, J., & Albert M. L. (1987). Perseveration in behavioral neurology. *Neurology, 37*, 1736–1741.

Shallice, T. (1982). Specific impairments of planning. *Philosophical Transactionis of the Royal Society of London, 298*, 199–209.

Shallice, T., & Burgess, P. W. (1991a). Deficits in strategy application following frontal lobe damage in man. *Brain, 114*, 727–741.

Shallice, T., & Burgess, P. (1991b). Higher-order cognitive impairments and frontal lobe lesions in man. In H. S. Levin, H. M. Eisenberg, & A. L. Benton (Eds.), *Frontal lobe function and dysfunction* (pp. 125–138). New York: Oxford University Press.

Shallice, T., & Evans, M. E. (1978). The involvement of the frontal lobes in cognitive estimation. *Cortex, 14*, 294–303.

Smith, A. (1984). Early and long-term recovery from brain damage in children and adults: Evolution of concepts of localization, plasticity, and recovery. In C. R. Almli & S. Finger (Eds.), *Early brain damage, Vol. 1: Research orientations and clinical observations* (pp. 299–324). New York: Academic Press.

Smith, M. L., & Milner, B. (1984). Differential effects of frontal-lobe lesions on cognitive estimation and spatial memory. *Neuropsychologia, 22*, 697–705.

Squire, L. S. (1982). Comparisons between forms of amnesia: Some deficits are unique to Korsakoff's syndrome. *Journal of Experimental Psychology: Learning, Memory, and Cognition, 8*, 560–571.

Stuss, D. T., & Benson, D. F. (1986). *The frontal lobes.* New York: Raven Press.

Stuss, D. T., Delgado, M., & Guzman, D. A. (1987). Verbal regulation in the control of motor impersistence: A proposed rehabilitation procedure. *Journal of Neurological Rehabilitation, 1*, 19–24.

Stuss, D. T., & Gow, C. A. (1992). "Frontal dysfunction" after traumatic brain injury. *Neuropsychiatry, Neuropsychology, and Behavioral Neurology, 5*, 272–282.

Terman, L. M., & Merrill, M. A. (1973). *Stanford-Binet Intelligence Scale. Manual for the third revision, Form L-M.* Boston: Houghton Mifflin.

Thorndike, R. L., Hagen, E. P., & Sattler, J. M. (1986). *Stanford-Binet Intelligence Scale: Fourth Edition.* Chicago: Riverside Publishing Company.

Wechsler, D. (1981). *WAIS-R Manual.* New York: Psychological Corporation.

Wechsler, D. (1987). *Wechsler Memory Scale-Revised.* San Antonio: Psychological Corporation.

Wechsler, D. (1991). *Wechsler Intelligence Scale for Children-Third Edition.* San Antonio: Psychological Corporation.

Zatorre, R., & McEntee, W. (1983). Semantic encoding deficits in a case of traumatic amnesia. *Brain and Cognition, 2*, 331–345.

4

Language Disorders

DAVID CAPLAN

Human language is a unique mental entity. It is a system of symbols that greatly enhances the ability of humans to represent aspects of the world, to think, and to communicate with each other. Language has a complex structure, and its use involves many diverse, interacting psychological operations. This chapter describes the progress that has been made in understanding language processing and its disorders, and presents an approach to the diagnosis of the most common of these disorders in acquired neurological disease in adults.

THE LANGUAGE CODE

Human language can be viewed as a code that links a set of linguistic forms to a number of aspects of meaning. The basic levels of the language code include the *lexical level,* the *morphological level,* the *sentential level,* and the *discourse level.*

The *lexical level* of language makes contact with concepts and categories. Lexical items designate concrete objects, abstract concepts, actions, properties, and relationships. The basic form of a simple lexical item consists of a phonological representation, or one that specifies the phonemes of the word and their organization into structures such as syllables (Halle & Vergnaud, 1987). The form of a word can also be represented orthographically, as a series of signs representing units of sound, or ideographically (Henderson, 1982). Simple words are assigned to different syntactic categories, such as nouns, verbs, or adjectives.

The *morphological level* of language allows words to be formed from other words. Derivational morphology tends to change the syntactic class of a word (e.g., the noun *destruction* is derived from the verb *destroy*) (Anderson, 1982). This allows

---

DAVID CAPLAN • Neuropsychology Laboratory, Massachusetts General Hospital, Boston, Massachusetts 02114.

Clinical Neuropsychological Assessment: A Cognitive Approach, edited by Robert L. Mapou and Jack Spector. Plenum Press, New York, 1995.

the meaning associated with a simple lexical item to be used as a different syntactic category without coining a huge number of new lexical forms (Williams, 1981). Other word formation processes (inflection) play roles in encoding syntactic relationships, such as subject–verb and adjective–noun agreement. English makes relatively little use of inflectional morphology compared to many other languages.

The *sentential level* of language expresses propositions that convey aspects of the structure of events in the world. The overall meaning of a sentence is determined by the way the meanings of simple and derived words combine in syntactic structures (e.g., noun phrase, verb phrase, or sentence) (Chomsky, 1965, 1981, 1986). Sentences expressing propositions are a crucial level of the language code because they make assertions about the world.

The propositional meanings conveyed by sentences are entered into higher order structures that constitute the *discourse level* of linguistic structure (Grosz, Pollack, & Sidner, 1989). Discourse includes information about the general topic under discussion, the focus of a speaker's attention, the novelty of the information in a given sentence, or the relationship of events and actions to each other. Information conveyed by the discourse level of language also serves to update an individual's knowledge of the world, for reasoning and planning action.

MODELS OF LANGUAGE PROCESSING

Current models of language processing subdivide functions such as reading, speaking, or auditory comprehension, into semi-indepenedent components or "modules." Each module is thought to perform a particular, highly specialized function in the overall system.

Information processing models of language are now widely expressed as flow diagrams that capture the sequence of operations of the different components performing a language-related task. Each of the major components of the language processing system activates the lexical, morphological, sentential, and discourse levels of the language code in the usual communication tasks. These tasks include speech, auditory comprehension, reading, and writing. This approach to defining language processing components groups together, into a single processor, different operations that all activate a similar type of linguistic representation in a given task. The major components of the language processing system for simple words are listed in Table 4.1, and the components of language processing for morphologically complex words and sentences are shown in Table 4.2. Figure 4.1 presents a model indicating the sequence of activation of components of the lexical processing system. Figure 4.2 presents a similar model of the processing system for morphologically complex words and sentences. Models of this general type can be developed in greater detail. For instance, in these tables and figures, the major processors involved in understanding auditorily presented words reflect a stage of acoustic–phonetic processing, a stage of activation of the forms of words, and a stage of activation of the meanings of words, but the operations of each of these components need to be described in considerably more detail.

TABLE 4.1. Summary of Components of the Language Processing System for Simple Words

Component	Input	Operation	Output
Auditory–oral modality			
Acoustic-phonological processing	Acoustic waveform	Matches acoustic properties to phonetic features	Phonological segments (phonemes, allophones, syllables)
Input-side lexical access	Phonological units	Activates lexical items in long-term memory on basis of sound; selects best fit to stimulus	Phonological forms of words
Input-side semantic access	Words (represented as phonological forms)	Activates semantic features of words	Word meanings
Output-side lexical access	Word meanings ("lemmas")	Activates the phonological forms of words	Phonological forms of words
Phonological output planning	Phonological forms of words (and nonwords)	Activates detailed phonetic features of words (and nonwords)	Speech
Written modality			
Written lexical access	Abstract letter identities	Activates orthographic forms of words	Orthographic forms of words
Lexical semantic access	Orthographic forms of words	Activates semantic features of words	Word meanings
Accessing orthography from semantics	Word meanings	Activates orthographic forms of words	Orthographic forms of words
Accessing lexical orthography from lexical phonology	Phonological representations of words	Activates orthographic forms of words from their phonological forms	Orthographic forms of words
Accessing sublexical orthography from sublexical phonology	Phonological units (phonemes, other units)	Activates orthographic units corresponding to phonological units	Orthographic units in words and nonwords
Accessing lexical phonology from whole-word orthography	Orthographic form of words	Activates phonological forms of words	Phonological forms of words
Accessing sublexical phonology from orthography	Orthographic units (graphemes, other units)	Activates phonological units corresponding to orthographic units	Phonological units in words and nonwords

TABLE 4.2. Summary of Components of the Language Processing System for Derived Words and Sentences (Collapsed over Auditory–Oral and Written Modalities)

Component	Input	Operation	Output
Processing affixed words			
Accessing morphological form	Word forms	Segments words into structural (morphological) units; activates syntactic features of words	Morphological structure; syntactic features
Morphological comprehension	Word meanings; morphological structure	Combines word roots and affixes	Meanings of morphologically complex words
Accessing affixed words from semantics	Word meanings; syntactic features	Activates forms of affixes and function words	Forms of affixes and function words
Sentence-level processing			
Lexico-inferential processing knowledge	Meanings of simple and complex words	Infers aspects of sentence meaning on basis of pragmatic plausibility	Aspects of propositional meaning (thematic roles; attribution of modifiers)
Syntactic comprehension	Word meanings; syntactic features	Constructs syntactic representation and combines it with word meanings	Propositional meaning
Construction of sentence form	Word forms; propositional meaning	Constructs syntactic structures; inserts word forms into structures	Sentence form (including positions of lexical items)

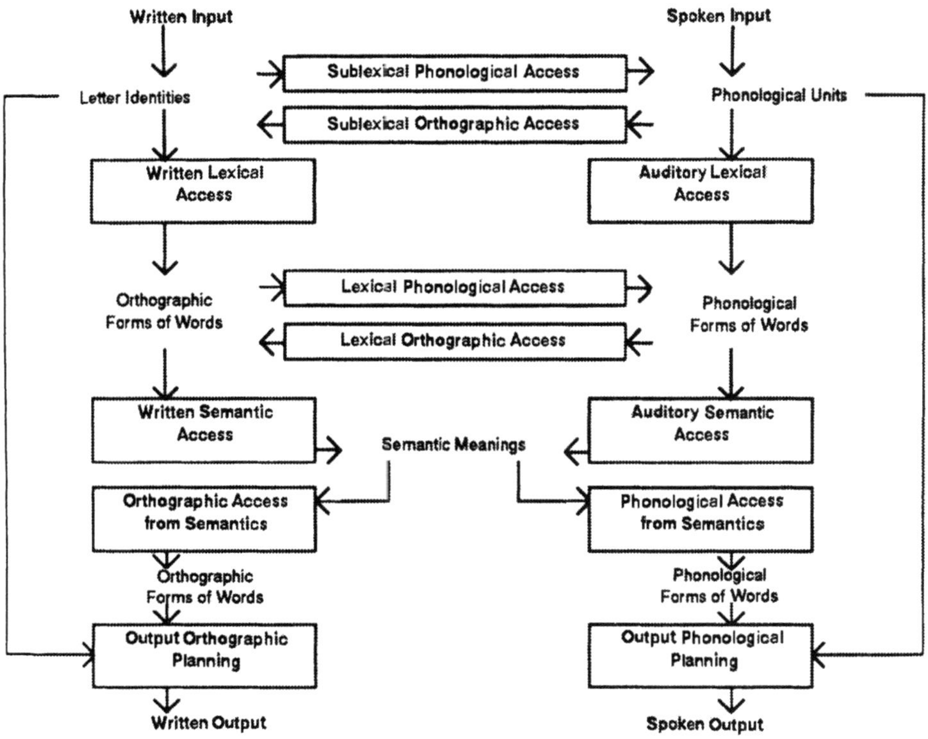

FIGURE 4.1. Diagrammatic representation of the sequence of activation of components of the processing system for single words. Processing components are presented in boxes in boldface; representations are presented in regular type. Arrows represent the flow of information (representations) from one processing component to another.

There are four important operating characteristics of the components of the language processing system.

First, each processor accepts only particular types of input and produces only specific types of output. For example, the processor that activates syntactic structures from auditory input may use as input many features derived from the speech signal, including the syntactic categories of the words presented to it, the meanings of these words, or intonational contours, but it does not make use of those acoustic properties that indicate that the speaker is a man or a woman. Fodor (1983) uses the term *encapsulation* to refer to this property of components of the language processing system. Similarly, the output of this processor is a syntactic structure—it is not a representation of the implications of a sentence. Fodor uses the term *domain specificity* to refer to this property.

Second, most processors are obligatorily activated when their inputs are presented to them. For instance, if the control and supervisory components of cognition lead us to attend to a sound that happens to be the word *elephant,* we must hear and understand that word; we cannot hear this sound as just a noise (Marslen-Wilson, 1987).

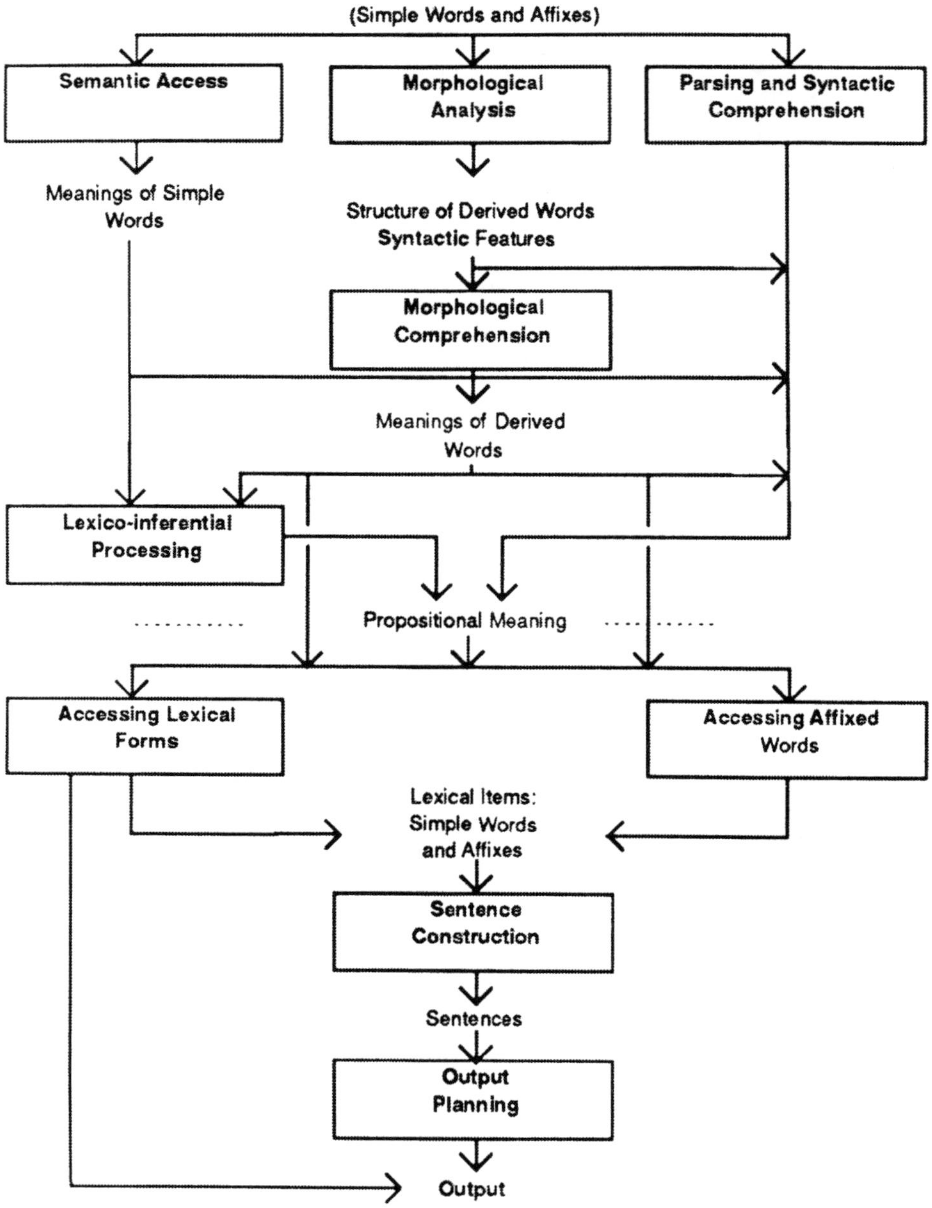

FIGURE 4.2. Diagrammatic representation of the sequence of operation of components of the language processing system for morphologically complex words and sentences. Processing components are presented in boxes in boldface; representations are presented in regular type. Arrows represent the flow of information (representations) from one processing component to another.

Third, language processors generally operate unconsciously. The unconscious nature of most of language processing can be appreciated by considering that when we listen to a lecture, have a conversation, read a novel, or engage in some other language processing task, we usually have the impression that we are understanding another person's meaning and producing linguistic forms appropriate to our intentions without paying attention to the details of the sounds of words or sentence structure.

Fourth and finally, components of the system operate remarkably quickly and accurately. For instance, it has been estimated that spoken words are usually recognized less than 125 milliseconds after their onset (Marslen-Wilson & Welsh, 1978; Tyler & Wessels, 1983). Similarly, normal word production in speech requires searching through a mental word-production "dictionary" of over 20,000 items, but still goes on at the rate of about three words per second, with an error rate of about one word misselected per million and another one word mispronounced per million (Levelt, 1989). The speed of the language processing system as a whole occurs because of the speed of each of its components, but also is achieved because of the massively parallel functional architecture of the system, which leads to many components of the system being simultaneously active.

The language processors can be used in different combinations to accomplish different language-related tasks such as auditory comprehension, reading, repeating what has been heard, or taking notes on a lecture. The use of these processors in these tasks is under the control of other cognitive systems, such as those that deploy and shift attention, search knowledge stored in memory, or match motivations to actions. Functional communication involving language occurs when people undertake language-related tasks to accomplish specific goals such as informing others, asking for information, or getting things done. The use of language is thus a special instance of intentional action.

DISORDERS OF PSYCHOLINGUISTIC PROCESSING

This chapter focuses on psycholinguistic disorders of language, that is, disorders that affect the language processors themselves. When neurological disease affects the forms and meanings that make up the language code, or disrupts the processors devoted to their activation, the ability to perform language-related tasks and to use language to accomplish goals is compromised. Therefore, an understanding of these disorders is important in the diagnosis and rehabilitation of patients with language impairments.

The term *aphasia* refers to any disturbance of the ability to use the language code for normal communication, due to central nervous system (CNS) disease. *Primary* aphasic disturbances affect the operation of one or more of the components of the language processing system directly. *Secondary* aphasic disturbances arise when disruptions of other cognitive functions lead to interference with the normal operation of one or more of the components of the language processing system. For reasons of space, only the literature on primary aphasic disturbances in the auditory–oral modality will be reviewed here.

Disturbances of Word Meanings

Most recent research on disturbances of word meanings in aphasia has focused on words that refer to objects. The meanings of these words are thought to be stored in a specialized semantic memory system (Tulving, 1972). Disturbances of word meanings for objects cause poor performance on word–picture matching and naming tasks (Warrington, 1975). However, the combination of deficits in word–picture matching and naming may be due to separate input- and output-side processing disturbances that affect word recognition and production (Howard & Orchard-Lisle, 1984). Deficits in naming and word–picture matching are more likely to result from a disturbance affecting concepts when (1) the patient makes many semantic errors in providing words to pictures and definitions, (2) he or she has trouble with word–picture matching with semantic but not phonological foils, (3) he or she fails on categorization tasks with pictures, and (4) the same words are affected in production and comprehension tasks (Hillis, Rapp, Romani, & Caramazza, 1990).

Semantic deficits may be modality-specific. Warrington (1975) first noted a discrepancy between comprehension of words and pictures in two dementing patients. Bub et al. (1988) have analyzed a patient, M.P., who showed very poor comprehension of written and spoken words but quite good comprehension of pictures.

Semantic disturbances may also be category-specific. Several authors have reported a selective semantic impairment of concepts related to living things and foods, as compared to human-made objects (Sartori & Job, 1988; Silveri & Gainotti, 1988; Warrington & Shallice, 1984). The opposite pattern has also been found (Warrington & McCarthy, 1983, 1987). Selective preservation and disruption of abstract versus concrete concepts, and of nominal versus verbal concepts, have also been reported (Miceli, Silveri, Villa, & Caramazza, 1984; Schwartz, Marin, & Saffran, 1979; Warrington, 1981; Zingeser & Berndt, 1988).

Disturbances of Oral Word Production

Disturbances affecting the oral production of single words are extremely common in aphasic patients. There are three basic disturbances affecting word production (other than semantic deficits): (1) disturbances in accessing the forms of words from concepts, (2) disturbances in planning the form of a word for articulation, and (3) disturbances of articulation.

A disturbance in activating word forms from concepts is manifested by an inability to produce a word from a semantic stimulus, such as a picture or a definition, coupled with intact processing at the semantic and phonological levels (determined by answering questions about pictures, picture categorization tests, and repetition). The form of a patient's errors is not a good guide to whether he or she has an impairment at this level of production, since disturbances in accessing word forms may appear in a variety of ways, ranging from pauses, to neologisms (complex sequences of sounds that do not form words), to semantic paraphasias (words related to the meaning of the target item). Rarely, patients show an inability to name objects presented in one modality only (Beauvois, 1982; Beauvois, Saillant, Meininger, & Lhermitte, 1978; Denes & Semenza, 1975; Lhermitte & Beauvois, 1973). These modality-specific naming disorders likely reflect a failure to transmit modality-specific semantic information to the processor responsible for activating the forms of words.

Disturbances of a patient's ability to convert the representation of the sound of a word into a form appropriate for articulatory production are usually manifested as phonemic paraphasias (substitutions, omissions, and misorderings of phonemes). Three features of a patient's performance suggest a disturbance in word sound planning. First, some phonemic paraphasias are closely related to target words (e.g., "befenit" for *benefit*) (Lecours & Lhermitte, 1969). Second, some patients make multiple attempts that come closer and closer to the correct form of a word (Joanette, Keller, & Lecours, 1980). Third, some patients make similar phonological errors in word repetition, word reading, and picture naming. Because the form of a word is presented to the output system in very different ways in these three tasks, the errors of such patients most likely arise in the process of planning the form of the word that is suitable for articulation (Caplan, Vanier, & Baker, 1986).

Patients with sound-planning problems are more affected on longer words and on words with consonant clusters (Kohn, 1984; Nespoulous, Joanette, Beland, Caplan, & Lecours, 1984). The frequency of occurrence of a word in the language has a variable effect on the occurrence of these types of errors (Garrett, 1982; Pate, Saffran, & Martin, 1987). Planning disturbances only rarely affect function words but more commonly affect nouns, verbs, and adjectives (Buckingham, 1979). Some patients have trouble planning the sounds of words only when words are inserted into sentences, making phonemic paraphasias in sentence production but not in naming or repetition tasks (Kohn, 1989).

Patients often have disturbances of articulation itself, as shown by abnormalities in the acoustic waveform they produce (Blumstein, Alexander, Ryalls, Katz, & Dworetzky, 1987; Blumstein, Cooper, Zurif, & Caramazza, 1977) and in the movement of the articulators in speech (Itoh, Sasanuma, & Hirose, 1980; Itoh et al., 1982; Schonle et al., 1987). Investigators have identified two major disturbances of articulation: dysarthria and apraxia of speech. Dysarthria is marked by hoarseness, excessive nasality, and slurred articulation, and is not significantly influenced by the type of linguistic material that the speaker produces or by the speech task (Darley, 1983). Apraxia of speech is marked by difficulty in initiating speech, searching for a pronunciation, better articulation for automatized speech (e.g., counting) than volitional speech, abnormal prosody, omissions of syllables in multisyllabic words, and simplification of consonant clusters (often by adding a short neutral vowel sound between consonants; Bowman, Hodson, & Simpson, 1980; Kent & Rosenbek, 1982).

Disturbances of Auditory Comprehension of Single Words

Disturbances affecting auditory comprehension of single words have been attributed to impairments of semantic concepts, as discussed above, and/or to an inability to recognize spoken words. The latter disturbances have, in turn, been thought to have two possible origins: disturbances affecting the recognition of phonemes in the acoustic signal, and disturbances affecting the ability to recognize words despite good acoustic–phonetic processing.

Disturbances of acoustic–phonetic processing may affect the ability to discriminate or to identify phonemes (Blumstein, Baker, & Goodglass, 1977), but it is unclear whether these disturbances lead to problems in recognizing or understanding spoken words. Several studies suggest that they do (Albert & Bear, 1974; Auerbach, Allard, Naeser, Alexander, & Albert, 1982; Caramazza, Berndt, & Basili, 1983; Saffran, Marin, & Yeni-Komshian, 1976), but other researchers have found weak correlations between comprehension capacities and phoneme discrimination capacities in aphasic patients (Basso, Casati, & Vignolo, 1977; Blumstein, Cooper, Zurif, & Caramazza, 1977; Miceli, Gainotti, Caltagirone, & Masullo, 1980). Blumstein, Cooper, Zurif, and Caramazza (1977) specifically concluded that phonemic processing disturbances could not be the main reason for Wernicke's aphasics' disturbances of auditory comprehension, as had been suggested by Luria (1973).

Many researchers believe that patients can have disturbances of word recognition despite good acoustic–phonetic processing. Such a disturbance was originally postulated by Wernicke (1974). However, there is no clear case of a patient who has intact acoustic–phonetic processing and who cannot recognize spoken words. The patient whose deficit comes closest to this is a case described by Berndt and Mitchum (1990). The patient could not identify spoken nonsense words (e.g., *bez*) as nonwords but could correctly identify and interpret real words.

Thus, the origin of many single-word comprehension problems remains unclear. Most of these problems appear to arise from a complex interaction of acoustic–phonetic disturbances, disturbances in recognizing spoken words, and disturbances affecting word meanings (Goodglass, Gleason, & Hyde, 1970).

Repetition of Single Words

Repetition of a word can be carried out in three ways (Marshall, 1987): (1) nonlexically, by repeating sounds without recognizing the word (as if one were imitating a foreign language); (2) lexically, by recognizing the stimulus as a word and uttering it without understanding it; and (3) semantically, by understanding the word and reactivating its form from its meaning. Any of these routes to repetition may be disturbed. For instance, Morton (1980) described a patient who could repeat only by the semantic route; this patient made many semantic paraphasias in repetition and could not repeat nonwords. McCarthy and Warrington (1984) have documented a double dissociation between good performance on repetition tasks that maximize semantic processing and those that minimize such processing. Patients with relatively isolated disturbances affecting the repetition of nonwords have been described (Caramazza, Miceli, & Villa, 1986), reflecting disruption of the nonlexical route. In most cases, patients have a more complicated picture, with lexical status (whether a stimulus is a word or a nonword), word frequency, and stimulus length affecting performance differently in different patients (Bub, Black, Howell, & Kertesz, 1987; Caplan et al., 1986; Miller & Ellis,

1987). Repetition of long words and nonwords stresses the language processing system and can reveal otherwise undetectable pathology.

Disturbances of Processing Morphologically Complex Words

The first modern studies that revealed a disturbance of processing morphological forms in single-word tasks were observations of the oral reading of complex words by patients with "deep dyslexia" (Coltheart, Patterson, & Marshall, 1980; see below). These patients make numerous derivational paralexic errors when reading (e.g., *write* → *wrote; fish* → *fishing; directing* → *direction*), and have particular difficulty with the recognition and anlaysis of written derived words (Badecker & Caramazza, 1987; Funnell, 1983; Job & Sartori, 1984; Patterson, 1980). A patient with similar difficulty affecting the auditory processing of words with inflectional but not derivational morphology has been described (Tyler & Cobb, 1987). Disturbances affecting morphological processing also appear in single-word production tasks (Miceli & Caramazza, 1988), even in patients who perform flawlessly on tasks that require recognition and comprehension of written morphologically complex words (Badecker & Caramazza, in press).

Disturbances affecting the production of morphologically complex words are most commonly seen in sentence production, where they are known as agrammatism and paragrammatism. The most noticeable deficit in agrammatism is the widespread omission of function words and affixes and the better production of common nouns (Menn, Obler, & Goodglass, 1990), which is always seen in the spontaneous speech of agrammatic patients, and often occurs in their repetition and writing as well. Patients in whom *substitutions* of these elements predominate, and whose speech is fluent, are called paragrammatic (Goodglass & Geschwind, 1976). Recent observations have emphasized the fact that these two patterns co-occur in many patients (Goodglass & Menn, 1985; Heeschen, 1985; Menn et al., 1990). They may result from a single underlying deficit that has different surface manifestations (Caplan, 1986; Grodzinsky, 1984).

Agrammatism and paragrammatism vary considerably, with different sets of words being affected or spared in different cases (Menn et al., 1990; Miceli, Silveri, Romani, & Caramazza, 1989). In some patients, there seems to be some regularity to the pattern of errors. For instance, English agrammatic patients frequently produce infinitives (e.g., *to walk*) and gerunds (e.g., *walking*) because these are the basic forms in English (Lapointe, 1983). In other cases, substitutions are closely related to the correct target (Miceli et al., 1989). In almost all cases, errors do not violate the word formation and the syntactic processes of the language (Kean, 1977). This suggests that most agrammatic and paragrammatic patients retain some knowledge of the rules of word and sentence formation, a feature that may be important in designing therapy.

Disorders of Sentence Production

When patients have disturbances with the production of simple or complex words, these problems almost always surface in sentence production as well. In addition, many patients have problems in the sentence-planning process itself. Agrammatism and paragrammatism are impairments of the ability to produce particular types of vocabulary elements in sentences. Two other disturbances of sentence production have been described: problems affecting the generation of syntactic form, and problems affecting the production of intonational contours.

Disorders of Syntactic Form Generation

Agrammatic patients usually produce only very simple syntactic structures. There are several reasons for this limitation. Ostrin, Schwartz, and Saffrin (1983) described four patients who could produce either an article and a noun (*the man*) or an adjective and a noun (*old man*), but not both (*the old man*). Since the patients produced either phrase on different attempts, Ostrin et al. concluded that they could not produce adequately complex syntactic structures for their thoughts. In a second study of the repetition abilities of six agrammatic subjects, Ostrin and Schwartz (1986) found that the patients tended to reproduce the order of nouns and verbs in the presented sentence, but made many syntactic errors, such as producing *The bicycle is riding by the boy* for *The bicycle is being ridden by the boy.* They argued that these performances resulted from an incomplete memory trace of the thematic roles of the noun phrases in the presented sentence (i.e., who was accomplishing or receiving an action). Saffran, Schwartz, and Marin (1980) suggested that more impaired patients lose the basic concepts of functional roles and/or cannot use even the basic word order of English to express these aspects of meaning.

The ability to express the thematic roles of noun phrases requires the ability to use verbs. McCarthy and Warrington (1985) described a patient whose category-specific degradation of the meaning of verbs resulted in almost no production of verbs in speech and limited the expression of functional roles for nouns. However, in a study by Miceli et al. (1984), patients' inability to produce verbs was only partially responsible for the shortened phrase length found in their speech. It thus appears that, in some patients, a disturbance affecting the ability to produce verbs affects the production of a normal range of syntactic structures, while, in others, at least some syntactic structures are built despite poor verb production. Yet other patients cannot produce normal syntactic structures despite relatively good verb production.

Several studies suggest that syntactic errors in sentence production differ in paragrammatic and agrammatic patients (Butterworth & Howard, 1987; Caplan, Kellar, & Locke, 1972; Ellis, Miller, & Sin, 1983). One type of error that has often been found in paragrammatism is a *blend,* in which the output seems to reflect a conflation of two different ways of saying the same thing (e.g., *They are not prepared to be of helpful,* a combination of *They are not prepared to be helpful* and *They are not prepared to be of help* (Butterworth & Howard, 1987). Butterworth (1982, 1985; Butterworth & Howard, 1987) has argued that the syntactic and morphological errors in paragrammatism result from the failure of these patients to monitor their speech production processes and their output. The complex disturbance that results from the combination of these deficits, disturbances in accessing and planning word forms, and impairments in producing morphologically complex words is known as *jargonaphasia* (Buckingham & Kertesz, 1976; Lecours & Rouillon, 1976).

Disorders of Prosody

Disturbances in prosody may be secondary to motor output disorders (Kent & Rosenbek, 1982; Monrad Krohn, 1947; Ryalls, 1982) or associated with other sentence production disorders (Danly, Cooper, & Shapiro, 1983; Danly & Shapiro, 1982). However, these disturbances may also occur in isolation. Shapiro and Danly (1985) reported that patients with anterior and central right-hemisphere lesions had a variety of disturbances of prosody in sentence production. These patterns occurred regardless of the emotion associated with a sentence, and thus are different from the aprosodias related to disturbances of emotional display that arise after right-hemisphere disease (Ross & Mesulam, 1979). Shapiro and Danly (1985) argued that some disorders of prosody reflect a primary disturbance of production of intonation in right-hemisphere-damaged patients, which differs as a function of lesion location in the hemisphere.

Disorders of Sentence Comprehension

There are many reasons why a patient might fail to understand the propositional content of a sentence. In addition to the carryover effect of disturbances affecting comprehension of simple and complex words, there are disturbances affecting the ability to understand aspects of propositional meaning despite good single-word processing.

The greatest amount of work in the area of disturbances of sentence comprehension has gone into the investigation of patients whose use of syntactic structures to assign meaning is not normal. Patients may have very selective disturbances affecting the use of particular syntactic structures or elements to determine the meaning of a sentence. For instance, one patient we studied could understand sentences with reflexive elements (*himself*) but not pronouns (*him;* Caplan & Hildebrandt, 1988). Other patients have virtually no ability to use syntactic structure at all, and rely on inferences based on their knowledge of the real world and their ability to understand some words in a sentence (Schwartz, Saffran, & Marin, 1980). Such a patient may understand a sentence like *The man ate the cake,* because he or she knows that men are animate and can eat and that cakes are inanimate and can be eaten, but not a sentence like *The man hugged the woman,* in which these semantic factors do not determine meaning (Schwartz et al., 1980). Finally, some patients can understand very simple syntactic forms, as in *The man hugged the woman,* but not more complex forms, such as *The woman was hugged by the man* (Caplan, Baker, & Dehaut, 1985).

Many clinicians attribute sentence comprehension disturbances to limitations in verbal short-term memory (STM). However, patients with STM impairments have been described who have excellent sentence comprehension abilities (Butterworth, Campbell, & Howard, 1986; McCarthy & Warrington, 1987). For instance, a patient of ours with an STM span of two to three items showed excellent comprehension of syntactically complex sentences, even under speeded response conditions (Waters, Caplan, & Hildebrandt, 1991). Though many STM patients have trouble in tasks in which the initial analysis of a sentence must be reviewed (Caplan & Waters, 1990), these disorders probably have little impact on comprehension.

A PSYCHOLINGUISTIC APPROACH TO THE ASSESSMENT OF LANGUAGE DISORDERS

The goal of a psycholinguistic assessment is to specify the types of linguistic representations (simple words, complex words, sentences, discourse) that are processed abnormally in each of the four major language-related tasks (speech, auditory comprehension, reading, writing). It should also attempt to identify selective impairments affecting each type of representation in each of these tasks, and the overall level of functioning of the patient with respect to each linguistic representation in each task. This effort will lead to a description of the patient's language disorder in relation to the major components of the language processing system. A psycholinguistic approach to diagnosing patients with language disorders will also identify compensations the patient makes to these impairments. Finally, this approach will provide a basis for grouping patients together who have similar psycholinguistically defined language disorders.

The obvious place to turn for assessment tools is existing aphasia batteries (Boston Diagnostic Aphasia Examination [BDAE]; Goodglass & Kaplan, 1972, 1983; the Western Aphasia Battery; Kertesz, 1979; Kertesz & Poole, 1974; the Porch Index of Communicative Ability [PICA]; Porch, 1971; the Auditory Discrimination Test; Wepman, 1958). However, for the most part, these batteries do not provide the basis for an analysis of patients' deficits in terms of language processing components. More specific tests, such as the Peabody Picture Vocabulary Test (Dunn, 1965), the Boston Naming Test (BNT; Kaplan, Goodglass, & Weintraub, 1983), or the Token Test (De Renzi & Vignolo, 1962) have similar limitations. For instance, the Token Test is often used as a test of syntactic comprehension. However, the test does not distinguish among problems in syntactic comprehension, in short-term memory, or in using the products of comprehension to plan actions. I do not wish to imply that all of these tests are completely unrevealing with respect to the language processing problems of a patient, but that they are very hard to use for this purpose. They only occasionally allow the clinician to identify the language processing components that are affected, and they never provide a systematic exploration of the nature of disturbances within a component. In addition, existing tests do not assess some important areas of language processing at all, such as comprehension and production of morphological structure.

The Psycholinguistic Assessment of Language

In response to the need for a psycholinguistically based general language assessment tool, a colleague, Daniel Bub, and I have created a psycholinguistically oriented language assessment battery, the Psycholinguistic Assessment of Langauge (PAL). The

PAL is currently being used for research purposes and may become available to clinicians in the next few years if it meets criteria for construct validity, sensitivity, and clinical applicability. It consists of 27 subtests (see Table 4.3), of which I here present those relevant to auditory–oral language processing at the word, word formation, and sentence levels. Each subtest contains items with different structural or categorical features, to assess the specificity of a deficit for particular stimulus types at each level of processing, as discussed above. Each subtest also contains items that vary in difficulty, to provide a measure of the extent to which a particular component is disturbed. To evaluate the integrity of a component of the language processing system, it is necessary to compare a patient's performance on several tests.

Because many of the tests in the battery involve matching language stimuli to pictures or producing language responses on the basis of pictorial stimuli, the first test on the battery is a screening test for the ability to identify pictures of objects. This test uses a pictorial forced-choice attribute-verification task to ascertain the subject's ability to extract semantic information from a picture. In this task, a patient must choose the one of two pictures that illustrates a feature of an object depicted in a third picture. Patients who show abnormalities that interfere with their ability to extract semantic information from pictures would be examined only on tests that do not make use of pictures.

The following provides a description of subtests relevant to auditory–oral language processing:

I. Auditory Comprehension

1. *The Single-Word Level*

Three proccessing components involved in single-word input processing are assessed: acoustic–phonetic processing, lexical access, and semantic access. The tests relevant to these components are:

(i) Test 1: PHONEME DISCRIMINATION

The ability to discriminate phonemes is tested by a same–different task with 40 pairs of monosyllabic nonwords (20 different and 20 identical trials). Different stimuli differ in a single phoneme with respect to place of articulation, manner of articulation, or voicing. The changed phoneme can occur in the initial or final position, either as a single consonant or as a member of a cluster. Consonants were chosen as the segments to be changed because they have been used more frequently than vowels in research on phonemic discrimination in aphasia.

(ii) Test 2: AUDITORY LEXICAL DECISION

Auditory lexical access is assessed using a lexical decision task for words and nonwords. The words consist of 40 concrete nouns. They vary in frequency (greater than 40/million or less than 5/million) and length (one syllable versus three or more syllables). Half of the foils are constructed by changing a single distinctive feature in a single phoneme in different syllabic positions of comparable words. The other 20 foils are created by changing the form of words matched to the

TABLE 4.3. Tests Used in the Psycholinguistic Assessment of Language (PAL) Battery

- I. Auditory–oral modality
  - A. Single-word processing
    - 1. Single-word input processing
      - Phoneme discrimination
      - Auditory lexical decision
      - Single-word auditory comprehension
      - (a) Word–picture matching
      - (b) Forced-choice attribute-verification procedure
      - (c) Relatedness judgment test for abstract words
    - 2. Single-word output processing
      - Word and nonword repetition
      - Picture homophone matching
      - Picture naming
  - B. Processing affixed words
    - 1. Input processing of affixed words
      - Auditory lexical decision for affixed words
      - Auditory comprehension of affixed words
      - (a) Word–picture matching
      - (b) Relatedness judgment
    - 2. Output processing of affixed words
      - Affixed word production
  - C. Sentence-level processing
    - 1. Sentence input processing
      - Constrained sentence comprehension
      - Syntactic comprehension
    - 2. Sentence output processing
      - Sentence production
- II. Written modality
  - A. Single-word processing
    - 1. Written single-word input processing
      - Written lexical decision
      - Written lexical comprehension
      - (a) Word–picture matching
      - (b) Forced-choice attribute-verification
      - (c) Relatedness judgment test for abstract words
    - 2. Written single-word output processing
      - Written naming
      - Writing to dictation
    - 3. Single-word written–oral transcoding
      - Oral reading
  - B. Processing affixed words
    - 1. Input processing of written affixed words
      - Lexical decision for written affixed words
      - Comprehension of written affixed words
    - 2. Output processing of written affixed words
      - Written affixed word production
  - C. Sentence-level processing
    - 1. Written sentence input processing
      - Constrained written sentence comprehension
      - Written syntactic comprehension
    - 2. Written sentence output processing
      - Written sentence production

positive targets so as to resemble possible words (e.g., *harpisform* from *harpsichord*); these stimuli were included because having only phonological foils sounded odd in pilot trials with normals. A yes/no (word/nonword) decision is required.

(iii) SINGLE-WORD AUDITORY COMPREHENSION

The PAL uses three means of assessing single-word comprehension: a word–picture matching test, a forced-choice attribute-verification procedure, and a relatedness judgment test for abstract words. These three tasks assess a subject's ability to map a word onto a picture and to recognize verbally presented features and synonyms of a word. Words that vary in animacy and abstractness are tested in different tasks. To test for a subject's consistency across different presentations of a given item, there is selective repetition of some words on the forced-choice attribute-verification task and the word–picture selection task (and also on the picture naming and written tasks described below).

(a) Test 3: *Word–picture matching*. In this task, 32 concrete nouns are presented auditorily, and the subject must select one of two pictures that matches the word. Foils are both semantically and visually similar to the targets (e.g., *deer* as target and *moose* as foil). Targets are of either high or low frequency and are either short (monosyllabic) or long (tri- or quadrisyllabic). They include examples from the categories of animals, fruits and vegetables, and tools.

(b) Test 4: *Forced-choice attribute-verification procedure*. In this task, 16 concrete nouns are presented auditorily, and three questions are asked regarding each noun. The questions require either a yes/no answer or the selection of one of two features (e.g., *Does a horse have fur or a hide?*). Three questions relate to physical and three to functional attributes. Nouns are from the categories of animals, fruits and vegetables, and tools, and vary in familiarity.

(c) Test 5: *Relatedness judgment test for abstract words*. A target word and two subsequent words are presented auditorily. The subject must select the word most closely related to the target (e.g., *strive—learn/try*). All targets are mono- and bisyllabic, but otherwise vary in frequency and syntactic category.

2. *The Word Formation Level*

The following subtests assess recognition and comprehension of morphologically complex words:

(i) Test 6: AUDITORY LEXICAL DECISION FOR AFFIXED WORDS

Recognition of derived words is assessed through a lexical decision task that tests a patient's ability to recognize derived words as well formed. Positive stimuli consist of high-frequency stems and affixes that are combined to form low-frequency morphologically complex words. Both derivational affixation and inflectional affixation are used. The positive stimuli thus consist of 24 words, 16 with derivational affixes (e.g., *happiness*) and eight with word-boundary inflectional affixes (e.g., *draws*), and an equivalent number of foils consisting of nonexistent derived forms (e.g., *detentive*). The stimuli are presented auditorily to the subject who must indicate whether or not each is a word.

(ii) AUDITORY COMPREHENSION OF AFFIXED WORDS

(a) Test 7: *Word–picture matching for affixed words*. Derived words are presented with a picture that conveys each word's meaning and a foil that reflects a different affix (e.g., the word *restless* is presented with a picture-pair showing a person who is restless [pacing] and one who is resting [sitting down relaxing]). Twenty words are presented auditorily, and the subject must select the appropriate picture. Words vary with respect to the nature of the affixation (derivational, inflectional).

(b) Test 8: *Relatedness judgment for affixed words*. A relatedness judgment task, similar to that used with abstract words, is used to assess patients' abilities to comprehend the meanings of affixes. A target affixed word is presented auditorily along with two affixed versions of another root (e.g., the target word *chosen* presented with the word pair *selection* and *selected*), and the subject must indicate which of the pair goes best with the target.

3. *The Sentence Level*

The battery assesses two ways that subjects comprehend sentences. The first, *lexico-inferential processing*, is the process whereby a subject infers aspects of sentence meaning from the meanings of words and his or her knowledge of the real world. This component of the comprehension system is tested by presenting sentences that are constrained by plausibility factors (e.g., *The dog ate the bone*) along with foils that contain an incorrect item (e.g., a picture of a dog eating a piece of meat). The second process, *parsing and syntactic comprehension*, involves the use of syntactic structure to determine propositional meaning. It is tested by presenting syntactically complex semantically reversible sentences (e.g., *The cat was scratched by the dog*) with foils that depict the opposite set of actors (e.g., a picture of a cat scratching a dog).

(i) Test 9a: CONSTRAINED SENTENCE COMPREHENSION

A sentence–picture matching test is used. Pictures consist of the correct interpretation and a foil that varies with respect to one of the words in the sentence (e.g., Target: *The car was waxed by the man;* Foil: *The car was washed by the man*). Twenty semantically irreversible sentences varying as to voice (active and passive) and nature of foil (e.g., verb, preposition) are presented auditorily. This test thus supplements the tests of single-word comprehension (Tests 3–5), which focus on nouns and adjectives. The subject must select the appropriate picture.

(ii) Test 9b: SYNTACTIC COMPREHENSION

Twenty semantically reversible sentences with four syntactic structures are presented in a sentence–picture matching test with correct pictures and syntactically incorrect foils (e.g., Target: *The man was pushed by the woman;* Foil: *The man pushed the woman*). Sentences are presented auditorily, and the subject must select the appropriate picture.

II. Oral Production

1. The Single-Word Level

Oral production of single words is divided into two components: accessing lexical phonological forms from the meanings of words, and planning phonological output. The following tasks are relevant to these components:

(i) Test 10: PICTURE HOMOPHONE MATCHING

A picture homophone matching task is used to assess a subject's ability to access lexical phonological representations from word meaning, despite any possible disruption of the ability to produce these representations orally. Thirty-two picture pairs are presented; half are homophones (*bat/bat*), and half differ by a single distinctive feature (*cat/can*). The subject must indicate whether the names of the pictures are homophones.

(ii) Test 11: WORD AND NONWORD REPETITION

As discussed above, repetition can be carried out by various mechanisms. The battery tests repetition of both words and nonwords. Twenty words, all common concrete nouns that vary in frequency and length, are presented auditorily, and the subject must repeat them. Twenty nonwords derived by changing multiple distinctive features in words comparable to the word stimuli are also presented auditorily, and the subject must repeat them.

In the repetition tasks, responses are classified into one of a number of major categories and are tallied: correct responses, phonetic (dysarthric and dyspraxic) errors, phonological errors (phonemic paraphasias and neologisms), semantically related errors (semantic paraphasias and circumlocutions), unclassifiable errors, and failures to respond.

(iii) Test 12: PICTURE NAMING

This task tests the ability both to access the name of an object and to produce it orally. Thirty-two line drawings of objects are presented for naming. The objects are the foils in the auditory word–picture matching test described above. The names are all common nouns, which vary as to semantic category, length, and frequency, as described above in the word–picture matching test. Errors are classified as phonetic, phonological, semantic, unclassifiable, and nonresponses, and are tallied. If a patient does not respond, he or she is asked to give the first sound of the word and the number of syllables in the word, as evidence of having accessed some aspect of the word's phonological form.

2. *The Affixed Word Level*

The goal of this section of the battery is to see whether a patient can produce appropriate morphologically complex forms on the basis of conceptual representations.

(i) Test 13: AFFIXED WORD PRODUCTION

A sentence completion task using a prespecified lexical item tests a patient's ability to produce appropriate morphological forms (e.g., COURAGE: If a man has a great deal of courage, we say, he is __________). Derivational (both word- and formative-boundary) and inflectional affixes are tested. The root is presented first, and then the sentence. The patient must complete the sentence with a morphological variant of the root (e.g., *courageous* in the example above). Thirty items are used in the test. Responses are scored correct if the production of the root and suffix are identifiable and correct.

3. *The Sentence Level*

The goal of the tasks described in this section is to determine a subject's ability to use specific syntactic structures to convey two aspects of propositional meaning: thematic roles and attribution of modification. These goals require a highly constrained task (in the same way as the production of affixed words requires such a task).

(i) Test 14: SENTENCE PRODUCTION

Pictures depicting actions are presented. The patient is asked to describe what is going on in the picture, mentioning the items designated by arrows and using a single sentence (he or she is told specifically that the word *and* cannot be used). Five syntactic structures conveying thematic roles and attribution of modification are targeted: actives (*The boy pushes the girl*); datives (*The boy gives the rattle to the baby*); passives (*The boy is pushed by the girl*); dative passives (*The rattle was given to the baby by the woman*); and subject–object relatives (*The girl pushing a cart is opening the door*).

To constrain production to these targets, the patient is instructed to (1) mention all the items that are designated, (2) begin with an item indicated by a dot next to the arrow, and (3) use the verb(s) provided by the examiner. For instance, a picture depicting a truck pushing a car is presented, and the patient's task is to describe the picture, mentioning both the car and the truck and using the word *car* as the first noun and the verb *push*. These constraints induce the patient to use a passive form.

Scoring of responses attributes credit for (1) producing the correct lexical items, (2) assigning the correct thematic role to each lexical item, and (3) using the correct aspects of sentence structure. Thus, a simple active sentence (e.g., *The boy pushed the girl*) can produce a score of four points (the two nouns produced correctly, and the two thematic roles, agent and theme, assigned to each of them correctly), whereas a dative passive (e.g., *The rattle was given to the baby by the woman*) can produce a score of nine points (three nouns, three correct thematic roles, and three syntactic markers: the passive form, the preposition *by* and the preposition *to*).

IDENTIFICATION OF DEFICITS IN LANGUAGE PROCESSING COMPONENTS

The PAL provides a database that allows the examiner to assess the integrity of the major components of the language processing system. Patients who do significantly less well than normal age-matched subjects with similar educational and socioeconomic backgrounds on a subtest of the PAL can be assumed to have some problem that prevents them from accomplishing that subtest. The analysis of the results obtained with the PAL is directed toward ascertaining how the pattern of tests on which a patient does well and poorly can be understood in terms of the integrity and impairment of the major language processing components.

To undertake this analysis, the examiner must first determine that major nonlinguistic factors are not affecting performance. The patient must be paying attention, be making a serious effort on the task, and be able to accomplish the actions needed for a subtest of the battery. Observation of the patient in the clinical setting, as well as more formal neuropsychological evaluations (including language assessment tests that focus on these capacities, such as the PICA), can help rule out these types of disturbances as the basis for a patient's abnormal performance. In general, it is also likely that a patient who cannot accomplish a handful of tests on a battery such as the PAL, but performs normally on many others, has a specific problem with these tests, not, for example, a general problem with attention.

If the examiner is confident that major nonlinguistic factors are not affecting performance, the pattern of performance on a series of tests gives an indication of what language processing components are affected. The examiner can attribute a *primary* deficit in a particular processing component to a patient if (and only if) (1) performance on the test(s) that requires that component is abnormal, and (2) the linguistic input to that component is intact (as judged by performance on other subtests). Thus, for instance, the Auditory Lexical Access component may be considered to be the locus of a deficit if (and only if) (1) performance on the auditory lexical decision test is abnormal, and (2) performance on the phonemic discrimination test is normal. It is inappropriate to conclude that a patient has a *primary* deficit in recognizing words if he or she cannot discriminate phonemes. The examiner can make the diagnosis of a *secondary* deficit in a language processing component when both performance on the test(s) that requires that component and performance on the subtests that assess processing of linguistic structures needed for the operation of the deficit component are abnormal. For instance, the Auditory Lexical Access component can be considered to be the locus of a deficit that is *secondary* to a disturbance of acoustic–phonetic processing if (1) performance on the auditory lexical decision test is abnormal, and (2) performance on the phonemic discrimination test is also abnormal.

In general, a patient's performance must be compared across several subtests to come to a decision as to which component of the language processing system is impaired. In Tables 4.4 and 4.5, I present the basic pattern of performance on the subtests of the PAL battery that can be taken as evidence for a primary deficit in each of language processing components I have described. This approach to attributing deficits in specific language processing components to a patient must be qualified by the recognition that a patient may fail on a subtest because of a highly specific cognition disturbance that is external to the linguistic processing demands of that subtest but that does not show up clearly in other tasks. For instance, failure on the homophone matching test (Test 10) may be due to an inability to *compare* two phonological representations, not to a failure to *activate* them. The possibility that failure of a patient on a

TABLE 4.4. Deficits in Auditory Comprehension, Defined by Performances on the PAL Battery[a]

Deficient component	Pattern of performance on subtest
A. Word level	
1. Acoustic–phonetic processing	*Abnormal performance on the phonemic discrimination test*
2. Auditory lexical access	Normal performance on the phonemic discrimination test
	Abnormal performance on the lexical decision task with words
3. Lexical semantic access	Normal performance on the phonemic discrimination test
	Normal performance on the lexical decision task with words
	Abnormal performance on any lexical comprehension test
B. Affixed word level	
1. Morphological analysis	Normal lexical access
	Abnormal performance on lexical decision for affixed words
2. Morphological comprehension	Intact single-word input processing
	Normal lexical decision for affixed words
	Abnormal performance on any test of affixed word comprehension
C. Sentence level	
1. Lexico-inferential comprehension	Normal lexical semantic access and morphological comprehension
	Abnormal performance on constrained sentence comprehension
2. Parsing and syntactic comprehension	Normal lexical semantic comprehension
	Normal lexical semantic access and morphological comprehension
	Normal performance on constrained sentence comprehension
	Abnormal performance on semantically unconstrained syntactically complex sentence comprehension

[a]Subtests on which the patient must perform normally are indicated in plain type. Subtests on which abnormal performance is criterial for the assignment of a particular deficit are in italics.

TABLE 4.5. Deficits in Oral Production, Defined by Performances on the PAL Battery[a]

Deficient component	Pattern of performance on subtest
A. Word level	
1. Accessing lexical phonological forms (from semantics)	Normal performance on picture comprehension screen *Abnormal performance on naming task* *Abnormal performance on homophone judgment task*
2. Phonological output planning	Normal performance on picture comprehension screen, homophone judgment, phonemic discrimination, auditory and written lexical decision *Phonemic paraphasias in naming, repetition, and oral reading tasks*
B. Affixed word level	
1. Accessing affixed words (from semantics)	Naming and repetition adequate for the patient's oral production of words to be recognized
C. Sentence level	
1. Expression of thematic roles	Normal word production in isolation Normal performance on affixed word production *Failure to produce word sequences that convey correct thematic roles on sentence production task*
2. Construction of syntactic structures	Normal word production in isolation Normal performance on affixed word production *Failure to produce complex structures (e.g., passives) on sentence production task*
3. Insertion of function words into syntactic structures	Normal word production in isolation Normal performance on affixed word production *Agrammatism and/or paragrammatism on sentence production task*
4. Insertion of content words into syntactic structures	Normal word production in isolation Normal performance on affixed word production *Anomia and/or phonemic paraphasias in content words on sentence production task*

[a]Subtests on which the patient must perform normally are indicated in plain type. Subtests on which abnormal performance is criterial for the assignment of a particular deficit are in italics.

subtest is due to these types of cognitive factors can be addressed in several ways. First, careful observation of each patient during testing can identify factors such as fatigue that can arise at one point in testing and thus lead to impaired performance on a given subtest. Second, comparisons across tests can serve to rule out several reasons for failure. For instance, a patient who fails on the lexical decision test for affixed words but performs well on the lexical decision test for simple words cannot have a general problem with nonlinguistic aspects of lexical decision tests (such as making decisions). As indicated in Tables 4.4 and 4.5, comparison across tests can also provide converging evidence regarding the deficit underlying poor performance on selected tests. For instance, in the example of homophone matching given above, a patient's performance on the tests of picture naming and word and nonword repetition can provide converging evidence regarding his or her ability to access phonology from semantics. An inability to produce words coupled with an intact ability to repeat them would be consistent with an inability to access phonology from semantics, also suggested by failure on homophone matching. Third, a patient's performance on these language tests can be compared with performance on other neuropsychological tests. This should serve to help decide whether some abnormal performances are due to extralinguistic factors, such as difficulty making comparisons or decisions.

CASE EXAMPLE OF DEFICIT ANALYSIS USING THE PAL

I shall illustrate the use of the PAL by briefly describing the performance of one patient, R.W., with respect to single-word processing.

R.W. was a 62-year-old, right-handed male who had a small stroke in May 1991. Magnetic resonance imaging revealed a small left temporo-parietal infarction. R.W. was a college graduate and had previously worked as an executive for a research corporation.

R.W. was tested on parts of the BDAE in June and again in August 1991. His output was described as fluent. He was considered to have mild-to-moderate impairments in auditory comprehension, which improved somewhat over that period of time. Written sentence comprehension was considered to be better than auditory sentence comprehension. Repetition was severely impaired at the word and sentence levels.

R.W. was tested on the BNT on several occasions. On June 24, 1991, he scored only 22/60; his errors consisted of phonemic errors, false starts, and occasional omissions. The BNT was repeated on July 25, 1991, and August 8, 1991, and R.W. scored 47/60 and 46/60, respectively.

R.W.'s performance on the single-word subtests of the PAL about 2 months after this event is summarized in Table 4.6.

TABLE 4.6. Performance of Patient R.W. on Selected Tests of Single-Word Processing of the PAL

Test	Score
I. Auditory comprehension	
Phoneme discrimination	35/40
Auditory lexical decision	73/80
Single-word auditory comprehension	
Word–picture matching	29/32
II. Oral production	
Picture homophone matching	20/20
Word and nonword repetition	2/40
Word and nonword reading	21/32 (words)
Picture naming	14/32
III. Written comprehension	
Written lexical decision	40/40
Single-word written comprehension	
Word–picture matching	32/32

At the level of input-side processing of auditorily presented single words, R.W. showed somewhat impaired performance on the test of phoneme discrimination (19/20 correct "same" and 14/20 correct "different" judgments). However his performances on auditory lexical decision (39/40 "yes" and 34/40 "no" responses correct) and auditory word–picture matching (29/32 correct selections) indicate that he nonetheless recognizes and comprehends auditorily presented words well. He was perfect at written lexical decision (40/40 items) and written word–picture matching (32/32 items), and answered 44/48 forced-choice questions about written words on the PAL. This indicates that he recognizes and comprehends written words normally.

R.W.'s output-side processing at the single-word level was abnormal. He made many errors in repetition, reading, and picture naming. He repeated only 2/20 words and 0/20 nonwords correctly. He read 21/32 words correctly, and there were no effects of frequency, length, or imageability, and a mild effect of regularity (13/16 regular words versus 8/16 irregular words) on his reading aloud performance. He named 14/32 pictures correctly. His errors on these three tasks were exclusively phonological, and consisted of misselection and misordering of phonemes and occasional syllable deletion and addition. There was no evidence of any misarticulation in his speech. R.W. performed perfectly on the picture homophone matching test, indicating that he was able to access many aspects of a word's form that he could not accurately produce.

These data on word production help to identify the locus of the functional disturbance in this patient. R.W. appears able to access the forms of words in the Output Phonological Lexicon, but is unable to utter these forms correctly. The difficulty he experiences does not appear to be one in which articulatory gestures are themselves abnormal, as in dysarthric or apraxic patients. Rather, it involves the selection and ordering of the phonemes in the words he produces. The location of this deficit is indicated in Figure 4.3.

Several features of the examination outlined above that are not found on standard aphasia examinations are crucial in establishing this deficit. These include the use of nonword stimuli in repetition and tests of reading aloud to establish the presence of an impairment in planning phonological representations, and the use of the picture hom-

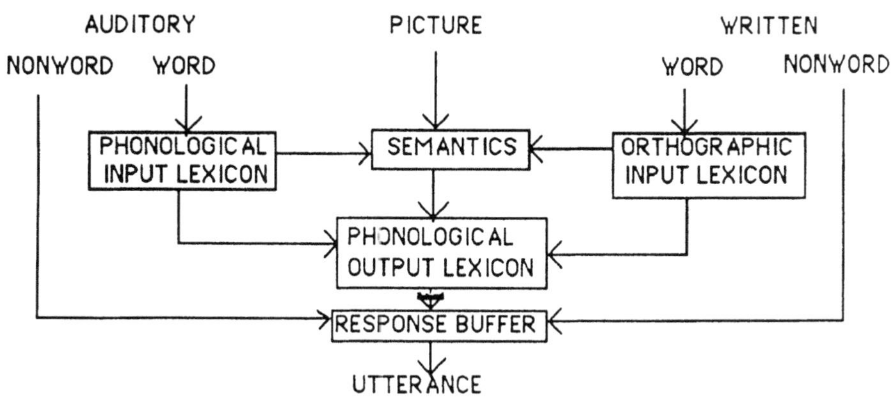

FIGURE 4.3. A model of the functional architecture of the word processing system showing the location of the deficit in case R.W.

ophone matching test to establish the ability to activate the lexical phonological representations of words. The use of phoneme discrimination tasks allows us to explain the increased difficulty the patient had with repetition compared to reading aloud. In addition to the use of these tests, this case analysis indicates the need to think about performances on specific tests in relationship to models of psycholinguistic processing.

This analysis of the deficit in R.W. also has implications for the nature of the word production process. First, it suggests that the process of accessing the representation of the sound pattern of a word in the Output Phonological Lexicon is at least partially separate from using that representation to plan articulatory gestures associated with producing that word. Several everyday observations indicate that a speaker must access a representation of the sound pattern of a word that is modified before it is actually articulated. Words can be uttered with varying intonation, at different loudness levels, in whispered form, and in many other ways that require very different articulatory gestures. It is unlikely that all of these articulatory forms are permanently stored for each word in a speaker's vocabulary; it is much more likely that a speaker accesses a standard form of a word, which is then modified as a function of speech characteristics. The minimal phonological information that must be lexically specified is that which allows the speaker to assign the spoken forms of each of the segments in the word in any discourse context. R.W.'s performances do not indicate what the nature of lexical phonological representations are, but the pattern does suggest that these representations are acted on by additional phonological planning processes before articulatory gestures are specified.

Second, these data suggest that the processes of reading aloud, repeating, and naming a picture all involve similar stages of speech production. Though there are differences in R.W.'s performances across these tasks, they can be explained by his other deficits and are outweighed by the similarities across tasks. The most striking task difference is that R.W. is worse at repetition than at either naming or reading aloud. This is most likely due to his mild impairment in phoneme discrimination. His errors on the three tasks are all similar in nature.

This case study illustrates the potential use of a psycholinguistically oriented battery such as the PAL. First, it has been possible to show that the errors R.W. made do not arise in input-side processing. Second, it has been possible to show that R.W. accesses phonological form from both input orthography and semantics. Third, it has been possible to show that R.W. retains the ability to access word forms in output tasks, and has trouble using these forms to select articulatory gestures. This degree of specificity in the analysis of a deficit is possible only with a battery such as the PAL.

Acknowledgments

This work was supported by a grant from the National Institute for Neurological Disease and Stroke (NS29101). I would like to thank the editors of this volume for their helpful comments on an earlier version of this chapter.

REFERENCES

Albert, M. L., & Bear, D. (1974). Time to understand: A case study of word deafness with reference to the role of time in auditory comprehension. *Brain, 97,* 373–384.

Anderson, S. R. (1982). Where's morphology? *Linguistic Inquiry, 13,* 571–612.

Auerbach, S. H., Allard, T., Naeser, M., Alexander, M. P., & Albert, M. L. (1982). Pure word deafness: Analysis of a case with bilateral lesions and a defect at the pre-phonemic level. *Brain, 105,* 271–300.

Badecker, W., & Caramazza, A. (1987). The analysis of morphological errors in a case of acquired dyslexia. *Brain and Language, 32,* 278–305.

Badecker, W., & Caramazza, A. (in press). Morphological composition in the lexical output system. *Cognitive Neuropsychology.*

Basso, A., Casati, G., & Vignolo, L. A. (1977). Phonemic identification defect in aphasia. *Cortex, 13,* 85–95.

Beauvois, M.-F. (1982). Optic aphasia: A process of interaction between vision and language. *Philosophical Transactions of the Royal Society of London B, 298,* 35–47.

Beauvois, M.-F., Saillant, B., Meininger, V., & Lhermitte, F. (1978). Bilateral tactile aphasia: A tactoverbal dysfunction. *Brain, 101,* 381–401.

Berndt, R. S., & Mitchum, C. C. (1990). Auditory and lexical information sources in immediate recall: Evidence from a patient with a deficit to the phonological short-term store. In G. Vallar & T. Shallice (Eds.), *Neuropsychological impairments of short-term memory* (pp. 115–144). Cambridge: Cambridge University Press.

Blumstein, S., Alexander, M. P., Ryalls, J. H., Katz, W., & Dworetzky, B. (1987). On the nature of the foreign accent syndrome: A case study. *Brain and Language, 31,* 215–244.

Blumstein, S. E., Baker, E., & Goodglass, H. (1977). Phonological factors in auditory comprehension in aphasia. *Neuropsychologia, 15,* 19–30.

Blumstein, S., Cooper, W. E., Zurif, E. B., & Caramazza, A. (1977). The perception and production of voice-onset time in aphasia. *Neuropsychologia, 15,* 371–383.

Bowman, C. A., Hodson, B. W., & Simpson, R. K. (1980). Oral apraxia and aphasic misarticulation. In R. H. Brookshire (Ed.), *Clinical aphasiology.* Minneapolis: B.R.K. Publishers.

Bub, D., Black, S., Hampson, E., & Kertesz, A. (1988). Semantic encoding of pictures and words: Some neuropsychological observations. *Cognitive Neuropsychology, 5,* 27–66.

Bub, D., Black, S., Howell, J., & Kertesz, A. (1987). Speech output processes and reading. In M. Coltheart, G. Sartori, & R. Job (Eds.), *The cognitive neuropsychology of language* (pp. 79–110). London: Lawrence Erlbaum.

Buckingham, H. W. (1979). Linguistic aspects of lexical retrieval disturbances in the posterior fluent aphasias. in H. Whitaker & H. Whitaker (Eds.), *Studies in neurolinguistics* (Vol. 4). New York: Academic Press.

Buckingham, H. W., & Kertesz, A. (1976). *Neologistic jargon aphasia.* Amsterdam: Swets & Zeitlinger.

Butterworth, B. (1982). Speech errors: Old data in search of new theories. In A. Cutler (Ed.), *Slips of the tongue in language production* (pp. 73–108). The Hague: Mouton.

Butterworth, B. L. (1985). Jargon aphasia: Processes and strategies. In S. Newman & R. Epstein (Eds.), *Current perspectives in dysphasia.* Edinburgh: Churchill Livingstone.

Butterworth, B., Campbell, R., & Howard, D. (1986). The uses of short-term memory: A case study. *Quarterly Journal of Experimental Psychology, 38,* 705–737.

Butterworth, B., & Howard D. (1987). Paragrammatisms. *Cognition, 26,* 1–38.

Caplan, D. (1986). In defense of agrammatism. *Cognition, 24,* 263–276.

Caplan, D., Baker, C., & Dehaut, F. (1985). Syntactic determinants of sentence comprehension in aphasia. *Cognition, 21,* 117–175.

Caplan, D., & Hilderbrandt, N. (1988). *Disorders of syntactic comprehension.* Cambridge, MA: Bradford Books.

Caplan, D., Kellar, L., & Locke, S. (1972). Inflection of neologisms in aphasia. *Brain, 95,* 169–172.

Caplan, D., Vanier, M., & Baker, C. (1986). A case study of reproduction conduction aphasia: I. Word production. *Cognitive Neuropsychology, 3*(1), 99–128.

Caplan, D., & Waters, G. S. (1990). Short-term memory and language comprehension: A critical review of the neuropsychological literature. In G. Vallar & T. Shallice (Eds.), *Neuropsychological impairments of short-term memory* (pp. 337–389). Cambridge: Cambridge University Press.

Caramazza, A., Berndt, R. S., & Basili, A. G. (1983). The selective impairment of phonological processing: A case study. *Brain and Language, 18,* 128–174.

Caramazza, A., Miceli, G., & Villa, G. (1986). The role of the (output) phonological buffer in reading, writing and repetition. *Cognitive Neuropsychology, 3,* 37–76.

Chomsky, N. (1965). *Aspects of the theory of syntax.* Cambridge, MA: MIT Press.

Chomsky, N. (1981). *Lectures on government and binding.* Dordrecht: Foris.

Chomsky, N. (1986). *Knowledge of language.* New York: Praeger.

Coltheart, M., Patterson, J., & Marshall, J. C. (1980). *Deep dyslexia.* London: Routledge & Kegan Paul.

Danly, M., Cooper, W., & Shapiro, B. (1983). Fundamental frequency, language processing, and linguistic structure in Wernicke's aphasia. *Brain and Language, 19,* 1–24.

Danly, M., & Shapiro, B. (1982). Speech prosody in Broca's aphasia. *Brain and Language, 16,* 171–190.

Darley, F. L. (1983). Foreword. In W. R. Berry (Ed.), *Clinical dysarthria.* San Diego: College Hill Press.

Denes, G., & Semenza, C. (1975). Auditory modality-specific anomia: Evidence from a case of pure word deafness. *Cortex, 11,* 401–411.

De Renzi, E., & Vignolo, L. A. (1962). The Token Test: A sensitive test to detect receptive disturbances in aphasics. *Brain, 85,* 665–678.

Dunn, L. M. (1965). *Expanded manual for the Peabody Picture Vocabulary Test.* Circle Pines, MN: American Guidance Service.

Ellis, A., Miller, D., & Sin, G. (1983). Wernicke's aphasia and normal language processing: A case study in cognitive neuropsychology. *Cognition, 15,* 111–144.

Fodor, J. A. (1983). *The modularity of mind.* Cambridge, MA: MIT Press.

Funnell, E. (1983). *Ideographic communication and word class effects in aphasia.* Unpubiished doctoral dissertation, University of Reading, England.

Garrett, M. F. (1982). Production of speech: Observations from normal and pathological language use. In A. W. Ellis (Ed.), *Normality and pathology in cognitive functions* (pp. 19–75). London: Academic Press.

Goodglass, H., & Geschwind, N. (1976). Language disorders (aphasia). In E. C. Carterette & M. Friedman (Eds.), *Handbook of perception.* New York: Academic Press.

Goodglass, H., Gleason, J. B., & Hyde, M. R. (1970). Some dimensions of auditory language comprehension in aphasia. *Journal of Speech and Hearing Research, 13,* 595–606.

Goodglass, H., & Kaplan, E. (1972). Boston Diagnostic Aphasia Examination booklet. *The assessment of aphasia and related disorders* (80 pages). Philadelphia: Lea & Febiger.

Goodglass, H., & Kaplan, E. (1983). *The assessment of aphasia and related disorders (2nd ed.).* Philadelphia: Lea & Febiger.

Goodglass, H., & Menn, L. (1985). Is agrammatism a unitary phenomenon? In M. L. Kean (Ed.), *Agrammatism* (pp. 1–26). London: Academic Press.

Grodzinsky, Y. (1984). The syntactic characterization of agrammatism. *Cognition, 16,* 99–120.

Grosz, B. J., Pollack, M. E., & Sidner, C. L. (1989). Discourse. In M. Posner (Ed.), *Foundations of cognitive science* (pp. 437–468). Cambridge, MA: MIT Press.

Halle, M., & Vergnaud, J.-R. (1987). *An essay on stress.* Cambridge, MA: MIT Press.

Heeschen, C. (1985). Agrammatism vs. paragrammatism: A fictitious opposition. In M.-L. Kean (Ed.), *Agrammatism* (pp. 207–248). London: Academic Press.

Henderson, L. (1982). *Orthography and word recognition in reading.* London: Academic Press.

Hillis, A., Rapp, B., Romani, C., & Caramazza, A. (1990). Selective impairment of semantics in lexical processing. *Cognitive Neuropsychology, 7,* 191–243.

Howard, D., & Orchard-Lisle, V. (1984). On the origin of semantic errors in naming: Evidence from the case of a global aphasic. *Cognitive Neuropsychology, 1*, 163–190.
Itoh, S., Sasanuma, S., & Hirose, H. (1980). Abnormal articulatory dynamics in a patient with apraxia of speech: X-ray microbeam observation. *Brain and Language, 11*, 66–75.
Itoh, M. Sasanuma, S., Tatsumi, I. F., Murakami, S., Fukusako, Y., & Suzuki, T. (1982). Voice onset time characteristics in apraxia of speech. *Brain and Language, 17*, 193–210.
Joanette, Y., Keller, E., & Lecours, A.-R (1980). Sequence of phonemic approximations in aphasia. *Brain and Language, 11*, 30–44.
Job, R., & Sartori, G. (1984). Morphological decomposition: Evidence from crossed phonological dyslexia. *Quarterly Journal of Experimental Psychology, 36A*, 435–458.
Kaplan, E., Goodglass, H., & Weintraub, S. (1983). *The Boston Naming Test*. Philadelphia: Lea and Febiger.
Kean, M.-L. (1977). The linguistic interpretation of aphasic syndromes: Agrammatism in Broca's aphasia, an example. *Cognition, 5*, 9–46.
Kent, R., & Rosenbek, J. (1982). Prosodic disturbance and neurological lesion. *Brain and Language, 15*, 259–291.
Kertesz, A. (1979). *Aphasia and associated disorders: Taxonomy, localization and recovery*. New York: Grune & Stratton.
Kertesz, A., & Poole, E. (1974). The aphasia quotient: The taxonomic approach to measurement of aphasic disability. *Canadian Journal of Neurological Sciences, 1*, 7–16.
Kohn, S. E. (1984). The nature of the phonological disorder in conduction aphasia. *Brain and Language, 23*, 97–115.
Kohn, S. (1989). The nature of the phonemic string deficit in conduction aphasia. *Aphasiology, 3*(3), 209–239.
Lapointe, S. (1983). Some issues in the linguistic description of agrammatism. *Cognition, 14*, 1–39.
Lecours, A. R., & Lhermitte, F. (1969). Phonemic paraphasias: Linguistic structures and tentative hypotheses. *Cortex, 5*, 193–228.
Lecours, A. R., & Rouillon, F. (1976). Neurolinguistic analysis of jargon aphasia and jargon agraphia. In H. Whitaker & H. Whitaker (Eds.) *Studies in neurolinguistics* (Vol. 2). New York: Academic Press.
Levelt, W. J. M. (1989). *Speaking: From intention to articulation*. Cambridge, MA: MIT Press.
Lhermitte, F., & Beauvois, M.-F. (1973). A visual-speech disconnexion syndrome: Report of a case with optic-aphasia, agnosic alexia and colour agnosia. *Brain, 96*, 695–714.
Luria, A. R. (1973). *The working brain*. New York: Basic Books.
Marshall, J. C. (1987). Routes and representations in the processing of written language. In E. Keller & M. Gopnik (Eds.), *Motor and sensory processes of language* (pp. 237–256). Hillsdale, NJ: Lawrence Erlbaum.
Marslen-Wilson, W. D. (1987). Functional parallelism in spoken word-recognition. *Cognition, 25*, 71–102.
Marslen-Wilson, W. D., & Welsh, A. (1978). Processing interactions and lexical access during word recognition in continuous speech. *Cognitive Psychology, 10*, 29–63.
McCarthy, R. A., & Warrington, E. K. (1984). A two-route model of speech productcion: Evidence from aphasia. *Brain, 107*, 463–485.
McCarthy, R., & Warrington, E. K. (1985) Category specificity in an agrammatic patient: The relative impairment of verb retrieval and comprehension. *Neuropsychologia, 23*, 709–727.
McCarthy, R., & Warrington, E. K. (1987). Understanding: A function of short-term memory? *Brain, 110*, 1565–1578.
Menn, L., Obler, L., & Goodglass, H. (1990). *A cross-language study of agrammatism*. Philadelphia: John Benjamins.
Micelli, G., & Caramazza, A. (1988). Dissociation of inflectional and derivational morphology. *Brain and Language, 35*, 24–65.
Miceli, G., Gainotti, G., Caltagirone, C., & Masullo, C. (1980). Some aspects of phonological impairment in aphasia. *Brain and Language, 11*, 159–169.

Miceli, G., Silveri, M. C., Romani, C., & Caramazza, A. (1989). Variation in the pattern of omissions and substitutions of grammatical morphemes in the spontaneous speech of so-called agrammatic patients. *Brain and Language, 36*, 447–492.

Miceli, G., Silveri, M., Villa, G., & Caramazza, A. (1984). On the basis for the agrammatic's difficulty in producing main verbs. *Cortex, 20*, 207–220.

Miller, D., & Ellis, A. W. (1987). Speech and writing errors in "neologistic jargonaphasia": A lexical activation hypothesis. In M. Coltheart, G. Sartori, & R. Job (Eds.), *The cognitive neuropsychology of language*. London: Lawrence Erlbaum.

Monrad Krohn, G. H. (1947). Prosody or altered "melody of language." *Brain, 70*, 405–423.

Morton, J. (1980). Two auditory parallels to deep dyslexia. In M. Coltheart, K. Patterson, & J. C. Marshall (Eds.), *Deep dyslexia* (pp. 189–197). London: Routledge & Kegan Paul.

Nespoulous, J. L., Joanette, Y., Beland, R., Caplan, D., & Lecours, A. R. (1984). Phonological disturbances in aphasia: Is there a "markedness" effect in aphasic phonemic errors? In F. C. Rose (Ed.), *Progress in aphasiology: Advances in neurology*. New York: Raven Press.

Ostrin, R., & Schwartz, M. F. (1986). Reconstructing from a degraded trace: A study of sentence repetition in agrammatism. *Brain and Language, 28*, 328–345.

Ostrin, R. K., Schwartz, M. F., & Saffrin, E. M. (1983). *The influence of syntactic complexity in the elicited production of agrammatic aphasics*. Paper presented at the Annual Meeting of the Academy of Aphasia, Minneapolis, MN.

Pate, D. S., Saffran, E. M., & Martin, N. (1987). Specifying the nature of the production impairment in a conduction aphasic: A case study. *Language and Cognitive Processes, 2*(1), 43–84.

Patterson, K. E. (1980). Derivational errors. In M. Coltheart, K. E. Patterson, & J. C. Marshall (Eds.), *Deep dyslexia* (pp. 286–306). London: Routledge & Kegan Paul.

Porch, B. E. (1971). *The Porch Index of Communicative Ability: Administration, scoring and interpretation*. Palo Alto, CA: Consulting Psychologists Press.

Ross, E., & Mesulam, M. (1979). Dominant language functions of the right hemisphere? Prosody and emotional gesturing. *Archives of Neurology, 36*, 144–148.

Ryalls, J. H. (1982). Note. Intonation in Broca's aphasia. *Neuropsychologia, 20*(3), 355–360.

Saffran, E. M., Marin, O., & Yeni-Komshian, G. (1976). An analysis of speech perception and word deafness. *Brain and Language, 3*, 209–228.

Saffran, E. M., Schwartz, M. F., & Marin, O. (1980). The word order problem in agrammatism II: Production. *Brain and Language, 10*, 263–280.

Sartori, G., & Job, R. (1988). The oyster with four legs: A neuropsychological study on the interaction of visual and semantic information. *Cognitive Neuropsychology, 5*, 105–132.

Schonle, T. W., Grabe, K., Wenig, P., Hohne, J., Schrader, J., & Conrad, B. (1987). Electromagnetic articulography: Use of alternating magnetic fields for tracking movements of multiple points inside and outside the vocal tract. *Brain and Language, 31*, 26–35.

Schwartz, M. F., Marin, O. S. M., & Saffran, E. M. (1979). Dissociations of language function in dementia: A case study. *Brain and Langauge, 7*, 277–306.

Schwartz, M., Saffran, E., & Marin, O. (1980). The word order problem in agrammatism I: Comprehension. *Brain and Language, 10*, 249–262.

Shapiro, B., & Danly, M. (1985). The role of the right hemisphere in the control of speech prosody in propositional and effective context. *Brain and Language, 25*, 19–36.

Silveri, M. C., & Gainotti, G. B. (1988). Interaction between vision and language in category specific semantic impairment for living things. *Cognitive Neuropsychology, 5*, 677–709.

Tulving, E. (1972). Episodic and semantic memory. In E. T. A. W. Donaldson (Ed.), *Organization of memory* (pp. 381–403). New York: Academic Press.

Tyler, L. K., & Cobb, H. (1987). Processing bound grammatical morphemes in context: The case of an aphasic patient. *Language and Cognitive Processes, 2*(3/4), 245–262.

Tyler, L., & Wessels, J. (1983). Quantifying contextual contributions to word-recognition processes. *Perception and Psychophysics, 34*, 409–420.

Warrington, E. K. (1975). The selective impairment of semantic memory. *Quarterly Journal of Experimental Psychology, 27*, 635–657.

Warrington, E. K. (1981). Neuropsychological studies of verbal semantic systems. *Philosophical Transactions of the Royal Society of London, B295*, 411–423.

Warrington, E. K., & McCarthy, R. (1983). Category specific access dysphasia. *Brain, 106*, 859–878.

Warrington, E. K., & McCarthy, R. (1987). Categories of knowledge: Further fractionation and an attempted integration. *Brain, 110*, 1273–1296.

Warrington, E. K., & Shallice, T. (1984). Category specific semantic impairments. *Brain, 107*, 829–853.

Waters, G. S., Caplan, D., & Hilderbrandt, N. (1991). On the structure of verbal short-term memory and its functional role in sentence comprehension: Evidence from neuropsychology. *Cognitive Neuropsychology, 8*, 81–126.

Wepman, J. M. (1958). *Auditory Discrimination Test.* Chicago, IL: Language Research Associates.

Wernicke, C. (1974). The aphasic symptom complex: A psychological study on a neurological basis. *Boston Studies in the Philosophy of Science, 4*, 34–97.

Williams, E. (1981). X features. In S. Tavakolian (Ed.), *Language acquisition and linguistic theory.* Cambridge, MA: MIT Press.

Zingeser, L. B., & Berndt, R. S. (1988). Grammatical class and context effects in a case of pure anomia: Implications for models of lexical processing. *Cognitive Neuropsychology, 4*, 473–516.

5

A Cognitive Neuropsychological Framework for Assessing Reading Disorders

GUILA GLOSSER and RHONDA B. FRIEDMAN

Reading is a learned skill that engages a complex set of cognitive procedures. By virtue of its complexity, it is vulnerable to disruption with many different kinds of brain damage. Reading impairment is characteristic of almost all patients with acquired aphasia (Goodglass & Kaplan, 1983), and reading disorders persist chronically in the overwhelming majority of these aphasic patients (Webb & Love, 1983). Detailed assessment of the pattern of acquired reading disturbance, or alexia, can be informative about the underlying neural dysfunction as well as the integrity of various component cognitive neuropsychological processes. Since reading is fundamentally a linguistic activity and is based on prior mastery of auditory language skills, it is possible to learn about the integrity and function of various components of the language processing system through careful analysis of reading performance. Reading also depends on visual processing. Visual letter and word identification pose many of the same problems as other types of patterns for the visual recognition system, so that the functions of certain visual processing mechanisms may also be revealed in the analysis of reading performance. Reading competence is a prerequisite for many adult functional activities; hence, comprehensive assessment of reading capabilities is important for predicting functional living skills.

We begin this chapter with an overview of the reading process as it is conceived currently within the field of cognitive neuropsychology. Figure 5.1 presents a generic model containing certain basic assumptions common to most current theories of the

GUILA GLOSSER • Department of Neurology, The Graduate Hospital, Philadelphia, Pennsylvania 19146. RHONDA B. FRIEDMAN • Department of Neurology, Georgetown University Medical Center, Washington, DC 20007.

Clinical Neuropsychological Assessment: A Cognitive Approach, edited by Robert L. Mapou and Jack Spector. Plenum Press, New York, 1995.

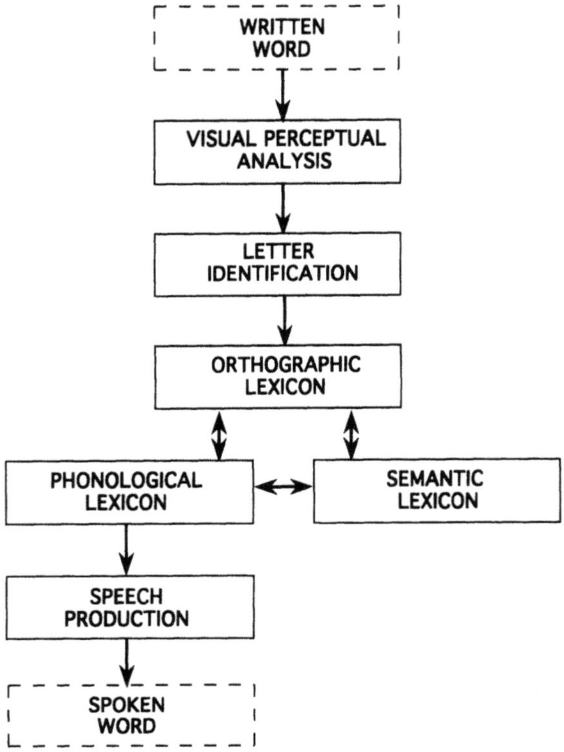

FIGURE 5.1. A generic model of the cognitive components entailed in single-word reading.

normal processes of single-word reading. Following review of this model, we show how this framework can be used to guide the systematic assessment of reading in brain-damaged adults. Finally, we illustrate the usefulness of this approach in the clinical diagnosis and treatment of alexia.

A MODEL OF NORMAL READING PROCESSES

The initial stage of reading involves *perceptual analysis* of the visual stimulus. This entails analysis of the physical characteristics of the written word such as its length and its location in space, especially in relation to other words. It leads to identifying individual letters of the written word and encoding the serial position and relative ordering of the letters in the word. *Letter identification* refers to coding the physical shapes of the letters into more abstract letter identities. All versions of a given letter (uppercase, lowercase, large, small, printed, and cursive) are coded identically (Coltheart, 1981; McClelland, 1976). Under normal circumstances, in the literate adult, this identification process occurs rapidly, automatically, and in parallel for all letters in a presented word (LaBerge & Samuels, 1974), as evidenced by the fact that in competent readers processing speed is unaffected by word length (Shiepers, 1980).

There is also an alternate visual analysis procedure, in which the letters are identified one by one, presumably in left-to-right order. This nonautomatic, serial processing strategy may be used by young children when learning to read. While it remains available to the practiced adult reader, it is not usually engaged.

Following visual perceptual analysis and letter identification, processing in reading proceeds to the *lexicons,* which consist of the stored memories of the *orthographic, phonological,* and *semantic* properties of all the words encountered previously by the individual. The orthographic lexicon is specific for processing *written* or orally spelled words, while the phonological and semantic lexicons are conceived to be modality-independent representations of lexical knowledge that are engaged in all types of oral and written language tasks.

The composite abstract letter strings generated by the letter identification process are first matched to representations of all previously encountered letter strings contained in the *orthographic lexicon.* These orthographic patterns are *not* visual templates of the overall shapes of words, but rather they are abstract representations of the orthographic composition of words (i.e., what letters each word contains and in what order). The same orthographic pattern would be accessed if the written word was presented in lowercase, uppercase, mixed case, or script writing. If the letter string activates an existing orthographic representation in memory, then the word is recognized as being familiar, part of the individual's sight reading vocabulary.

From activation of the orthographic system, processing proceeds in two directions. One path leads to activation of the codes in the *phonological lexicon,* which specify the pronunciations of letter strings. In many models of reading (Glushko, 1979; Kay & Marcel, 1981; Seidenberg & McClelland, 1989), including the one adopted here, all pronounceable letter strings, both words and nonwords, are read using the same lexical phonological mechanism.[1] When a word is viewed, orthographic units corresponding to that word, plus (to a lesser extent) orthographically similar words, are activated. For example, viewing the word *cake* would result in activation of orthographic units that are shared by words like *lake, cape,* and *coke.* Only the word *cake* corresponds to all of the activated orthographic units. Thus, under normal circumstances the word *cake* receives maximal activation in the phonological lexicon.

Likewise, pseudowords activate orthographically similar real-word patterns. For example, presentation of the pseudoword *tace,* activates orthographic units consistent with words such as *take, lace,* and *ace.* These orthographic units, in turn, activate corresponding phonological units. The combined units do not correspond exactly with

[1]An alternate account of pseudoword reading maintains that there exists a nonlexical phonological reading route consisting of a specialized set of procedures for converting orthographic units (graphemes) into sounds (phonemes). The conversion procedures are assumed to depend on a system of "rules." These spelling-to-sound correspondence rules indicate which sounds are appropriate for which letter(s) (Venezky, 1970). The nonlexical phonological reading route is considered to be specialized for the processing of legally spelled pronounceable pseudowords (and under certain circumstances it may also support reading of real words). For a more complete discussion of this postulated reading mechanism and its role in certain alexic disorders, the reader is referred to Morton and Patterson (1980). Humphreys and Evett (1985) provide a comprehensive review of the controversy regarding the posited existence of the "third" nonlexical phonological reading route.

any real word. Rather, the pattern of activated phonological units specifies a novel pronunciation that is a pseudoword.

Once a word's pronunciation is determined, it may be pronounced directly if the task is oral reading. The phonological code also may be used to activate the word's meaning in the semantic lexicon, just as it does when one listens to spoken language.

In the second reading pathway, the orthographic pattern activates the word's meaning directly. When pronunciation of the written word is not required (silent reading), its meaning can be accessed through the *semantic lexicon* without necessarily activating phonological representations. The notion that a semantic code can be activated without phonological mediation is supported by the observation that we can readily distinguish the meanings of homophones such as *son* and *sun* (Barron & Baron, 1977). There is a bidirectional flow of information between the semantic and phonological lexicons, so that once the semantic code is retrieved, it can also activate the phonological code, as occurs when we name a picture.

One final component that needs to be considered in charting the procedures necessary for *oral* reading is a mechanism for speech production. Once a composite phonological code for the written words has been assembled or accessed in the lexicon, it must be programmed for actual speech output. All tasks requiring an articulatory response—naming, repetition, and oral reading—rely on the same output mechanisms.

DISTURBED READING PROCESSES IN THE ALEXIAS

Using the model just described, we turn now to a discussion of the ways that reading has been observed to break down in brain-damaged adults. In each case, we relate observed alexic symptoms to disruption of, or impaired access to, one or more processing mechanisms contained within the presented model of reading processes.

Disturbances in Visual Perceptual Analysis

The most common type of perceptual disturbance results in *neglect alexia* (Kinsbourne & Warrington, 1962), which consists of failure to identify letters at one end of the word. In neglect alexia, as in other forms of visual neglect, the inattention is most often to elements in left visual space, that is, the leftmost letters in words. When patients with left neglect alexia are asked to read written words presented vertically, neglect is not seen (Behrmann, Black, & Bub, 1990). When words are presented in a manner such that the beginning of the word appears on the right and the end is on the left, neglect again appears on the left; the end of the word is now misread (Ellis, Flude, & Young, 1987). Such neglect errors in reading occur irrespective of hemianopic defects (i.e., blindness in one visual field). The majority of errors in left neglect alexia involve substitutions of letters at the beginning of words, so that the overall length of the word is usually preserved (Ellis et al., 1987). Also, it has been found that the severity of neglect depends on the lexical status of the presented letter string, so that fewer neglect errors are produced for reading real words as compared to nonwords (Sieroff, Pollatsek, & Posner, 1988). Failure to process the leftmost portions of words, therefore, cannot be attributed to complete absence of elementary sensory information that should affect all types of visual stimuli equally; rather, neglect alexia appears to reflect variable allocation of attention in extrapersonal space.

Another, much less common form of disrupted visual perceptual analysis results in *attentional alexia* (Shallice & Warrington, 1977). Recall that during the initial perceptual analysis of the written stimulus, individual words are segregated from neighborhood words on the page. If this process is not successful, letters from adjacent words might "migrate" and result in letter intrusions. Attentional alexia is manifested as a disturbance in reading multiword displays, while single-word reading remains intact. The underlying problem that causes this disorder is thought to be a deficit in selective attention (Shallice & Warrington, 1977).

Disturbance in Accessing Orthographic Representations

Letter-by-letter reading, also called "alexia without agraphia," is the reading disorder seen when orthographic representations remain intact but cannot be accessed normally from the printed word. Although letter-by-letter readers have great difficulties recognizing written words, they decode orally spelled words normally. Such patients also show a pronounced effect of word length in reading; words with more letters are read more slowly and less reliably than short words. It has been postulated that letter-by-letter reading reflects a disconnection between the parallel letter identification mechanism and the orthographic lexicon, thereby forcing reliance on a slower mechanism of sequential processing of individual letters (Patterson & Kay, 1982). Alternately, it has been hypothesized that letter-by-letter reading results from disruption in the mechanisms for identifying individual letters and other nonlinguistic visual forms rapidly and automatically (Friedman & Alexander, 1984; Wallace & Farah, 1990). The cognitive impairment in letter-by-letter reading, therefore, appears to involve disruption in or output from the mechanism for letter identification.

Disturbance of Orthographic Representations

The transfer of information from the visual perceptual processing system to the language system takes place through the orthographic lexicon. When orthographic patterns themselves are disturbed, the resulting reading disorder is *surface alexia* (Patterson, Marshall, & Coltheart, 1985). This alexia is manifested in difficulties decoding words with less frequently occurring or "irregular" spelling-to-sound correspondences. Reading of words (and pseudowords) with regular correspondence between orthography and phonology is better preserved (but usually not completely intact). There is also a tendency to produce "regularization" errors. These consist of pronunciations that are incorrect but plausible, as they conform to the more frequent spelling-to-sound correspondence patterns (e.g., pronouncing *pint* to rhyme with *mint*).

It has been postulated that surface alexia results from failure to adequately activate familiar word patterns in the orthographic lexicon (Friedman, 1988; Patterson et al., 1985). Disruption in this automatic lexical recognition mechanism results in an attempt to read all words as if they are unfamiliar pronounceable letter strings, like pseudowords. Defective activation of entries in the orthographic lexicon is more likely to disrupt the assembled pronunciations of those word patterns in the orthographic lexicon with the fewest "neighbors" sharing common orthographic and phonological features. Words with highly predictable or regular letter-to-sound correspondence (and pseudowords that are by definition regular in their spelling-to-sound correspondence) are most likely to be pronounced correctly, even with incomplete activation of orthographic word forms. For words such as *bake* that have many orthographically and phonologically related neighbors, only one possible pronunciation is activated through the lexical phonological processing system described earlier. These words are read with a high degree of accuracy. Words with mildly irregular spelling-to-sound correspondences (e.g., the word *fear* may be pronounced to rhyme with either *near* or *bear*) will be read less accurately when both correct and incorrect orthographic entries are partially activated, but no single entry gains more prominent activation. This situation is also more likely to yield pronunciations that are frequently occurring but incorrect (i.e., "regularization errors"). Unique words with very irregular spellings like *yacht* have no orthographic neighbors that may enhance the probability of activating the correct phonological code. These words are most likely to be misread. Indeed, Shallice, Warrington, and McCarthy (1983) demonstrated that "very irregular" words are more difficult for surface alexic patients than "mildly irregular" words. Thus, the two basic characteristics of surface alexia—impaired reading of words with more irregular spellings, and regularization errors—may be explained by impaired access to or processing within the orthographic lexicon.

Orthographic paralexic errors, where a response word sharing most of the letters with the target stimulus is substituted (for example, reading *symphony* as "sympathy"), are sometimes taken to indicate impairment in the activation of lexical entries in the orthographic lexicon (Marshall, 1984). While this may be an adequate explanation in certain cases of alexia, Friedman, Ween, and Albert (1993) argue persuasively that orthographic paralexias may have many possible sources, and only sometimes reflect specific impairments within the orthographic lexicon.

Disturbance in Semantic Processing

Some of the most compelling evidence for the notion that there are two independent routes for processing written words, a semantic one and a phonological one, comes from the findings that certain brain-damaged patients can read aloud without comprehending what is read, while other patients comprehend written words without being able to pronounce them. The former pattern exemplifies a disorder in semantic processing.

Patients with the diagnosis of probable Alzheimer's disease have been shown to retain the ability to read aloud all types of real words (including words with highly irregular spelling-to-sound correspondences), along with most types of pseudowords, well into the later stages of their disease (Friedman et al., 1992; Schwartz, Saffran, & Marin, 1980). Oral reading is preserved in these patients, despite their inability to comprehend the meanings of written or spoken words. Some investigators (e.g.,

Nebes, 1989; Ober & Shenaut, 1990) have argued that these patients are impaired in accessing what appear to be intact representations in their semantic lexicon. Others have presented evidence to suggest that impaired semantic processing of oral and written language in Alzheimer's disease is due to disrupted organization within the semantic lexicon itself (Glosser & Friedman, 1991; Huff, Corkin, & Growden, 1986; Martin & Fedio, 1983). In either case, as long as the phonological lexical processing route remains operational, demented patients can use this alternate means for accessing the pronunciations of words and for *reading without meaning.*

Disturbance in Accessing Phonological Representations

It has been suggested that *phonological alexia* (Beauvois & Derouesne, 1979) reflects disrupted direct access to phonological representations in the face of intact processing through the semantic lexical route (Friedman, 1988). Information from the orthographic lexicon cannot access the phonological lexicon directly. Phonological representations are accessed only indirectly after words are processed first through the semantic lexicon. Pronunciations for words that do not have representations in the semantic lexicon, therefore, are inaccessible to such patients. Oral reading of unfamiliar pronounceable letter strings (pseudowords) and morphemes that serve primarily syntactic functions and have low semantic value (functor words) is compromised in patients with phonological alexia (Patterson, 1982). The modality-specific processing deficit characteristic of some patients with phonological alexia who do not have accompanying aphasic syndromes suggests that the reading disorder in these cases involves impaired access to, rather than disruption of, phonological lexical codes.

Disturbance of the Phonological Representations

In some cases (Friedman & Kohn, 1990), phonological alexia is seen in the context of cross-modal impairments in phonological processing, such as in conduction aphasia. This symptom cluster suggests that the disruption lies within the phonological lexicon itself. As disturbance in the phonological lexicon becomes more severe, patients may produce neologisms in spontaneous speech and repetition as well as producing errors in oral reading, yet they may continue to understand the meanings of written words quite well (Caramazza, Berndt, & Basili, 1983). The preserved comprehension of word meanings indicates that orthographic input is processed normally through a functional semantic lexicon. The inability to read aloud, along with impaired repetition and neologistic naming, suggests that the codes necessary to achieve correct pronunciations for words are not being properly activated within the phonological lexicon.

Simultaneous Disruptions in Multiple Components of the Reading System

Discussion of the acquired alexias would not be complete without review of *deep alexia* (Coltheart, 1980). Deep alexia is considered to be a multicomponent disorder (Shallice & Warrington, 1980). Unlike the reading disorders described above, in which only one cognitive component may be disturbed, deep alexia is believed to involve simultaneous disturbance in more than one component of the reading system. Understanding this disorder is important for appreciating the complexities of other multicomponent reading disorders. The defining characteristic of deep alexia is the production of semantic paralexias in oral reading. A semantic paralexia is a word that is not related to the target orthographically or phonologically, but is related to the target semantically (e.g., *lion* is read as "tiger"). When reading out loud, patients who make semantic paralexic errors also invariably demonstrate an inability to read pronounceable pseudowords; greater difficulties reading abstract, nonimageable words as compared with reading concrete words; a "part-of-speech effect" that consists of a gradient of difficulty reading words belonging to different syntactic classes (nouns and adjectives are read better than verbs, which are, in turn, read better than function words); derivational and inflectional errors that are manifested in substitutions, additions, or omissions of bound syntactic morphemes; and orthographic paralexias (Coltheart, 1980).

Recent conceptions view deep alexia as a variant of phonological alexia (Glosser & Friedman, 1990). In common with phonological alexia, deep alexia involves impairment in accessing phonological lexical representations directly from orthographic input, so that pseudowords cannot be read and function words are read poorly. Reading proceeds only through the semantic lexicon. In deep alexia, unlike in phonological alexia, there appears to be an impairment in semantic processing in addition to disrupted access to the phonological lexicon. With impaired access to, organization of, or retrieval of word meanings in the semantic lexicon, those lexical items with less richly developed networks of semantic associations (abstract nouns, verbs, and functors) are most vulnerable (Friedman & Glosser, 1990). Disturbed access to representations in the semantic lexicon can also result in loss of the selectivity by which specific lexical items are activated. Sometimes semantically related content words that are closely linked in the semantic associative network are inadvertently activated, resulting in semantic paralexias (Friedman & Glosser, 1990). This account explains the symptom cluster associated with deep alexia by postulating impairments in *both* semantic and phonological lexical processing components.

We have argued (Glosser & Friedman, 1990) that cases of deep alexia, and those with other multicomponent reading disorders, may present with a range of relative impairments in the different affected components of the reading system. In the example of deep alexia, depending on the severity of the semantic processing impairment, there may be more or less difficulty reading abstract nouns and different rates of semantic paralexias. Different degrees of impairment in component processes yield a continuum of related, but not necessarily identical, alexic disorders.

Recognizing that reading disorders can result from different patterns of graded impairments in different component reading processes is especially important in the clinical setting. Models that recognize continuities between different reading disorders and heterogeneity in the behavioral presentations of related reading problems are likely to be most useful for guiding clinical assessment and treating individual patients. For discussions of other examples of multicomponent or combination alexic disorders, the reader is referred to Friedman and Hadley (1992) and Friedman, Ween, and Albert (1993).

ASSESSING COMPONENTS OF THE READING SYSTEM

Having described a theoretical model of the normal reading process and having reviewed how specific impairments in components of this cognitive model result in the major types of acquired reading disorders, we proceed to discuss clinical methods for assessing the integrity of component cognitive processes.

Visual Processing

To determine the integrity of the peripheral components of the reading system that are specialized for analyzing visual inputs, certain nonlinguistic visual capacities must be assessed along with evaluation of letter identification skills. Visual scanning procedures requiring symbol or line cancellation (Albert, 1973; Weintraub & Mesulam, 1985) and line bisection tasks (Schenkenberg, Bradford, & Ajax, 1980) can reveal visual neglect disorders. Visual attention disorders revealed by these assessment methods may not result in gross neglect errors in reading, but such visual processing problems may disrupt reading performance in a more covert manner. Frank visual neglect in reading is determined most directly by analyzing the spatial location of errors within words. In normal reading, errors tend to occur principally for letters in the (rightmost) end and in the middle of the written word (Shankweiler & Lieberman, 1972). Omission and substitution errors occurring for the leftmost portions of words indicate a disturbance in visual attention. Also, when there is a substantial advantage for reading single words presented vertically as compared to the standard horizontal presentation, visual neglect must be considered to be a significant factor that may be disrupting reading performance.

Impairment in letter identification may be assessed explicitly by having the patient name individual letters, distinguish correct from mirror-reversed letters, and match upper- to lowercase letters and letters written in different fonts. These tasks of explicit letter identification may be failed for a variety of reasons while implicit letter identification remains intact (Friedman, 1981). To test for implicit identification, the patient may be asked to distinguish real words from orthographically illegal, nonpronounceable letter strings. Success in this task requires some (covert) knowledge of letter identities.

The letter-by-letter reader may be identified by obvious attempts to name letters of a word one at a time. An effect of word length is a reliable marker of this disorder. Decreased accuracy or speed of reading long versus short words may indicate a breakdown in the parallel processing of visually presented letters, and a reliance on the slower mechanism that processes visual input serially.

Peripheral alexic disorders are usually revealed in one of the aforementioned manipulations. Such manipulations tend to produce negligible effects on reading in the normal population, and thus are diagnostically specific. Suspicion that a reading disorder is due to defective visual perceptual analysis can be confirmed by demonstrating that orally spelled words are well recognized, in contrast to defective recognition of visually presented letter patterns.

Orthographic Processing

Variation in oral reading associated with manipulations in the regularity of spelling-to-sound correspondence is the critical marker for the reading disorders classed under the broad category of surface alexia. When a specific impairment in reading words with irregular spellings is seen for moderate and high-frequency items, in addition to low-frequency words, a comprehensive assessment of other symptoms associated with surface alexia should be undertaken. Such an assessment may clarify the locus of the cognitive defect for the particular alexic patient.

The typical surface alexic patient comprehends words as they are sounded out, so that an incorrect pronunciation of an irregularly spelled word results in activation of an incorrect semantic representation (e.g., the word *bear* is understood to be an alcoholic beverage). These patients have an impairment in accessing the correct orthographic pattern. A lexical decision task may be used to confirm this locus of impairment. The individual is required to decide whether a presented letter string is a real word or not (latency to respond and response accuracy can both be measured). Items should include real words with irregular spelling-to-sound correspondence (e.g., *pint*) and pseudowords that are homophonic with real words (e.g., *boal*). Failure to recognize real words with exceptional spellings as familiar letter patterns, or acceptance of pseudohomophones as real words, indicates disturbed access to orthographic lexical representations. Accuracy on untimed lexical decision tasks for words of high to moderate frequency is quite high normally (greater than 90%), even among patients with significant aphasia, so that the slightest deficit in performance on such tasks may be considered significant. Poor detection of low-frequency words must be interpreted cautiously, however, as it may reflect low education and premorbid vocabulary. In individuals with well-developed vocabularies, selective impairments in recognizing low-frequency words as familiar letter patterns may indicate milder disturbance in accessing orthographic word patterns.

Some surface alexic patients can process written words correctly for meaning and in lexical decision tasks; their deficit is strictly in the oral reading of irregularly spelled words. Unlike patients with other forms of surface alexia, these patients can disambiguate the meanings of homophones that are orthographically and semantically distinct. These patients appear to have difficulty activating correct phonological representations despite intact activation of orthographic (and corresponding semantic) representations. The problem, then, may be a failure to activate phonological codes specific to individual words, so the patient is forced to pronounce all written words as if they are pseudowords. This type of surface alexic patient tends to have problems accessing phonological representations from other modalities as well (Kay & Patterson, 1985). If a patient shows an effect of spelling regularity in oral reading but performs well on tests of written homophone comprehension, tests of naming should be given and spontaneous speech should be examined to determine if there is a cross-modal impairment in phonological activation.

Phonological Processing

Phonological processing of written words is assessed most directly by pseudoword reading tests. Since pseudowords have no representation in the orthographic or semantic lexicons, their pronunciation can only be assembled by drawing on information in the phonological lexicon (or, by some accounts, grapheme–phoneme correspondence rules). Pseudoword reading that is disproportionately impaired in comparison with real (content) words is the hallmark of a disturbance in accessing phonological representations.

Impaired use of the phonological processing route may be specific to reading, or it may represent a more general problem in phonological processing. Additional tests may help tease apart these possibilities. If the problem is restricted to phonological processing of written information, then functor word reading will be poor, and function word substitution errors (e.g., reading *them* as "in") will be produced (Friedman, in press), but pseudoword repetition should not be affected.

Impaired pseudoword repetition suggests a more general problem in phonological processing. Such a general processing deficit will often also be manifested in a syllable length effect. Words with more syllables will present more difficulty for reading and repetition than words with fewer syllables, when letter length is kept constant (Friedman & Kohn, 1990).

Semantic Processing

Semantic processing is assessed traditionally using word–picture matching tasks to evaluate single-word comprehension. A written word is matched to an array of presented objects or pictures, or a picture may be matched to an array of words. Such tasks require that written words be processed for meaning, while at the same time other response demands (such as speaking) are minimized. Task difficulty may be increased by employing distractor items that are closely related to the target stimulus in terms of meaning (Butterworth, Howard, & McLoughlin, 1984). Patients with semantic processing impairments tend to have the greatest difficulties distinguishing among items belonging to the same superordinate semantic category as compared to items drawn from different semantic categories. Poor comprehension of low imageability–low operativity (Gardner, 1973; Gardner & Zurif, 1975) words is also a characteristic of milder forms of disrupted semantic lexical processing. To test comprehension of substantive words that are not high-imageability picturable nouns, various semantic decision tasks may be used. In the odd-man-out procedure, for example, the word that does not belong with or differs in meaning from other presented words must be identified. In a category decision procedure, patients are required to judge if presented words belong to a designated semantic category.

When semantic processing is disturbed in the presence of impaired phonological processing, word class effects in oral reading may result. Words with less stable or less accessible representations in the semantic lexicon are read more poorly (i.e., verbs and abstract nouns are read less reliably than concrete nouns). As the semantic processing impairment becomes more severe, semantic paralexias appear as well. Patients with this constellation of symptoms of deep alexia are nearly always aphasic as well as alexic and demonstrate significantly impaired naming and auditory comprehension (Marshall & Newcombe, 1977). For all patients with suspected or known impairments in semantic processing of written words, semantic processing of oral language should be investigated carefully by testing auditory comprehension in parallel with the evaluation of reading comprehension.

Speech Production

Disturbance at the stage of motor output should disrupt verbal responses on all reading and oral language tasks in a qualitatively similar manner, regardless of input and central processing requirements. Phonological errors (literal paraphasias) occur most commonly and are seen across a variety of language tasks; successful word production often is related to word length (shorter words are more likely to be pronounced correctly); and usually speech production errors are recognized by the patient spontaneously (although these mistakes cannot always be self-corrected). If the disturbance is confined to output mechanisms, performance should be normal on tasks that do not require verbal response. Pronunciations and meanings of presented words will be recognized normally, for example, when tested using a multiple-choice format. Unlike the disorders that affect the central components of lexical processing, there should be no effects of word frequency, imageability, and grammatical class on reading and other language performances when the locus of impairment is confined to the stage of speech production.

Interpretation of Paralexias

Most types of paralexic errors are not by themselves diagnostic of particular alexic disorders or disruption in specific components of the reading system. Careful analyses of the types of paralexias produced by the patient in oral reading tasks in relation to other reading and language performances, however, are fruitful in determining the locus of disturbance in the reading system.

As noted earlier, orthographic paralexias are extremely common and are seen in association with all alexia types. Orthographic paralexias produced in letter-by-letter readers may be due to loss of orthographic information when serially decoded letter strings must be kept in working memory temporarily until the full word is processed. Orthographic paralexias can also reflect impaired activation of word patterns in the orthographic lexicon as in surface alexia. Deep and phonological alexic patients also produce orthographic paralexias, but these may arise from disruption within the semantic lexicon. Such patients produce more orthographic errors for words that are nonimageable or abstract as compared with concrete words (Morton & Patterson, 1980).

Semantic paralexias reflect disruption in semantic processing, but, as demonstrated by Friedman and Perlman (1982), these errors may have different sources. In cases where semantic errors are seen in word reading, but the same referent can be named normally when depicted in a picture, the semantic paralexic errors are taken to be the result of a problem in retrieving (presumably intact) representations in semantic memory. In other cases, semantic substitutions (paralexias) in reading are associated with semantic substitutions (paraphasias) when naming the corresponding object, indicating that the semantic representation itself, or its ability to access the appropriate phonological representation, may be disturbed.

Derivational and inflectional paralexic errors reflect impairment in processing grammatical markers. When such errors are seen in isolation in reading, but not in speech, they are taken to reflect disrupted access from orthography to (nonsemantic) phonological lexical representations. When these errors occur in association with paragrammatic or agrammatic speech, they may be due to a more pervasive disturbance in grammatical processing.

Finally, it should be emphasized that in many cases paralexias may have several simultaneous causes. For example, derivational/inflectional errors usually are related to the target not only in base meaning but also in the orthography (e.g., *dangerous* read as "danger"). Sometimes orthographic errors combine with semantic errors to produce a novel paralexic response (e.g., *even* read as "night").

Special Issues in Assessing Reading Skills

Implicit in the preceding discussion is the idea that an adequate assessment of reading skills requires concurrent assessment of certain oral language and visual processing abilities. The reader is referred to the chapter by Caplan (Chapter 4, this volume) for discussion of relevant psycholinguistic assessments of oral language disorders that complement the cognitive assessment of reading dysfunction.

The interpretation of a deficit in reading performance often can only be made with reference to oral language abilities. Impaired reading comprehension in the context of a generalized auditory comprehension disorder, for example, suggests a cross-modal lexical semantic processing deficit, such as that associated with Wernicke's aphasia. In such instances, the reading disorder must be addressed as part of a generalized linguistic disturbance diagnostically and therapeutically. On the other hand, impaired reading comprehension in the context of spared auditory comprehension suggests that the dysfunction is specific to the process by which the written word form gains access to central lexical semantic processing components. Similarly, an impairment in oral reading that is seen in the context of normal or near normal naming, repetition, auditory comprehension, and writing indicates a defect in the early stages of analysis of visual inputs or in the transfer of information from the visual modality to central language processing components. In general, cross-modal deficits on tasks that presumably draw on the same processing components (e.g., repetition, oral reading, and naming all depend on activating information in the phonological lexicon) suggest an impairment *within* the processing component, whereas modality-specific deficits (e.g., defective oral reading but spared repetition) tend to implicate a disorder in *accessing* certain processing components.

These kinds of distinctions are extremely important when developing therapeutic programs geared to remediating reading or oral language problems. They are especially relevant in situations where reading might be used to circumvent a defect in auditory comprehension. If the assessment leads to the conclusion that there is loss of specific knowledge or a specific procedure within one of the central processing components, it may be necessary to develop ways by which other processors or procedures can be engaged to achieve the same functioning goal. On the other hand, if the processing component is determined to be intact but access to it is blocked, then one might explore other routes that may be used to access the functioning processing component.

Assessment of reading performance would be incomplete without some gauge of the individual's functional/adaptive reading skills. Sentence and paragraph reading have typically been excluded from consideration in developing cognitive models such as the one reviewed above. While it is assumed that sentence and paragraph reading draw on many of the same components used in single-word reading, it is thought that because of their complexity, the former tasks also draw on numerous other nonlinguistic cognitive sytems (e.g., memory, attention, executive control, and higher level inferential programs), and thus are unlikely to be explained by specifying the architecture of a cognitive system specialized for processing written language. Although assessment of sentence- and paragraph-reading abilities may not be informative about the specific location of neurological or cognitive dysfunction, it is important for determining the extent to which a patient can read for pleasure or to achieve functional goals.

ASSESSMENT INSTRUMENTS

Unfortunately, well-standardized test batteries validated in neurological populations do not exist currently for conducting the types of reading assessments outlined above in the clinical setting (but see Chapter 9, by Kay and Franklin, in this volume, for discussion of new tests currently being developed). While clinical assessments may be guided by the principles we have been discussing, the actual methods and tests that are used still must be borrowed from other disciplines:

- Portions of standardized aphasia tests are quite useful. For example, the Symbol Matching subtest from the Boston Diagnostic Aphasia Examination (BDAE; Goodglass & Kaplan, 1983) may be used to quantify impairments in visual orthographic analysis, and Comprehension of Oral Spelling, another subtest of the BDAE, may be used to help identify letter-by-letter readers.
- Certain tests intended for assessing developmental reading disorders also contain standardized measures useful in the componential analysis of reading processes. As an example, the Word Attack subtest of the Woodcock Reading Mastery Test-Revised (Woodcock, 1987) yields a normatively based estimate of pseudoword reading abilities that may be compared to the individual's real-word read-

ing level as assessed on the Word Identification subtest from the same reading battery. Since there is considerable variation within the normal population in terms of real-word and pseudoword reading abilities, it is especially important to use normatively based tests to compare reading skills for different stimuli before establishing that there is a specific cognitive defect.

- In other cases, standardized tests are not necessary to determine that performance is defective. Some simple manipulations that otherwise should not affect reading performance can yield important clues as to the locus of underlying dysfunction. For example, an obvious effect of changing the orientation of written words on reading performance is diagnostic of a disturbance in visual input analysis that requires no additional psychometric assessment.
- There are some tests designed to assess symptoms specific to certain acquired reading disorders. For example, the National Adult Reading Test (Nelson, 1982) assesses oral reading of words with irregular spellings to achieve an estimate of premorbid sight vocabulary in patients who are otherwise demented (Blair & Spreen, 1989; Nelson & O'Connell, 1978). The Reading Comprehension Battery for Aphasia (LaPointe & Horner, 1979) includes a single-word reading comprehension subtest that employs semantically related distractors and a written synonym recognition subtest. Both tasks are useful for assessing impairments in single-word reading comprehension using a response mode that minimizes the potential confounding effects of peripheral output disorders.
- A variety of tests exist that can be used to assess functional reading capacities. Some are more appropriate for quantifying abilities within the lower range of function. Tests such as the Reading Comprehension Battery for Aphasia, for example, employ stimuli that are very familiar in everyday settings. Other tests, such as the Gates-MacGinities Reading Tests (MacGinitie & MacGinitie, 1989), the Gray Oral Reading Test-Revised (Wiederholt & Bryant, 1986), and the Woodcock-Johnson Tests of Achievement (Woodcock & Johnson, 1989), are geared for higher functioning patients and assess abilities that may be relevant for more demanding educational/occupational performances.

CASE STUDIES

Two cases will be presented to illustrate application of the principles outlined above. The first case (Glosser & Friedman, 1990) focuses on assessment issues and methods for a patient with symptoms of deep alexia, while the second case describes the formulation and implementation of cognitively based treatment for a patient with alexia without agraphia (Friedman et al., 1993; Lott, Friedman, & Linebaugh, 1994).

A Case of Deep Alexia

This 23-year-old, right-handed accountant suffered a closed head injury in a motor vehicle accident and sustained hematomas in the right frontal and left temporal lobes.

Evaluation of a residual fluent aphasia and alexia was conducted over the course of several weeks beginning about 1 month postinjury.

Semantic paralexias were first observed during administration of the BDAE. The production of semantic paralexias, of course, constitutes the core symptom in the syndrome of deep alexia. Initially, the reading evaluation focused on assessing each of the expected co-occurring symptoms of deep alexia (Coltheart, 1980).

Pseudoword reading was assessed using the list of pronounceable nonwords from the Word Attack subtest of the Woodcock Reading Mastery Test-Revised (Woodcock, 1987). Only 1 of the 20 presented nonwords was read correctly. This result suggested an inability to access phonological representations directly from orthography. Repetition of single real words and pseudowords was essentially without error, however, indicating that the phonological lexicon was relatively intact, as it could be accessed by auditory, but apparently not by visual, inputs.

Pseudoword reading was then compared with real-word oral reading to determine if, as would be expected in deep alexia, phonological representations for some real words might be accessed indirectly through the semantic lexicon. On the Wide Range Achievement Test-Revised (WRAT-R; Jastak & Wilkinson, 1984), single-word oral reading was scored at about a third-grade level. While this level of performance is certainly below estimated premorbid abilities, it was markedly higher than pseudoword reading, which was assessed to be below levels expected in first-grade readers.

To assess the effects of imageability and part of speech on oral reading, a published list of words used by Saffran, Bogyo, Schwartz, and Marin (1980) was administered. This list contains short (four-letter) concrete nouns, abstract nouns, and functors that are matched in terms of word frequency. Eighty-two percent of the concrete nouns but only 40% of the abstract nouns and 34% of the functors were read correctly. These results demonstrated effects of both imageability and part of speech on oral reading, findings that would be compatible with the notion that the patient was attempting to process all written words exclusively through a defective semantic reading system.

Responses obtained on all of the single- (real) word reading tasks were combined to conduct a qualitative analysis of the errors. Of the 58 paralexic errors, 14% were semantic paralexias; 5% were real-word responses with no obvious semantic or orthographic relation to the target; 5% were orthographically and semantically related to the target; 52% were orthographic paralexias; 9% were derivational/inflectional paralexias; and 16% were other errors such as nonword and multiword responses. The pattern of reading errors closely matched that expected in deep alexia. Consistent with the diagnosis of deep alexia, this patient's oral reading performance displayed no effects of word length and regularity of the spelling-to-sound correspondence.

A comprehensive neuropsychological evaluation indicated serious language impairments, but nonverbal visuospatial processing and memory abilities were generally intact. In particular, there was no evidence for disturbed visual scanning or visual neglect. A subset of stimuli from the single-word reading tasks was presented in vertical orientation, to assess whether disturbance in peripheral visual processing might contribute to reading performance. Manipulations of the visual characteristics of target words had *no* effect on reading accuracy. On the BDAE, symbol discrimination (matching letters and words written in different fonts and scripts) and letter naming were performed without error, also suggesting intact letter identification.

Characterization of the aphasia accompanying alexia is critical for evaluating the integrity of those central processing components that are shared in both oral and written language functions. Assessment in this case of deep alexia focused on the integrity of the phonological and semantic processors by determining whether these could be accessed through the auditory modality.

The patient's retained ability to repeat pseudowords and also real words suggested that phonological representations in the lexicon were relatively intact. Single-word comprehension was assessed extensively to determine the integrity of semantic lexical processes as accessed through both auditory and visual modalities. Written word–picture matching and auditory word–picture matching tasks from the BDAE were performed at essentially identical levels of mild to moderate impairment. A direct comparison of single-word auditory and reading comprehension was undertaken using the Peabody Picture Vocabulary Test-Revised (PPVT; Dunn & Dunn, 1981). In the standard administration, consisting of auditory presentation of words that are to be matched to pictures, this test generates age-corrected standard scores and percentile scores, as well as developmental age ratings. Visual presentation of stimulus words from the alternate form of the PPVT stimulus words normally yields a small decrement in absolute accuracy when compared to auditory presentation (Glosser, Roeltgen, & Friedman, 1991). Comparisons of age ratings for comprehension of PPVT stimuli presented auditorily and in written form with age ratings for single-word oral reading abilities on the WRAT suggested that for this deep alexic patient, oral reading capacities remained quite impaired (at or below a 9-year-old level) and comprehension of written words was substantially better (well above a 10-year-old level) but still not at levels expected based on auditory comprehension skills (at or above a 16-year-old level).

The results of these analyses taken together were consistent with a hypothesized impairment in central lexical semantic processing. Word meanings were not being accessed normally apparently through either the visual or auditory modalities. Lexical semantic information, nonetheless, was accessed more reliably than lexical phonological information, as evidenced by the apparently greater facility in comprehending the meanings of written words than reading them out loud.

Longitudinal monitoring revealed that over an 8-month period the pattern of the patient's reading disorder evolved from a deep alexia to a pattern that most closely approximated phonological alexia. Subsequent evaluations used the same tasks and procedures as those reported for the initial evaluation so that quantitative and qualitative changes could be monitored objectively. Semantic paralexic errors and the effects of part of speech and imageability on oral reading disappeared completely in follow-up examinations, but the patient continued to demonstrate a persistent but attenuated deficit in pseudoword reading.

Over time, the focus of the assessments was broadened to include a delineation of the patient's *functional* reading abilities, in addition to identifying the locus of cognitive impairment underlying the alexia. At 8 months postonset, numerous errors were made in reading aloud paragraphs at about a third-grade level of difficulty on the Gray

Oral Reading Test-Revised (Wiederholt & Bryant, 1986). By contrast, comprehension and retention of information gained through silent reading of connected narratives was substantially better, with virtually no errors occurring on questions about information contained in paragraphs at about a 10th-grade level of difficulty. No further changes in oral reading capacities were found in a subsequent examination, but reading comprehension skills continued to improve, so that at 15 months postinjury the patient's understanding of written texts was comparable to his estimated premorbid abilities.

The serial examinations indicated that despite apparently persistent impairments in phonological processing of written words, problems in semantic lexical processing resolved almost completely. Eventually the patient was able to use a recovered semantic processing system to read for meaning at functional levels that were adequate for return to professional employment as a tax auditor. Since correlations between the severity of neuropsychological impairment and adaptive functions are often imperfect, it is important to assess both aspects of behavior in a comprehensive evaluation of a reading disorder.

Treatment for Alexia Based on a Cognitive Neuropsychological Analysis

This 67-year-old, right-handed, college-educated, retired printer suffered an intracerebral hemorrhage in the left temporal-parietal region approximately 1 year prior to initiation of treatment. In addition to a residual aphasia, there was persistent lower right homonymous quadrantonopia. A language evaluation 2 months after the cerebrovascular accident revealed a performance profile on the BDAE consistent with a transcortical sensory type of aphasia. The language disorder was characterized by moderate anomia, good repetition, mild auditory comprehension deficits, and a moderate to severe alexia with less severe agraphia.

Characteristics of letter-by-letter reading were evident in the pretreatment evaluation 14 months postonset. Recognition of oral spelling and spelling production were performed substantially better than oral reading for single words (91% and 97% versus 25% correct) and pseudowords (75% and 95% versus 0% correct). Similarly, comprehension as assessed by presenting PPVT stimuli as spoken words (84% correct) or orally spelled words (67%) was substantially better than presentation of these stimuli as written words (38% correct). Attempts to read using a letter-by-letter strategy, however, were largely unsuccessful due to severely impaired letter-naming abilities.

A cognitive analysis suggested that the primary disturbance involved impaired activation of the orthographic lexicon through the visual, but not the auditory, modality. Unforunately, because of disrupted letter identification, this patient could not adopt the strategy of reading by naming individual letters out loud, which is successfully used by other patients to circumvent the problem in automatic parallel processing of visual inputs characteristic of this type of alexia. A treatment to enhance letter identification was designed with the goal of developing a functional letter-by-letter reading strategy.

Treatment focused on improving letter naming. A combined tactile–kinesthetic approach was chosen in which the patient was trained to copy letters onto his own palm and subsequently to name them out loud. In this way, multisensory information might be used to improve letter naming, thereby allowing this patient to use a letter-by-letter strategy.

Letters were divided into two sets of increasing difficulty based on the patient's accuracy in naming letters in a pretest. For each letter set, two lists of words composed of letters from that set were created. One served as a training list, and the second as a control list to assess generalization of the treatment effect. The word lists were matched for part of speech, length, word frequency, and number of orthographically related real-word neighbors.

Study of treatment efficacy followed a multiple baseline design (Hersen & Barlow, 1976). Six baseline sessions were followed by 60 one-hour therapy sessions consisting of sequentially administered treatment phases using the lists of increasing difficulty, and then there were assessments of treatment maintenance at 1, 4, and 8 weeks posttreatment. In each phase of treatment, training continued until at least 90% accuracy was achieved in two consecutive therapy sessions.

The data presented in Table 5.1 indicate that treatment resulted in substantial improvement of reading accuracy on both the training lists (by 54%) and the generalization lists (by 37%), and that some improvement on the two lists was also maintained for 2 months following treatment. The effect of treatment was very specific and was evident only when the trained tactile–kinesthetic strategy was actually applied. Performance on a 32-word list that had been read with 25% accuracy pretreatment improved to an accuracy of 66% posttreatment when the hand-tracing strategy was used. Reading accuracy when the patient was not allowed to use the trained strategy showed no improvement over pretreatment accuracy (22% correct).

The therapy devised for this patient with alexia without agraphia was guided by a cognitive neuropsychological model of the reading process. A componential analysis first determined that information in the central lexicons was intact and accessible through the auditory modality, but inaccessible through the visual modality. An additional impairment in visual letter identification prevented this patient from using an alternative strategy in which written words are identified from their individual letters. Treatment focused on developing means for accessing intact knowledge through alternative sensory modalities, and this resulted in the transformation of a severely alexic patient into a letter-by-letter reader.

TABLE 5.1. Percentage of Words Read Correctly during Each Phase of Treatment to Increase Letter-by-Letter Reading Accuracy

	Baseline	Treatment[a]	Maintenance[b]
Training lists	39	93	63
Generalization lists	41	78	70

[a]Mean percentage of correct reading responses in the final two sessions of each treatment phase.
[b]Percentage of correct reading responses at 8 weeks posttreatment.

REFERENCES

Albert, M. L. (1973). A simple test of visual neglect. *Neurology, 23,* 658–664.

Barron, R. W., & Baron, J. (1977). How children get meaning from printed words. *Child Development, 48,* 586–594.

Beauvois, M. F., & Derouesne, J. (1979). Phonological alexia: Three dissociations. *Journal of Neurology, Neurosurgery and Psychiatry, 42,* 1115–1124.

Behrmann, M., Black, S. E., & Bub, D. (1990). The evolution of pure alexia: A longitudinal study of recovery. *Brain and Language, 39,* 405–427.

Blair, J. R., & Spreen O. (1989). Predicting premorbid IQ: A revision of the National Adult Reading Test. *The Clinical Neuropsychologist, 3,* 129–136.

Butterworth, B., Howard, D., & McLoughlin, P. (1984). The semantic deficit in aphasia: The relationship between semantic errors in auditory comprehension and picture naming. *Neuropsychologia, 22,* 409–426.

Caramazza, A., Berndt, R. S., & Basili, A. G. (1983). The selective impairment of phonological processing: A case study. *Brain and Language, 18,* 128–174.

Coltheart, M. (1980). Deep dyslexia: A review of the syndrome. In M. Coltheart, K. Patterson, & J. C. Marshall (Eds.), *Deep dyslexia* (pp. 22–47). London: Routledge & Kegan Paul.

Coltheart, M. (1981). Disorders of reading and their implications for models of normal reading. *Visible Language, 15,* 245–286.

Coltheart, M., & Funnell, E. (1987). Reading and writing: One lexicon or two. In A. Allport, D. G. Mackay, W. Prinz, & E. Scheerer (Eds.), *Language perception and production* (pp. 313–339). New York: Academic Press.

Coltheart, M., Patterson, K., & Marshall, J. C. (1987). Deep dyslexia since 1980. In M. Coltheart, K. Patterson, & J. C. Marshall (Eds.), *Deep dyslexia* (pp. 407–451). London: Routledge & Kegan Paul.

DePartz, M. P. (1986). Re-education of a deep dyslexic patient: Rationale of the method and results. *Cognitive Neuropsychology, 2,* 149–177.

Dunn, L. M., & Dunn, L. M. (1981). *Peabody Picture Vocabulary Test-Revised.* Circle Pines, MN: American Guidance Service.

Ellis, A. W., Flude, B. M., & Young, A. W. (1987). "Neglect dyslexia" and the early visual processing of letters in words and nonwords. *Cognitive Neuropsychology, 4,* 439–464.

Friedman, R. B. (1981). Preservation of orthographic knowledge in aphasia. *Brain and Language, 14,* 307–314.

Friedman, R. B. (1988). Acquired alexia. In F. Boller & J. Grafman (Eds.), *Handbook of neuropsychology* (Vol. 1, pp. 377–391). Amsterdam: Elsevier.

Friedman, R. B. (in press). Two types of phonological alexia. *Cortex.*

Friedman, R. B., & Alexander, M. P. (1984). Pictures, images and pure alexia: A case study. *Cognitive Neuropsychology, 1,* 9–23.

Friedman, R. B., Beeman, M., Lott, S. N., Link, K., Grafman, J., & Robinson, S. (1993). Modality-specific phonological alexia. *Cognitive Neuropsychology, 10,* 549–568.

Friedman, R. B., Ferguson, S., Robinson, S., & Sunderland, T. (1992). Dissociation of mechanisms of reading in Alzheimer's disease. *Brain and Language, 43,* 400–413.

Friedman, R. B., & Glosser, G. (1990). *The structure of the semantic lexicon: Implications for a theory of deep alexia.* Presented at the Academy of Aphasia, Baltimore, MD.

Friedman, R. B., & Hadley, J. A. (1992). Letter-by-letter surface alexia. *Cognitive Neuropsychology, 9,* 185–208.

Friedman, R. B., & Kohn, S. E. (1990). Impaired activation of the phonological lexicon: Effects upon oral reading. *Brain and Language, 38,* 278–297.

Friedman, R. B., & Perlman, M. B. (1982). On the underlying causes of semantic paralexias in a patient with deep dyslexia. *Neuropsychologia, 20,* 559–568.

Friedman, R. B., & Robinson, S. R. (1991). Whole-word training therapy in a stable surface alexic patient: It works. *Aphasiology, 5,* 1–7.

Friedman, R. B., Ween, J. E., & Albert, M. L. (1993). Alexia. In K. M. Heilman & E. Valenstein (Eds.), *Clinical neuropsychology* (3rd ed., pp. 37–62). New York: Oxford University Press.
Gardner, H. (1973). The contribution of operativity to naming in aphasic patients. *Neuropsychologia, 11*, 213–220.
Gardner, H., & Zurif, E. (1975). "Bee" but not "be"; oral reading of single words in aphasia and alexia. *Neuropsychology, 13*, 181–190.
Glosser, G., & Friedman, R. B. (1990). The continuum of deep/phonological alexia. *Cortex, 26*, 343–359.
Glosser, G., & Friedman, R. B. (1991). Lexical but not semantic priming in Alzheimer's disease. *Psychology and Aging, 6*, 522–527.
Glosser, G., Roeltgen, D., & Friedman, R. B. (1991). Hyperlexia: A case of reading without meaning. *Journal of Clinical and Experimental Neuropsychology, 13*, 54.
Glushko, R. J. (1979). The organization and activation of orthographic knowledge in reading aloud. *Journal of Experimental Psychology: Human Perception and Performance, 5*, 674–669.
Goodglass, H., & Kaplan, E. (1983). *The assessment of aphasia and related disorders.* Philadelphia: Lea & Febiger.
Hersen, M., & Barlow, D. H. (1976). *Single case experimental designs: Strategies for studying behavior change.* Oxford: Pergamon Press.
Huff, F. J., Corkin, S., & Growden, J. H. (1986). Semantic impairment and anomia in Alzheimer's disease. *Brain and Language, 28*, 235–249.
Humphreys, G. W., & Evett, L. J. (1985). Are there independent lexical and nonlexical routes in word processing? An evaluation of the dual-route theory of reading. *Behavioral and Brain Sciences, 8*, 689–740.
Jastak, S., & Wilkinson, G. S. (1984). *Wide Range Achievement Test-Revised.* Wilmington, DE: Jastak Associates.
Kay, J., & Marcel, A. (1981). One process, not two, in reading aloud: Lexical analogies do the work of non-lexical rules. *Quarterly Journal of Experimental Psychology, 33A*, 397–413.
Kay, J., & Patterson, K. E. (1985). Routes to meaning in surface dyslexia. In K. E. Patterson, J. C. Marshall, & M. Coltheart (Eds.), *Surface dyslexia* (pp. 79–104). London: Lawrence Erlbaum.
Kinsbourne, M., & Warrington, E. K. (1962). A variety of reading disability associated with right hemisphere lesions. *Journal of Neurology, Neurosurgery and Psychiatry, 25*, 339–344.
LaBerge, D., & Samuels, S. J. (1974). Toward a theory of automatic information processing in reading. *Cognitive Psychology, 6*, 293–323.
LaPointe, L. L., & Horner, J. (1979). *Reading Comprehension Battery for Aphasia.* Tigard, OR: C. C. Publications.
Lott, S. N., Friedman, R. B., & Linebaugh, C. W. (1994). Rationale and efficacy of a tactile–kinesthetic treatment for alexia. *Aphasiology, 8*, 181–195.
MacGinitie, W. H., & MacGinitie, R. K. (1989). *Gates-MacGinities Reading Tests.* Chicago: Riverside Publishing Company.
Marshall, J. C. (1984). Towards a rational taxonomy of the acquired dyslexias. In R. N. Malatesha & H. A. Whitaker (Eds.), *Dyslexia: A global issue* (pp. 211–232). The Hague: Martinus Nijhoff.
Marshall, J. C., & Newcombe, F. (1977). Variability and constraint in acquired dyslexia. In H. Whitaker & H. A. Whitaker (Eds.), *Studies in neurolinguistics* (Vol. 3, pp. 257–286). New York: Academic Press.
Martin, A., & Fedio, P. (1983). Word production and comprehension in Alzheimer's disease: The breakdown of semantic knowledge. *Brain and Language, 19*, 124–141.
McClelland, J. L. (1976). Preliminary letter identification in the perception of words and nonwords. *Journal of Experimental Psychology: Human Perception and Performance, 2*, 80–91.
Morton, J., & Patterson, K. E. (1980). A new attempt at an interpretation, or, an attempt at a new interpretation. In M. Coltheart, K. Patterson, & J. C. Marshall (Eds.), *Deep dyslexia* (pp. 91–118). London: Routledge & Kegan Paul.
Nebes, R. D. (1989). Semantic memory in Alzheimer's disease. *Psychological Bulletin, 106*, 377–394.
Nelson, H. E. (1982). *National Adult Reading Test.* Windsor, England: NFER-Nelson Publishing Company.

Nelson, H. E., & O'Connell, A. (1978). Dementia: The estimation of premorbid intelligence levels using the New Adult Reading Test. *Cortex, 14,* 234–244.

Ober, B. A., & Shenaut, G. K. (1990). Automatic versus controlled priming in Alzheimer's disease: A synthesis of current findings. *Journal of Clinical and Experimental Neuropsychology, 12,* 79.

Patterson, K. E. (1982). The relation between reading and phonological coding: Further neuropsychological observation. In A. W. Ellis (Ed.), *Normality and pathology in cognitive functioning* (pp. 77–111). London: Academic Press.

Patterson, K. E., & Kay, J. (1982). Letter-by-letter reading: Psychological description of a neurological syndrome. *Quarterly Journal of Experimental Psychology, 34A,* 411–441.

Patterson, K. E., Marshall, J. C., & Coltheart, M. (Eds.). (1985). *Surface dyslexia.* London: Lawrence Erlbaum.

Saffran, E. M., Bogyo, L. C., Schwartz, M. F., & Marin, O. S. M. (1980). Does deep dyslexia reflect right hemisphere reading? In M. Coltheart, K. Patterson, & J. C. Marshall (Eds.), *Deep dyslexia* (pp. 381–406). London: Routledge & Kegan Paul.

Schenkenberg, T., Bradford, D. C., & Ajax, E. T. (1980). Line bisection and unilateral visual neglect in patients with neurologic impairment. *Neurology, 30,* 509–517.

Schwartz, M. F., Saffran, E. M., & Marin, O. S. M. (1980). Fractionating the reading process in dementia: Evidence for word-specific print-to-sound associations. In M. Coltheart, K. Patterson, & J. C. Marshall (Eds.), *Deep dyslexia* (pp. 259–269). London: Routledge & Kegan Paul.

Seidenberg, M. S., & McClelland, J. L. (1989). A distributed, developmental model of word recognition and naming. *Psychological Review, 96,* 523–568.

Shallice, T., & Warrington, E. K. (1977). The possible role of selective attention in acquired dyslexia. *Neuropsychologia, 15,* 31–41.

Shallice, T., & Warrington, E. K. (1980). Simple and multiple component central dyslexic syndromes. In M. Coltheart, K. Patterson, & J. C. Marshall (Eds.), *Deep dyslexia* (pp. 119–145). London: Routledge & Kegan Paul.

Shallice, T., Warrington, E. K., & McCarthy, R. (1983). Reading without semantics. *Quarterly Journal of Experimental Psychology, 35A,* 111–138.

Shankweiler, D., & Lieberman, I. W. (1972). Misreading: A search for cues. In J. F. Kavanagh & I. G. Mattingly (Eds.), *Language by ear and by eye.* Cambridge, MA: MIT Press.

Shiepers, C. (1980). Response latency and accuracy in visual word recognition. *Perception and Psychophysics, 27,* 71–81.

Sieroff, E., Pollatsek, A., & Posner, M. I. (1988). Recognition of visual letter strings following injury to the posterior visual attention system. *Cognitive Neuropsychology, 5,* 427–449.

Venezky, R. L. (1970). *The structure of English orthography.* The Hague: Mouton.

Wallace, M. A., & Farah, M. J. (1990). *Pure alexia as a visual impairment: A reconsideration.* Presented at the Academy of Aphasia, Baltimore, MD.

Warrington, E. K., & Shallice, T. (1980). Word-form dyslexia. *Brain, 103,* 99–112.

Webb, W. G., & Love, R. J. (1983). Reading problems in chronic aphasia. *Journal of Speech and Hearing Disorders, 48,* 164–171.

Weintraub, S., & Mesulam, M. M. (1985). Mental state assessment of young and elderly adults in behavioral neurology. In M. M. Mesulam (Ed.), *Principles of behavioral neurology* (pp. 71–123). Philadelphia: F. A. Davis.

Wiederholt, J. L., & Bryant, B. R. (1986). *Gray Oral Reading Tests.* Austin, TX: Pro-Ed.

Woodcock, R. W. (1987). *Woodcock Reading Mastery Tests-Revised.* Circle Pines, MN: American Guidance Service.

Woodcock, R. W., & Johnson, M. B. (1989). *Woodcock-Johnson Tests of Achievement.* Allen, TX: DLM Teaching Resources.

6

Assessment of Visuocognitive Processes

DANIEL X. CAPRUSO, KERRY deS. HAMSHER, and ARTHUR L. BENTON

HISTORICAL INTRODUCTION

> I would still advocate the view I brought forward in the *Lancet* that the right cerebral hemisphere is the seat of perception. (Jackson, 1875/1958, p. 59)

The specialized role of the posterior right hemisphere in visual perception was first advanced by John Hughlings Jackson in 1864. Twelve years later, Jackson (1876/1958) described a patient whose course of illness confirmed his speculations about the lateralization of higher visual function. The clinical onset of illness in Jackson's patient was marked by a sudden episode of spatial disorientation. Although the patient had resided in the same neighborhood for 30 years, she could not find her way to a nearby park that she had visited frequently. Jackson observed that his patient suffered from what he called "imperception": the inability to recognize objects, persons, and places. Within months, the patient developed a left hemiplegia and rapidly deteriorated to coma and death. Autopsy revealed a large tumor in the posterior right hemipshere, with two smaller tumors in close proximity.

In the century and more that has passed since Jackson's classic observations, a mass of clinical and scientific evidence (reviewed in Benton, 1985b) has demonstrated that the perception of visual patterns and spatial relationships is a specialized function of the posterior right hemisphere of the human brain. More recently, it has been determined that there are two anatomically distinct visual subsystems operating in the human brain as well as in nonhuman primates, and that these two subsystems perform qualitatively different functions.

DANIEL X. CAPRUSO • Department of Neurology, State University of New York at Buffalo, Buffalo, New York 14203. KERRY deS. HAMSHER • Department of Neurology, University of Wisconsin Medical School, Milwaukee, Wisconsin 53233-1325. ARTHUR L. BENTON • Departments of Neurology and Psychology, University of Iowa, Iowa City, Iowa 52242.

Clinical Neuropsychological Assessment: A Cognitive Approach, edited by Robert L. Mapou and Jack Spector. Plenum Press, New York, 1995.

THE DUALITY OF VISUAL PERCEPTION

> These results can be taken as evidence for a pathological differentiation of the effects of the anatomical lesion, and point to the independence of various perceptual abilities. We have to differentiate between: (1) sensation of brightness; (2) sensation of color, of quality; (3) sensation of movement or change; and (4) visual acuity, which is the basis for form vision. *All these systems demonstrate their relative independence of each other through the different forms of their respective visual fields.* (Poppelreuter, 1917/1990, p. 36)

Poppelreuter's conclusion that the perception of form, color, and movement could be dissociated in the visual fields of World War I veterans suffering penetrating missile wounds led him to speculate that these functions were served by different areas of the brain. This fractionation of visual functions was further elucidated by Newcombe and Russell (1969), who provided clear evidence of a dissociation between visuoperceptual ("pattern analysis") and visuospatial ability in the human brain. Their patients were World War II veterans suffering from focal, penetrating missile wounds who were tested on a visuoperceptual (closure) and visuospatial (maze learning) task. Patients with left-hemisphere lesions did not differ from controls, whereas the right-hemisphere lesion group was inferior to the left-hemisphere lesion group on both tasks. Within the right-hemisphere group they culled out several who manifested a "double dissociation" between visuoperceptual and visuospatial performance: those individuals with defective visuoperceptual performance retained relatively preserved visuospatial ability, whereas those individuals with defective visuospatial performance retained relatively preserved visuoperceptual ability. Individuals performing most defectively on the visuoperceptual task had lesions in the region of the right posterior temporal lobe, with involvement of the temporo-parietal-occipital junction. Individuals performing most defectively on the visuospatial task had superior right parietal lesions in close proximity to the longitudinal (interhemispheric) fissure, usually with occipital involvement.

Newcombe and Russell's demonstration of the dissociation of visuoperceptual and visuospatial functioning in humans was paralleled by the discovery of two separate higher visual systems in nonhuman primates (Newcombe, 1985). Lesion and electrophysiological experiments in primates disclosed that visual object discrimination and processing of visual space could be selectively disrupted by focal lesions in different areas of the cerebrum (e.g., Cowey & Gross, 1970; Iwai & Mishkin, 1968; Pohl, 1973), a phenomenon that has been referred to as the "what versus where" distinction (Maunsell, 1987; Ungerleider & Mishkin, 1982; but see Ettlinger, 1990, for a critical review of this concept).

In nonhuman primates, both the visuoperceptual and visuospatial systems derive their input from the photoreceptors, but these systems exhibit segregation as early as the ganglion cell level of the retina (Livingstone & Hubel, 1988). The two visual systems remain almost completely segregated from their relay centers in discrete cell layers of the lateral geniculate nucleus to their representation in multiple retinotopic maps in the occipital cortex. The visuoperceptual system is referred to as the "parvocellular" system because it arises from the dorsal layers of the lateral geniculate nucleus, which contain relatively small neurons. The visuospatial system is referred to as the "magnocellular" system because it arises from the ventral layers of the lateral geniculate nucleus, which contain relatively large neurons. Although both systems are represented in many of the same cortical areas, they retain their segregation by synapsing in separate cortical cell layers. For example, although both the visuoperceptual and visuospatial systems course from the lateral geniculate nucleus to the primary visual cortex in the occipital lobe, the visuoperceptual system synapses in cell layer 4C-beta, whereas the visuospatial system synapses in cell layer 4C-alpha.

The ultimate destination of the visuoperceptual system is the inferior temporal cortex, whereas the ultimate destination of the visuospatial system is the posterior parietal cortex. As described in Table 6.1, the two visual systems are not only anatomically segregated, they are physiologically distinct in their specialization for the processing of the qualities of objects, or conversely, their location in space. Demonstrations of the dissociation between visuoperceptual and visuospatial processing may be apparent in some patients suffering focal brain lesions (e.g., Newcombe, Ratcliff, & Damasio, 1987), and in normal subjects using experimental techniques (Livingstone & Hubel, 1987, 1988). For example, the spatial qualities of stimuli tend to be neutralized when stimuli are made equiluminant. Because it can process only luminance contrast, and not color, the magnocellular system is unable to process the spatial information inherent in colored but equiluminant stimuli. The parvocellular system is able to process the color information in the equiluminant stimuli, but lacks the specialized capacity to process the spatial aspects of visual material.

DISORDERS OF VISUAL PERCEPTION

Disorders of Visuoperceptual Functioning

Primary Sensory Impairment

The ability to perform simple visual discriminations for single stimulus attributes such as size, brightness, and length is relatively resistant to the effects of focal, unilateral lesions of the human brain (Bisiach, Nichelli, & Spinnler, 1976; Taylor & Warrington, 1973; Warrington & Rabin, 1970). Although there is a trend for patients with posterior right-hemisphere lesions to perform less well than other lesion groups on these tasks, this trend is neither statistically nor clinically reliable (Benton, 1985b). Thus, visuoperceptual disorders occurring in the context of right-hemisphere disease are not the result of elementary deficits in visual sensation or acuity. As Warrington (1982) has pointed out, the visuoperceptual deficit syndrome that may result from a focal hemispheric lesion is often not apparent when objects are seen under good viewing conditions and viewed from angles that provide maximal visual information. These visuoperceptual disorders may become manifest only when objects are transformed by an unusual angle or view, or when the amount of visual information they contain is degraded, or reduced through shadowing. The syndrome of visual object agnosia is an exception to this rule.

TABLE 6.1. Features of the Visuoperceptual and Visuospatial Systems[a]

	Visuoperceptual	Visuospatial
	Retina	
Ganglion cell type	P	M
Dendritic fields	Limited	Extensive
Cell bodies	Small	Large
Axonal conduction	Slow	Fast
	Lateral geniculate nucleus	
Cell types	Parvocellular	Magnocellular
Anatomic location	Dorsal Geniculate	Ventral Geniculate
Electrophysiology		
Response latency	Long	Short
Response length	Sustained	Transient
Sensitivity		
Spectral	Color selective	Color-blind
Contrast	Low	High
	Cerebral cortex	
Cortical areas	Inferior Temporal	Posterior Parietal
Receptive fields		
Include fovea	100%	60%
Relative size	Small	Large
Bilateral inputs	60%	40%
Electrophysiology		
Response latency	Long	Short
Response length	Sustained	Transient
Sensitivity		
Spectral	Color selective	Color-blind
Contrast	Low	High
Temporal resolution	Slow	Fast
Response selectivity		
Stimulus attributes	Complex Texture Shape	Simple Depth Motion
Face and hand selective cells present	Yes	No

[a]This table summarizes findings reported by Chagas, Gattass, & Gross, 1985; Desimone, Schein, Moran, & Ungerleider, 1985; Gross et al., 1985; Livingstone & Hubel, 1987, 1988; Maunsell, 1987; Ungerleider & Mishkin, 1982; Wise & Desimone, 1988.

Visual Agnosia

Visual Object Agnosia

The clinical syndrome Jackson described as "imperception" was experimentally induced in dogs by Hermann Munk (cited in Benton, 1978). After surgical destruction of the convex surfaces of the occipital lobes, Munk observed that the dogs were capable of spatial navigation, but no longer responded in a meaningful way to familiar objects such as their human master, the sight of a whip with which they had been trained, or a bowl of food. Munk described this condition as "mindblindedness," and he proposed that the dogs "see, but do not understand."

Munk's findings received clinical support in 1890 from Lissauer (cited in Benton, 1978), who described in detail a patient whose deficits closely resembled those of Munk's dogs. Lissauer also introduced a distinction between "apperceptive" and "associative" contributions to visual recognition, the former involving derangement of visuoanalytic processing, and the latter involving derangement of semantic or functional identification. Subsequently, Freud (1891/1953) introduced the term *agnosia* (from the Greek "not knowing") to describe the deficits of patients who had specific difficulties in recognizing familiar objects, persons, and places. Modern nomenclature discards the terms *imperception* and *mindblindedness,* but retains Freud's *agnosia* to describe deficits in recognition. Lissauer's conceptual dichotomy is also retained, in that agnosias are described as either apperceptive or associative in nature, even though, as Benton (1990) has pointed out, Lissauer thought in terms of the contributions of two separate processes to a single visual syndrome. Currently, many investigators accept Teuber's (1965) position that the concept of agnosia should be restricted to an inability to appreciate an object's meaning in the context of normal perception. Thus, only the associative, or semantic, form of the syndrome is considered to constitute a "pure" agnosia.

Prosopagnosia

> Gazing in a mirror, he described the delineaments of what he saw, but could not recognize the face as his [own]. (Critchley, 1953, p. 293)

Although the inability to recognize familiar faces had been described as a specific syndrome by Quaglino and Borelli in 1867, the now familiar term *prosopagnosia* to describe this deficit was introduced much later by Bodamer in 1947. Visual object agnosia is always accompanied by prosopagnosia, although prosopagnosia may exist independently of a general visual object agnosia. These patients are unable to recognize the faces of immediate family members, although they may achieve recognition of familiar persons on the basis of voice, clothing, or gait. As described above by Critchley (1953), one of Bodamer's patients even failed to recognize himself in a mirror. Bodamer saw prosopagnosia as a highly selective perceptual deficit confined to the recognition of the human face. This concept cannot account for the fact that prosopagnosic patients are almost always unable to identify the meaning of other objects, such as abstract symbols.

It is clear that the deficit underlying prosopagnosia is not simply a failure to appreciate the visual configuration of the human face. Warrington and James (1967) and Benton and Van Allen (1972) demonstrated that patients afflicted with prosopagnosia may perform quite adequately on formal tests calling for the discrimination of unfamiliar faces.

Prosopagnosia has been explained as a highly selective memory disorder (e.g., Warrington & James, 1967), or alternatively, as an inability to appreciate the individual identity of a given item within a general category (Damasio, Damasio, & Van Hoesen, 1982; Whitely & Warrington, 1977). Many prosopagnosic patients may recognize a face as being a face, but the specific features of that face fail to activate the individual memories associated with a given person. This conceptualization may be applicable to some prosopagnosic patients, who cannot, for example, recognize their own automobiles (Damasio et al., 1982), although there are other prosopagnosic patients who are able to recognize their personal belongings when they are placed among similar items owned by others (De Renzi, 1986).

The fact that correlated deficits in memory, perception, and symbolic thought may all be present or absent in a particular patient with prosopagnosia led Benton (1980, 1985a, 1990) and De Renzi (1986) to suggest that there may be distinctly different types of prosopagnosia. Also, there is considerable variability in the phenomenological descriptions of faces provided by patients with the disorder. The majority are able to describe faces accurately, but some patients perceive the faces as distorted, or with morbid affective features (e.g., the "prosopometamorphopsia" described by Critchley, 1953).

Faust (cited from Benton, 1985b), Hécaen and Angelergues (1962), and Meadows (1974) attributed prosopagnosia to right inferior occipital lesions because of the strong association of the disorder with left superior quadrantanopsia. However, cases coming to autopsy have revealed bilateral disease (Benton, 1979, 1985b; Damasio et al., 1982). Neuroimaging data on living prosopagnosic patients supported this view of the anatomic correlates of the disorder, such that bilateral mesial temporo-occipital lesions were seen as necessary for the development of disorder (Damasio & Damasio, 1983; Damasio et al., 1982). More recently, Benton (1990) has suggested that in light of new reports of prosopagnosia in which neuroimaging data, and even a single autopsied case, demonstrated unilateral right-hemisphere disease, perhaps the view that bilateral lesions are a necessary condition for prosopagnosia should be revisited. Although the recognition of familiar faces is a process involving both hemsipheres, a unilateral right temporo-occipital lesion may be necessary and sufficient for the onset of prosopagnosia.

In a recent series of positron emission tomography (PET) studies, Sergent and colleagues (Sergent, Ohta, & McDonald, 1992; Sergent & Signoret, 1992) demonstrated that prosopagnosia may best be thought of as a disorder in which facial processing may be deranged at any one of a number of anatomic and functional modules. The results of their functional imaging studies suggest that the right lingual and fusiform gyri are involved in processing the configurational invariants of a face. The right hippocampal gyrus may associate the perceptual invariants of the face with relevant biographical information about that face, with the anterior temporal lobe bilaterally extracting further biographical information that is not exclusively activated by facial information. A lesion at any one of these anatomic and functional modules may potentially yield prosopagnosia. Although the left hemisphere contributes to facial processing, its role is seen as limited, and a single right-hemisphere lesion is viewed as necessary and sufficient to cause prosopagnosia.

The discovery of face and hand selective cells in the lateral inferior temporal cortex of the macaque (Gross, Desimone, Albright, & Schwartz, 1985) supports the notion that the perception of faces holds a special place in cognition (Benton, 1980, 1990). Investigators have found that these neurons demonstrate response selectivity for faces viewed at a particular angle of regard, with electrophysiological responding decreased by removing individual features of the stimulus face, such as an eye (Gross et al., 1985). Rearrangement of the internal configuration of the face reduces responding to the level of spontaneous firing. In humans, lesions to the medial, rather than the lateral, inferior temporal cortex tend to be crucial in producing prosopagnosia (Sergent & Signoret, 1992).

Discrimination of Unfamiliar Faces

Tasks calling for the discrimination of unfamiliar faces were developed to investigate the mechanisms of prosopagnosia (Benton, 1980). Yet, as mentioned above, investigators subsequently discovered that many prosopagnosic patients performed adequately on these tasks, whereas a high rate of impairment was seen in patients with focal neurological disease but who did not manifest prosopagnosia (Benton & Van Allen, 1968; Warrington & James, 1967). A recent study (Capruso, Hamsher, Levin, & Barr, 1993) using the Facial Recognition Test has reconfirmed that the discrimination of familiar faces (U.S. presidents) remains preserved in the overwhelming majority of patients with right-hemisphere lesions, even though approximately one-half of these same patients performed defectively in discriminating unfamiliar faces.

The Facial Recognition Test (Benton, Hamsher, Varney, & Spreen, 1983) has, in particular, been the subject of a series of experiments aimed at determining the relationship between neurological variables, locus of lesion, and visuoperceptual performance. The task, illustrated in Figure 6.1, has three components: matching of identical front-view faces, matching of faces transformed by angle of view, and matching of faces transformed by shadowing. Hamsher, Levin, and Benton (1979) found that defective performance in discrimination of unfamiliar faces is common only in patients with right-hemisphere lesions, and in aphasic patients with left-hemisphere lesions who also have impairment in language comprehension. The frequency of defective performance was higher in both these groups when the lesion was located in the posterior portion of the hemisphere. The performance of patients with left-hemisphere lesions who were nonaphasic, or who were aphasic but without language comprehension defects, did not differ from normal controls.

The finding that a minority of individuals with left-hemisphere disease perform defectively on the Facial Recognition Test was further investigated by Capruso and Risser (1992). They found that those patients with left-hemisphere lesions (n = 18) performing defectively were able to match identical front-view faces at satisfactory

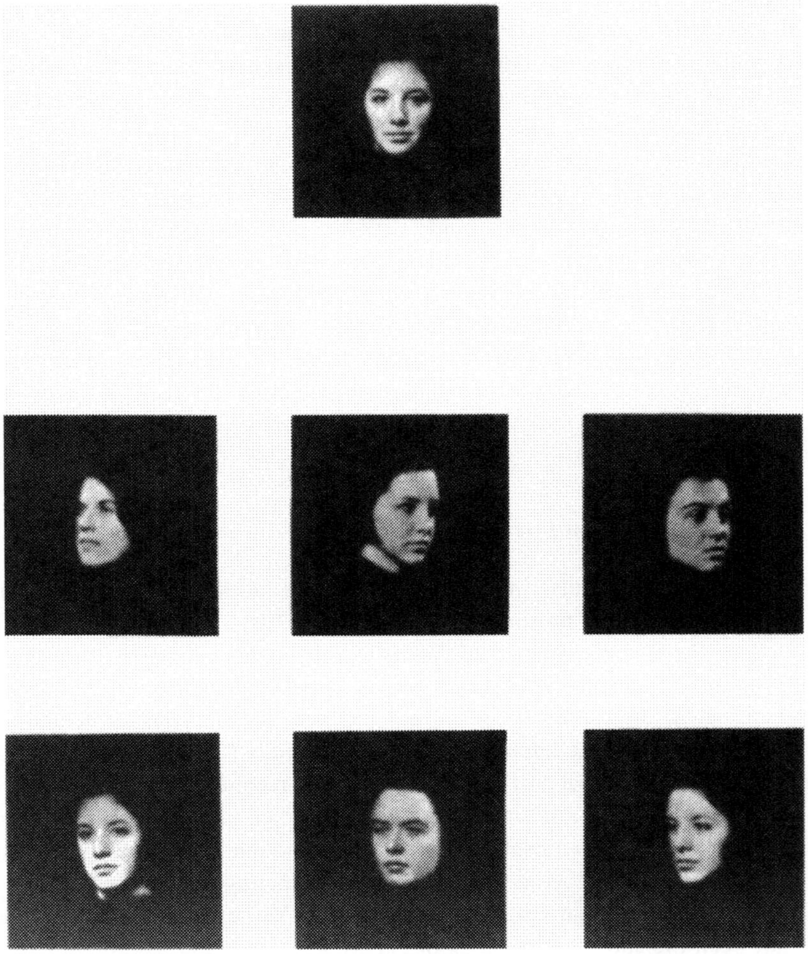

FIGURE 6.1. Angle transformation item from the Facial Recognition Test. The task is to match the face at top with three faces from the array at bottom. From Benton, A. L., Hamsher, K. deS., Varney, N. R., & Spreen, O. (1983). *Contributions to neuropsychological assessment: A clinical manual.* New York: Oxford University Press. Copyright © 1983 by Oxford University Press, Inc. Reprinted by permission.

levels. However, 48% of patients with right-hemisphere lesions (n = 27) showed significant impairments in matching identical front-view faces, as well as in matching faces transformed by angle or shadow configuration. This finding confirms Benton's (1967) observation that, although a minority of patients with left-hemisphere disease will perform at defective levels on some tasks of complex visual perception, the severity of deficit is typically much greater in patients with right-hemisphere disease.

Levin, Grossman, and Kelly (1977) found that closed head injury patients with coma durations of less than 24 hours had a relatively low rate of defective performance (12%) on the Facial Recognition Test. In contrast, those patients with coma durations greater than 24 hours had a significantly higher rate of impairment (50%), suggesting that visuoperceptual deficits in head-injured patients are associated with substantial and diffuse cerebral damage. An association between aphasic disturbance and impairment in facial discrimination was also seen in seriously head-injured patients. Of those patients without neurological signs of brainstem trauma, the presence of an aphasic disturbance on formal testing was associated with poorer facial discrimination performances.

Visual Analysis

Discrimination of Overlapping Figures. An example of this type of task is provided in Figure 6.2. The discrimination of overlapping figures was introduced by Poppelreuter (1917/1990) as a brief method for the study of visual analysis. Since that time, overlapping figures have been used in a number of investigations of patients with focal brain lesions. Patients with right-hemisphere lesions have been observed to manifest particularly poor performances (De Renzi & Spinnler, 1966), as have patients with lesions in the posterior areas of the brain in general (Masure & Tzavaras, 1976).

Discrimination of Hidden Figures. The visual analysis of geometric figures for the extraction of an "embedded" target stimulus was introduced by Gottschaldt (cited in Benton, 1985b), and a more widely used version of the task was introduced by Thurstone (1944). An example of this type of task is provided in Figure 6.3. Performance on extracting embedded figures is affected by lesions of either hemisphere (Corkin, 1979; Teuber, Battersby, & Bender, 1960). Aphasic patients (Russo & Vignolo, 1967) tend to have severe difficulties on these tasks. Patients with frontal lobe lesions (Teuber, Battersby, & Bender, 1951) and patients with Korsakoff's psychosis (Talland, 1965) also tend to manifest significant difficulties with the detection of embedded figures, perhaps due to impairment in disengaging and shifting perceptual sets.

Visual Synthesis

Closure Tasks. "Closure" tasks require that patients identify a single object that has been obscured by exaggerated shadowing and loss of contour cues. Of these tasks, the Mooney faces test (1956) has been the subject of the most clinical investigation. A sample item is provided in Figure 6.4. Both Newcombe (1969) and Lansdell (1970) demonstrated that this closure task is most sensitive to lesions of the right temporal lobe. Despite the fact that Mooney's test uses faces as stimuli, the task apparently has little relation to the Facial Recognition Test (Newcombe et al., 1987). In fact, the correlation between the Mooney faces and the Benton faces is on the order of $r = .04$ for patients with right-hemisphere disease (Wasserstein, Zappulla, Rosen, Gerstman, & Rock, 1987). The Street Gestalt Completion Test (Street, 1931) is another closure test using a variety of nonfacial objects as stimuli, and patients with lesions of the right hemisphere have been shown to be selectively impaired (Benton, 1985b).

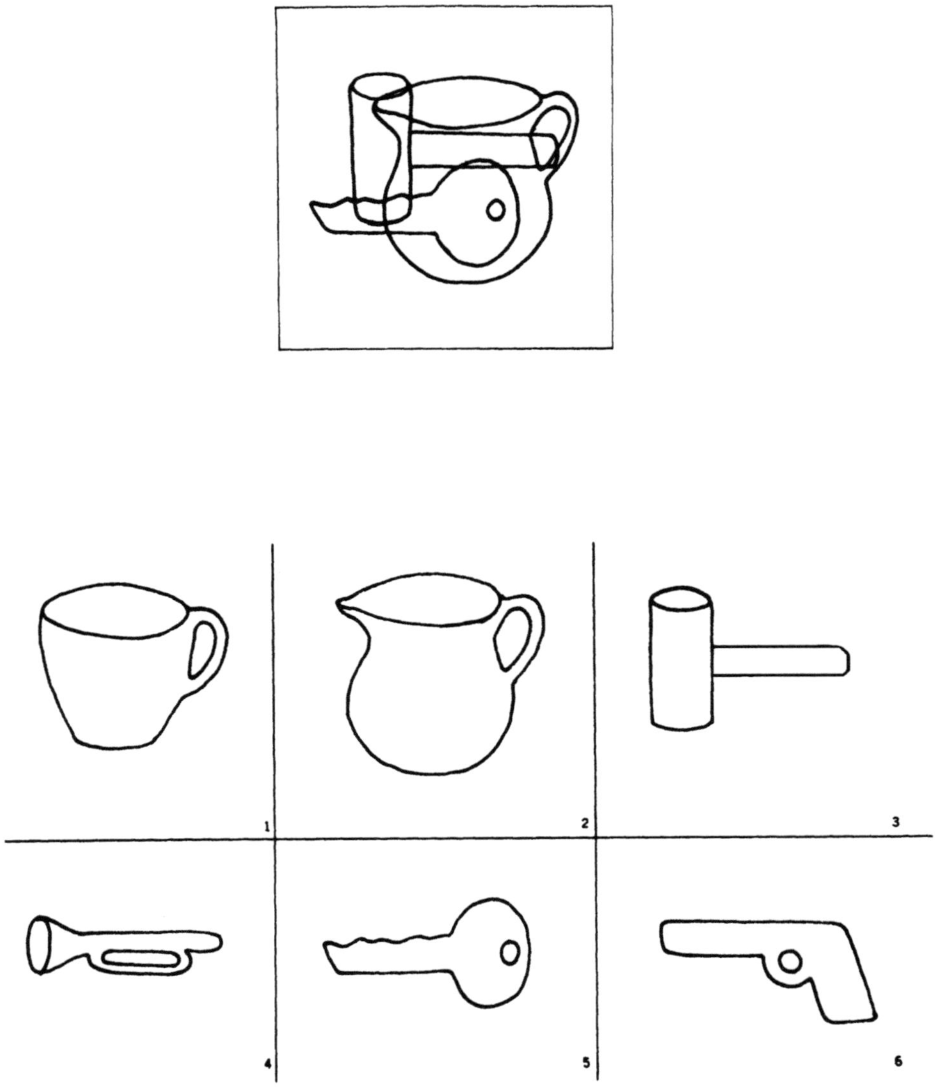

FIGURE 6.2. Overlapping figure task. From Ayres, A. J. (1972). *Sensory integration and praxis tests.* Copyright © 1972 by Western Psychological Services. Reprinted by permission of the publisher, Western Psychological Services, 12031 Wilshire Boulevard, Los Angeles, California 90025.

Visual Organization. The organization of fragmented objects into a perceptual whole may be measured by such tasks as the Object Assembly subtest of the Wechsler Adult Intelligence Scale-Revised (WAIS-R; Wechsler, 1981) and the Hooper Visual Organization Test (Hooper, 1983). Object Assembly has the advantage of placing no demands on naming ability, but demands constructional ability. In contrast, the Hooper places no demands on motoric or constructional ability, but demands naming ability. However, there is little evidence that this task assesses constructional or spatial ability, not does it appear sensitive to focal brain lesions (Spreen & Strauss, 1991).

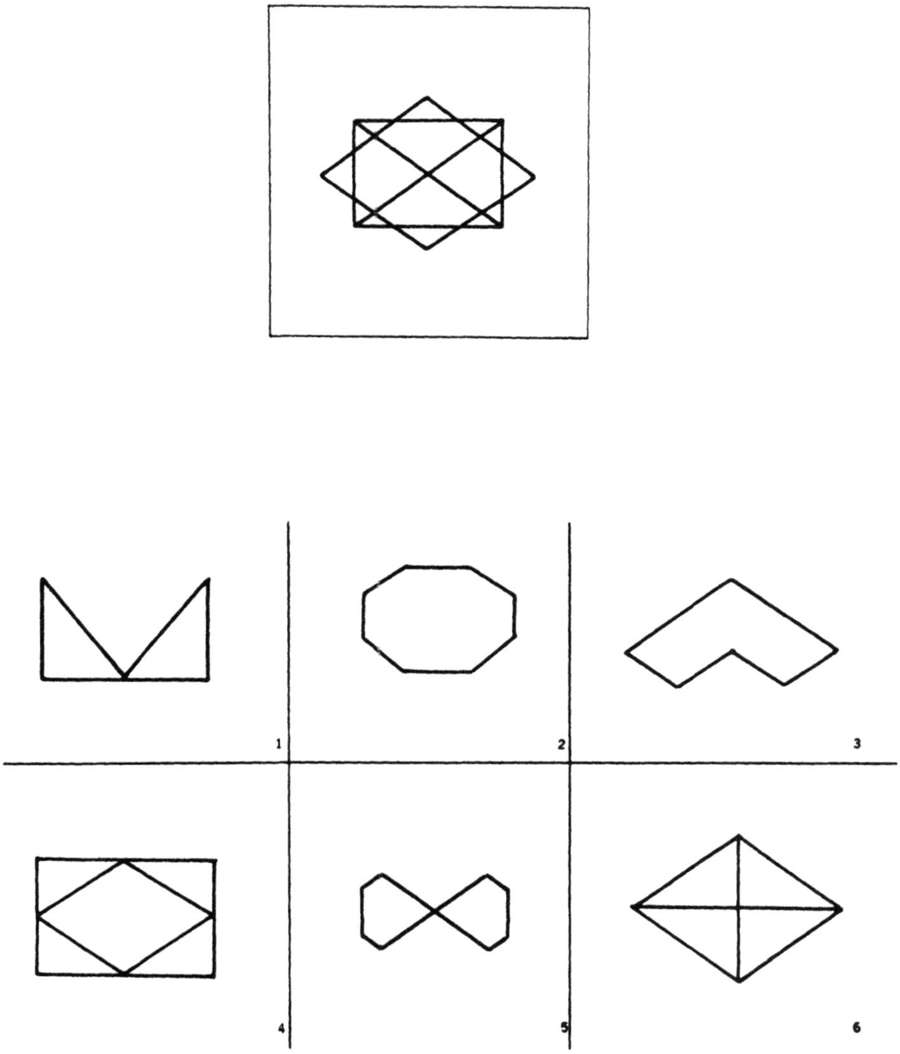

FIGURE 6.3. Hidden figures task. From Ayres, A. J. (1972). *Sensory integration and praxis tests.* Copyright © 1972 by Western Psychological Services. Reprinted by permission of the publisher, Western Psychological Services, 12031 Wilshire Boulevard, Los Angeles, California, 90025.

Visual Integration of a Complex Scene. The ability to perceive and appreciate the individual elements of a complex perceptual array, while failing to comprehend the percept's obvious relationship with other closely situated stimuli, has been reported in several case studies (Kinsbourne & Warrington, 1962, 1963; studies cited in Farah, 1990). This clinical phenomenon was termed "simultanagnosia" by Wolpert (cited in Benton, 1985b). It is most clearly seen when patients are presented with a dramatic picture in which several interrelated activities are depicted (e.g., the "Cookie Theft" picture from the Boston Diagnostic Aphasia Examination; Goodglass & Kaplan, 1983). The patient described as having simultanagnosia will only be able to identify

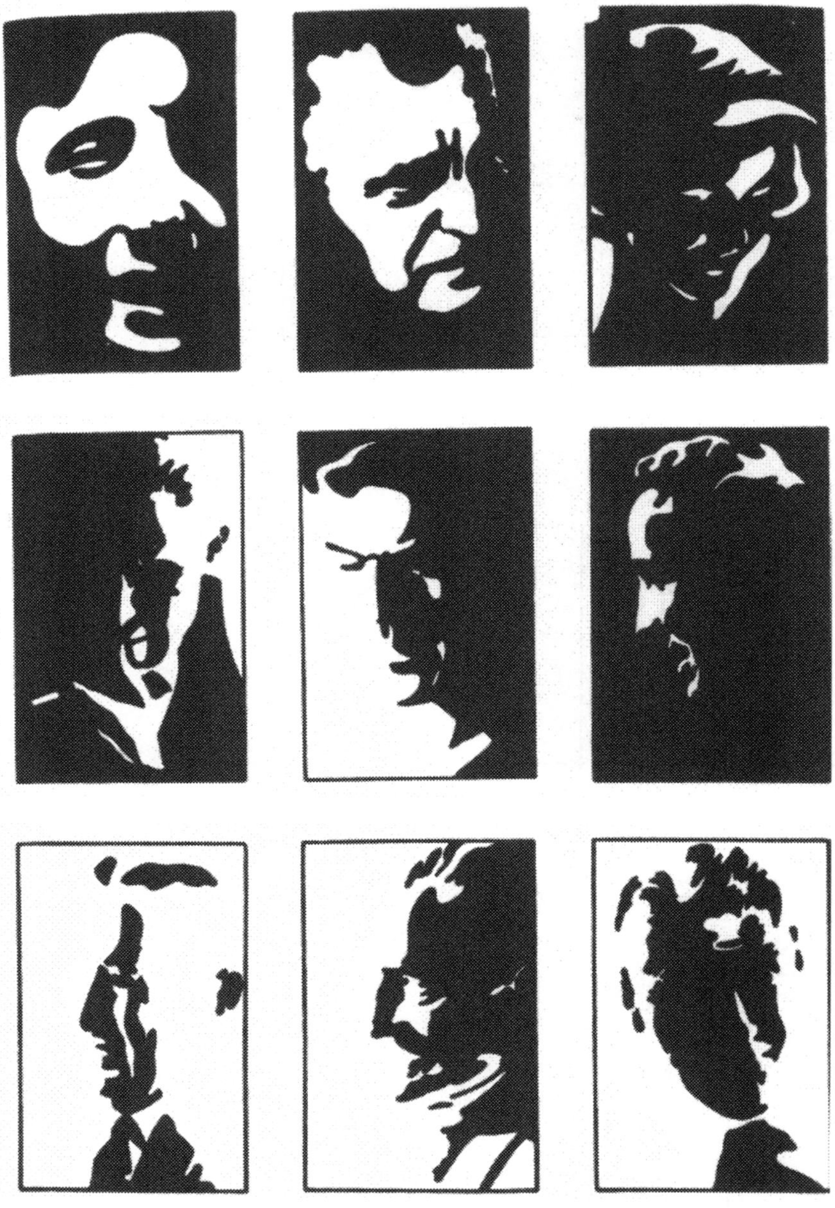

FIGURE 6.4. Closure test item. The task is to identify the gender of the face, and whether the face is that of a child, a young man or woman, or an old man or woman. From Mooney, C. M. (1956). Closure with negative after-images under flickering light. *Canadian Journal of Psychology, 10,* 191–199. Copyright © 1956 by Canadian Psychological Association. Reprinted by permission.

the parts in the scene and not the overall meaning (gestalt). As Farah (1990) has emphasized, this disorder is best understood as a disorder of selective visual attention, rather than of form perception.

Color Perception

Color vision is clearly a function of the visuoperceptual system and is segregated from visuospatial processing (Livingstone & Hubel, 1987, 1988). The parvocellular layers of the lateral geniculate nucleus, which innervate the cortical systems mediating form vision, project to the spectrally sensitive "blob" and "interblob" systems. The blob system responds selectively to the quality (hue) of colors. The interblob system is functionally capable of processing both form and color contrast, but does not respond selectively to the quality of colors. The ultimate projection area of the blob system is in the temporo-occipital cortex. The magnocellular system, which mediates visuospatial ability, is, in fact, color-blind. Deficits in color appreciation may involve perceptual, linguistic, or associational domains of cognition (Benton, 1985b).

Achromatopsia. Achromatopsia describes a deficit in color perception resulting from an acquired brain lesion. In this way achromatopsia is distinguished from the color vision deficits that are caused by congenital or acquired disease affecting the spectrally sensitive photoreceptors and photopigments in the retina. De Renzi and Spinnler (1967) found that 23% of their patients with right-hemisphere lesions and 12% of their patients with left-hemisphere lesions had some degree of impairment in color perception as measured by performance on the Ishihara plates, perhaps in part due to achromatic perceptual factors. Among individuals with right-hemisphere lesions, deficits in color perception were associated with visual field defects (and therefore posterior lesions). Among those with left-hemisphere lesions, deficits in color perception were associated with aphasia. Although abnormal color perception may be apparent in a substantial minority of patients with unilateral right-hemisphere lesions (De Renzi & Spinnler, 1967; Scotti & Spinnler, 1970), impairment in color perception severe enough to warrant the diagnosis of achromatopsia is relatively rare. As Damasio and Damasio (1983) point out, the rarity of achromatopsia is related to the type of lesion needed to produce selective loss of color vision. A lesion in the inferior temporo-occipital junction (fusiform gyrus) is required, sparing both the optic radiations and the primary visual cortex. A bilateral lesion in this crucial area will produce "full" achromatopsia in both visual fields, whereas a unilateral lesion may produce a "hemiachromatopsia" affecting only the contralateral visual field. Zeki (1973, 1983) has identified a seemingly homologous area in the temporal lobe of the macaque that also contains a high proportion of color-selective neurons.

Color Anomia. Deficits in color naming or in identifying colors to command are strongly associated with the presence of aphasic disorders (Benton, 1985b). However, De Renzi and Spinnler (1967) identified patients with left-hemisphere disease who suffer color anomia, despite otherwise preserved general naming ability and intact color perception. They also determined that color anomia may accompany defective color perception in some nonaphasic individuals with right-hemisphere disease. Selective anomias for color have been reported as part of the syndrome of alexia without agraphia that can result from lesions of the left occipital lobe and splenium of the corpus callosum (Geschwind & Fusillo, 1964, 1966; Gloning, Gloning, & Hoff, 1968).

Color Association. Deficits in color cognition, independent of impairments in both color perception and color naming ability, may be demonstrated by having patients color with crayons or colored pencils black and white drawings of objects that are distinctively colored in the environment, such as a banana (De Renzi & Spinnler, 1967). Using this method, De Renzi and Spinnler found deficits in color association in approximately 50% of aphasic patients. Varney (1982) had patients match black and white drawings of distinctively colored objects with a multiple-choice array of colors. He found that deficits in color association were invariably associated with alexia, although alexic deficits were often seen independently of color association deficits. The strong relationship between deficits in color association, aphasia, and, especially, alexia implies that left-hemisphere lesions may result in impairment of conceptual processes that seemingly require little or no language ability for their performance (De Renzi, Faglioni, Scotti, & Spinnler, 1972; De Renzi & Spinnler, 1967).

Disorders of Visuospatial Functioning

Balint-Holmes Syndrome

Badal, Balint, and Holmes (cited in Benton, 1982) each produced separate but similar clinical descriptions of patients who manifested a profound visuospatial disorder that would come to be known as the Balint, or Balint-Holmes syndrome. The syndrome consists of the symptom tetrad of oculomotor apraxia (psychic paralysis of gaze), misreaching (optic ataxia, visuomotor apraxia or ataxia), impaired visual attention (simultanagnosia), and defective judgment of distances (De Renzi, 1982; Newcombe & Ratcliff, 1989). The spatial disturbance in these patients may be so severe that they collide with large objects in their path. Balint-Holmes syndrome has typically been associated with bilateral parietal lesions. Damasio and Benton (1979) concluded that the superior parietal lobule was the crucial lesion site, and this is consistent with the work of Mountcastle and his colleagues (1975), who found electrophysiological evidence that the superior parietal lobule of the monkey contains neurons that prepare and guide attention to points in space, and coordinate arm movements to spatial targets (objects of regard).

Visual Neglect

Inattention to stimuli occurring in the visual space opposite the side of a brain lesion is known as visual neglect or extinction. It can occur in the context of the more pervasive hemispatial neglect syndrome involving the sensory modalities of vision, audition, and tactile (somatosensory) perception (Heilman, Watson, & Valenstein,

1985). When the visual neglect syndrome is associated with tactile or somatosensory neglect (somatoagnosia) it may present quite dramatically, with patients failing to shave one side of the face or failing to dress one side of the body. That visual neglect is a disorder of attention and awareness, and not simply sensory impairment, is made apparent by several observations (Heilman et al., 1985; Poppelreuter, 1917/1990). Many patients with hemianopia scan and attend to the contralateral hemispace (Rosenberger, 1974), whereas some without visual field defects may neglect contralateral hemispace (McFie, Piercy, & Zangwill, 1950). Bisiach and Luzzatti (1978) found that patients with unilateral lesions may neglect one side of a familiar scene, even when they are imaging the scene. Neglect may be multimodal in that patients may ignore visual events, sounds, and somesthetic stimulation on the side contralateral to the lesion (De Renzi, Faglioni, & Scotti, 1970; Farah, Wong, Monheit, & Morrow, 1989; Heilman, Bowers, Coslett, & Watson, 1983).

Neglect occurs more frequently and with greater severity following unilateral right-hemisphere lesions than following unilateral left-hemisphere lesions (Albert, 1973; Gainotti, Messerli, & Tissot, 1972). This finding is consistent with other speculations that the right hemisphere may be specialized for both spatial and visuoattentional functioning. Lesions producing neglect have often been localized to the inferior parietal lobule (Brain, 1941; Heilman, Watson, Valenstein, & Damasio, 1983). However, it has been demonstrated that a multiplicity of lesion sites including the mesencephalic reticular formation (Watson, Heilman, Cauthen, & King, 1973), dorsolateral frontal lobe and cingulate gyrus (Damasio, Damasio & Chui, 1980; Heilman & Valenstein, 1972), thalamus (Watson & Heilman, 1979), and putamen may be contributory in the development of the neglect syndrome. Kertesz and Dobrowlski (1981) actually found a greater tendency toward neglect in patients with right frontal lesions than in patients with right parietal lesions. The increasing recognition of the role of frontal lobe lesions in neglect is consistent with evidence that spatial processing is mediated by a highly integrated neural system involving both prefontal and parietal areas (Selemon & Goldman-Rakic, 1988).

Stereopsis

An object viewed in near-space will produce an image on noncorresponding points of the left and right retina. Stereopsis describes the process through which the brain detects this retinal disparity and uses it to judge the depth of the object in space. The closer an object, the greater the degree of retinal disparity.

There are two types of stereopsis. "Local" stereopsis, or stereoacuity, demands the point-to-point matching of the retinal images produced by a well-defined object to arrive at a depth judgment for that object. Impairment of local stereopsis is found in a small minority of patients following lesions of either hemisphere (Hamsher, 1978a). "Global" stereopsis demands the fusion of an array of seemingly random points on two retinas into a single image with different levels of depth (Julesz, 1971). Forms may then be discriminated in the spatially resolved image according to their position in depth. A number of investigators (Benton & Hécaen, 1970; Carmon & Bechtoldt, 1969; Hamsher, 1978a) have found that although patients with left-hemisphere lesions who have adequate stereoacuity perform normally on tests of global stereopsis, patients with right-hemisphere lesions demonstrate a high rate of defective performance on these global stereoscopic tasks, while performing normally on tests of local stereopsis. Rizzo and Damasio (1985, cited in Livingstone & Hubel, 1987) found that occipito-parietal lesions in humans produced impairments in stereoacuity, although a recent study documented impairments in global stereopsis following right temporal lobectomy in seizure patients (Ptito, Zatorre, Larson, & Tosoni, 1991).

Experiments in the macaque (Poggio, 1984) have revealed a concentration of neurons sensitive to binocular disparity in the V2 retinotopic map in the occipital lobe (Brodmann's area 18). Even small lesions of this area produce considerable impairment of stereopsis (Cowey & Wilkinson, 1991). Lesions of the superior colliculus and its rostrally adjacent pretectum may also impair stereopsis through derangement of ocular convergence (Lawler & Cowey, 1986).

Anomalous Contour Illusions

Anomalous or subjective contour illusions are one of the most powerful demonstrations that perception is an active and organizing process of the human brain. These illusions are produced when a group of figures have interposition cues appearing as anomalies in their contours, causing the brain to perceive an opaque form in the foreground whose edges would overlap the other figures and thereby perceptually "explain" the anomalous contours (Kanizsa, 1986). An example is provided in Figure 6.5. Anomalous contour illusions are so potent that their edges appear to differ in brightness from the background of the illusion. Hamsher (1978b) found that in patients with right-hemisphere lesions, failure to perceive anomalous contours was associated with impairments in global stereopsis. This finding indicates that the right hemisphere is specialized not only for the perception of depth using retinal disparity cues for complex forms, but also for the perception of depth using monocular tasks in which the illusion of space is created using simple figure/ground effects. Stereopsis and anomalous contour illusions are neutralized under conditions of equiluminance, again indicating that illusions of spatial depth are a function of the magnocellular–parietal system, which cannot operate without luminance contrast. The parvocellular–temporal system, which can process equiluminant stimuli, cannot register the depth information that stereoscopic and anomalous contour illusions provide.

Visuospatial Judgment of Direction

Tasks requiring the judgment of line orientation are among the purest measures of visuospatial functioning (De Renzi, 1985). The evolution of judgment of line orientation from laboratory technique to clinical test also provides a clear example of the interplay between experimental and clinical techniques in neuropsychology (Benton, 1978). A number of investigators (Benton, Hannay, & Varney, 1975; De Renzi, Faglioni, & Scotti, 1971; Fontenot & Benton, 1972; Warrington & Rabin, 1970) had used Judgment of Line Orientation tasks as an experimental technique, and the results had consistently demonstrated significant deficits in performance in patients with right-

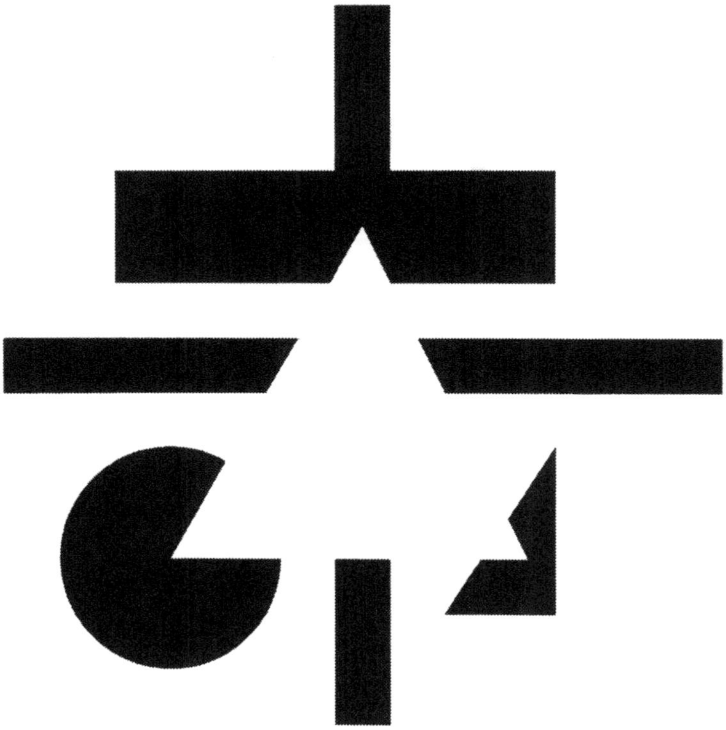

FIGURE 6.5. Anomalous contour illusion. The task is to name or trace the figure that appears in the center. From Hamsher, K. deS. (1978). Stereopsis and the perception of anomalous contours. *Neuropsychologia, 16*, 453–459. Copyright © by Pergamon Press, Ltd. Reprinted by permission.

hemisphere lesions when compared to patients with left-hemisphere lesions. Benton, Varney, and Hamsher (1978) introduced a brief, standardized version of the line orientation task. A sample item is provided in Figure 6.6. Judgment of Line Orientation demonstrated a high rate of defective performance (75%) following posterior right-hemisphere lesions, but showed preservation of performance in all but a minority (10%) of patients with left-hemisphere lesions. This finding has been replicated in several clinical studies (Levick, 1982; Trahan, 1991), and increases in right-hemisphere cerebral blood flow have been observed during performance of the Judgment of Line Orientation task (Deutsch, Bourbon, Papanicolaou, & Eisenberg, 1988).

Masure and Benton (1983) found that of left-handed or ambidextrous patients with focal brain lesions, 6/8 with right-hemisphere lesions and 0/7 patients with left-hemisphere lesions performed defectively on Judgment of Line Orientation. In Masure and Benton's sample, three patients had right-hemisphere lesions and aphasia, thus demonstrating that language functions were represented in the right hemisphere. All three patients performed defectively on Judgment of Line Orientation, suggesting that the right hemisphere is specialized for visuospatial functioning even in those patients with atypical language lateralization.

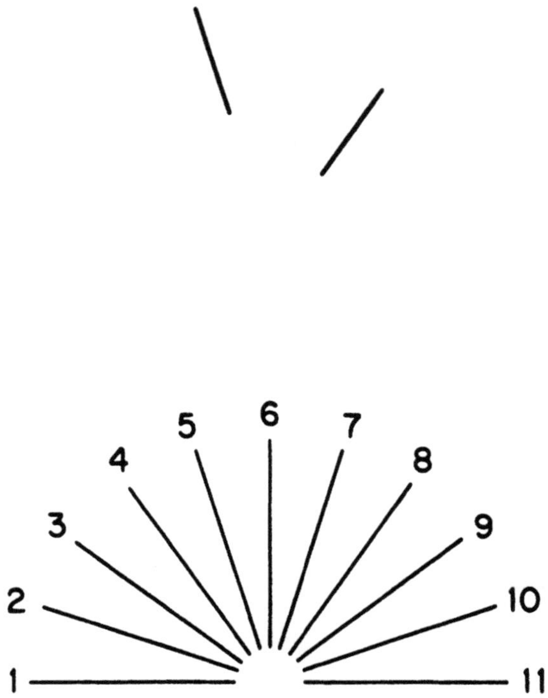

FIGURE 6.6. Item from Judgment of Line Orientation. The task is to match the two lines at top with the two lines in the array that point in the same direction and are in the same position on the page. Either verbal or pointing responses may be used. From Benton, A. L., Hamsher, K. deS., Varney, N. R., & Spreen, O. (1983). *Contributions to neuropsychological assessment: A clinical manual.* New York: Oxford University Press. Copyright © 1983 by Oxford University Press, Inc. Reprinted by permission.

A dissenting note was sounded by Mehta, Newcombe, and Damasio (1987). They reported that in select groups of World War II veterans the mean performance on Judgment of Line Orientation in those with left-hemisphere penetrating missile wounds was significantly worse than that of their controls, whereas the mean performance of those with right-hemisphere missile wounds was not. All groups in this study were of uncommonly high intelligence and appeared to have performed within the normal range on this task, thereby obscuring the meaning of their results. Hamsher, Capruso, and Benton (1992) administered Judgment of Line Orientation to 56 patients with unilateral lesions documented by computerized tomography (CT) or magnetic resonance imaging (MRI) to reexamine the relationship between unilateral hemispheric lesions and visuospatial judgment. This study replicated the findings of Benton et al. (1978) of a high rate of defective performance following right-hemisphere lesions, with a significantly lower rate of defective performance among those with left-hemisphere lesions. Although the mean performance of aphasic patients was significantly worse than that of nonaphasic patients, only a minority of aphasic patients performed defectively, demonstrating the relative preservation of performance on this task in the context of aphasia.

Topographic Disorientation

The inability to navigate familiar surroundings was a symptom shown by one of Jackson's patients (1876/1958), and similar cases have been thoroughly reviewed by De Renzi (1982). As he points out, this deficit may be better described as "topographic amnesia" in patients whose deficits appear to stem from a memory disorder specific to spatial schema. Others have been described as manifesting "topographic agnosia" in that they fail to recognize familiar landmarks (Paterson & Zangwill, 1945). De Renzi (1982) concludes that either spatial memory or landmark recognition deficits may be responsible for topographical disorientation, depending on the specific case. De Renzi notes a strong association between topographical disorientation and lesions of the right hemsiphere, involving either the hippocampus or the posterior cerebral areas. Impairment on navigational tasks without a memory component may be observed in patients with lesions of either parietal lobe (Semmes, Weinstein, Ghent, & Teuber, 1955).

Visuoconstructive Ability

In 1912, Kleist (cited in Benton, 1982) introduced the term *constructional apraxia* to describe disturbances in assembling or drawing objects, in the context of otherwise intact motor performance. Visuoconstructive ability may be measured using a variety of tasks. The patient may be required to produce a two-dimensional drawing either on command or in imitation of a model. Two-dimensional models or patterns may also be reproduced through the manipulation of sticks or blocks. Critchley (1953) observed that patients performing adequately on two-dimensional tasks may display striking abnormalities on tasks demanding construction in three dimensions. For this reason, Benton and Fogel (1962) developed, standardized, and normed the Three-Dimensional Block Construction task illustrated in Figure 6.7.

The diversity of visuoconstructive tasks that have been employed led Benton (1985b) to note the differing demands these tasks place on sustained attention, motor skills, spatial judgment, and for some, intellectual ability. In fact, Benton (1973) found correlations of relatively modest magnitude among visuoconstructive tasks of varying format. Stick constructions, WAIS Block Designs, and Three-Dimensional Block Constructions were intercorrelated in the range of *phi*(100) = .32 to .39. In contrast, graphomotor design copying tasks were intercorrelated in the range of *phi*(100) = .24 to .28 with the other constructional tasks, suggesting that graphomotor design copying tasks may represent a distinct type of visuoconstructive performance. Kleist (1922, cited in Benton, 1982) proposed that the parieto-occipital area of the left hemisphere was the site of lesion producing constructional apraxia. Nevertheless, the preponderance of subsequent research has demonstrated that constructional disability is more frequently seen in patients with right-hemisphere lesions than in patients with left-hemisphere lesions (e.g., Benton, 1973, Benton & Fogel, 1962; Hécaen, Ajuriaguerra, & Massonet, 1951; McFie, Piercy, & Zangwill, 1950; Paterson & Zangwill, 1944; Piercy & Smyth, 1962). Moreover, it has been repeatedly demonstrated that although

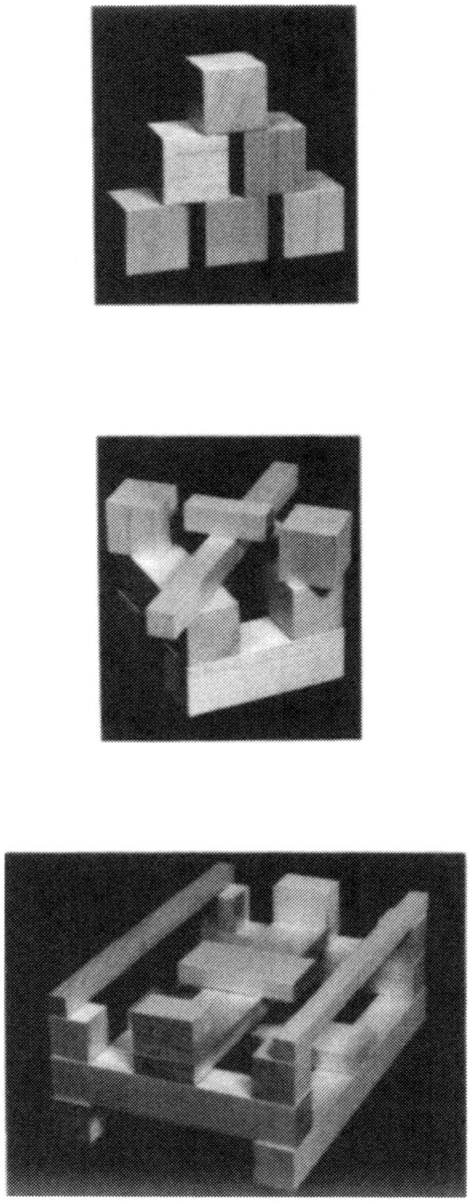

FIGURE 6.7. Stimulus models from the Three-Dimensional Block Construction test. The task is to construct a copy of the model from a selection of blocks provided by the examiner. From Benton, A. L. Hamsher, K. deS., Varney, N. R., & Spreen, O. (1983). *Contributions to neuropsychological assessment: A clinical manual.* New York: Oxford University Press. Copyright © 1983 by Oxford University Press, Inc. Reprinted by permission.

there are a substantial minority of patients with left-hemisphere lesions who show a degree of visuoconstructive disability, patients with right-hemisphere lesions typically demonstrate a severity of deficit beyond that of patients with left-hemisphere lesions (Benton, 1967, 1973). An exception to this rule may be seen in performances on the Wechsler Block Design task. Benton (1967) noted that on the Wechsler Block Design test, left- and right-hemisphere groups tend to show an equal frequency and severity of deficit. Benton interpreted this finding as support for the notion that the Wechsler Block Design task, which demands the assembly of a design from a schematic model under speeded conditions and involves the use of a greater number of diverse cognitive resources (visual analysis, visual synthesis, spatial and planning ability) than other constructional tasks, is therefore more sensitive to lesions of either hemisphere.

Visuoconstructive disability is most commonly associated with lesions in the posterior parietal area (Critchley, 1953; Hécaen, Penfield, Bertrans, & Malmo, 1956; Newcombe, 1969). However, visuoconstructive disability may also result from lesions in the frontal lobes (Benton, 1968), perhaps in some cases due more to deficits in planning ability than spatial impairment (Gainotti, 1985; Luria & Tsvetkova, 1964).

Because of the complexity of the responses involved and the latitude afforded to patients in the method by which they may perform constructional tasks, qualitative analysis of performance can be of particular clinical usefulness. The WAIS-R Block Design task often yields different error patterns depending on the laterality of the cerebral lesion (Critchley, 1953; Kaplan, 1990). A clinical illustration is provided in the case studies at the end of this chapter.

The nature of the basic disability causing defective visuoconstructive performances has been the subject of considerable debate. Kleist (1934, cited in Benton, 1967) saw visuoconstructive disability as an executive deficit resulting from disconnection of the visual association areas in the occipital and posterior parietal cortices from the anterior motor and premotor areas. Kleist's conception prefigured Geschwind's (1965) later examples of "disconnection syndromes." Kleist believed that constructional apraxia existed independently of either visuospatial deficit or motor disability, and that instead the phenomenon represented a failure in integration of these two intact abilities. Subsequent investigators (Arrigoni & De Renzi, 1964; Dee, 1970; Piercy & Smyth, 1962) have demonstrated that visuoconstructive disability is almost always associated with a more general visuoperceptual or visuospatial impairment. A number of investigators (Duensing, 1953, cited from Benton, 1982; Costa & Vaughan, 1962; Ettlinger, Warrington, & Zangwill, 1957) have proposed that an executive or apractic form of constructional impairment may be observed following left-hemisphere lesions (corresponding to the concept of constructional apraxia advanced by Kleist), whereas a perceptually based constructional impairment may be observed following right-hemisphere lesions. Although some studies have supported this distinction, a greater number have not (Gainotti, 1985). Also, the association between perceptual deficits and visuoconstructive disability has been observed to have equivalent magnitude in patients with either left- or right-hemisphere lesions (Arena & Gainotti, 1978; Dee, 1970; Piercy & Smyth, 1962).

VISUAL DISORDERS IN PATIENTS WITH DIFFUSE OR DEGENERATIVE BRAIN DISEASE

Thus far, this chapter has focused almost exclusively on patients suffering from focal brain disease from etiologies such as stroke, tumor, or penetrating missile wound. Attention will now turn to visuoperceptual, visuospatial, and visuoconstructive performance in patients suffering from diffuse and/or degenerative brain disease.

Alcohol Abuse

A number of investigators (e.g., Parsons & Farr, 1981; Tarter & Edwards, 1985) have found relative deficits on nonverbal tasks, particularly on the WAIS-R Performance scale, in alcoholic patients. Some (Jones, 1971; Jones & Parsons, 1972; Parsons & Leber, 1981) have hypothesized that alcohol abuse may cause disproportionately severe dysfunction in the right hemisphere. This position has engendered considerable controversy (Ryan & Butters, 1982; Walsh, 1985), as it is difficult to understand why a toxicometabolic condition should affect one hemisphere more than the other. Typically, critics have pointed out that many perceptual–constructional tasks, such as those found in the WAIS-R Performance scale, are speeded whereas those in the Verbal scale are not.

Toxicometabolic Confusional States

Lee and Hamsher (1988) found that patients suffering from nonalcoholic toxicometabolic confusional states showed a particularly high frequency of defective performance on visuospatial and visuoconstructive tasks, relative to equally challenging verbal tasks. Lee and Hamsher's use of unspeeded tasks, and the comments of patients perplexed by their own difficulties on such seemingly familiar tasks as Three-Dimensional Block Construction, suggest that the differential novelty of perceptual tasks was not the determining factor in poor performance. They propose that increased difficulties with perceptual tasks may have been caused by the fact that these tasks generally demand fine judgments in comparing similar and easily confused stimuli, thus making these patients susceptible to the deficits in self-monitoring that commonly accompany diffuse toxicometabolic conditions of the brain.

Dementia

Deficits in visuoperceptual and visuospatial functioning are common in patients with dementia (Eslinger & Benton, 1983; Freedman & Dexter, 1991; Ska, Poissant, & Joanette, 1990). Yet, orientation and memory tasks typically provide much greater sensitivity for the purpose of detecting early cognitive demise in patients with primary (e.g., Alzheimer's disease) and secondary (e.g., multi-infarct disease) neurodegenerative disorders. For example, the rate of defective performance on the Benton Visual Retention Test was 66% for patients with mild to moderate dementia of varying etiologies, whereas only 23% of these patients performed defectively on the Facial Recognition Test, with 32% performing defectively on Judgment of Line Orientation (Eslinger, Damasio, Benton, & Van Allen, 1985).

In the context of a severe dementia of either vascular or degenerative etiology, perceptual deficits severe enough to warrant the diagnosis of agnosia may be commonly observed. However, profound deficits of recognition are not characteristic of mild to moderate dementia.

Impairment of Three-Dimensional Block Construction, which makes no apparent demands on language and memory functions and only mild demands on attentional and motor functions, may also be found in dementia. Benton and Fogel (1962) observed that 25% of patients with focal neuropsychological deficits performed defectively on the Three-Dimensional Block Construction task, as compared with a 60% rate of defective performance in patients with dementia.

Alzheimer's Disease

In Alzheimer's disease, the primary visual cortex remains relatively free of neurofibrillary tangles, whereas their density increases geometrically in progression toward the visual association cortices (Brun & Englund, 1981; Lewis, Campbell, Terry, & Morrison, 1987). Consistent with this histological finding, visual fields remain intact or relatively preserved in Alzheimer's disease, while the ability to perform higher visual functions deteriorates (Mendez, Mendez, Martin, Smyth, & Whitehouse, 1990). A recent study by Cronin-Golumb et al. (1991) compared the visual functions of healthy elderly against patients with mild to severe Alzheimer's disease. Neurological and neuro-ophthalmological examination disclosed a general lack of abnormalities of the eye and cranial nerves in comparison with the normal patients, and the two groups did not differ in visual acuity. The patients with Alzheimer's disease performed more poorly than elderly controls on tests of tritanomalous (blue) color vision, stereoacuity, and contrast sensitivity. The findings suggest that deficits on complex visual tasks can be found in Alzheimer's patients, and that these deficits may reflect intellectual compromise or degeneration in the visual association cortices.

Parkinson's Disease

A number of investigations have demonstrated that visuoperceptual, visuospatial, and visuoconstructive deficits may accompany Parkinson's disease (Huber, Shuttleworth, & Paulson, 1986; Levin, Llabre, & Weiner, 1989; Mohr, Litvan, Williams, Fedio, & Chase, 1990; Mortimer, Pirozzolo, Hansch, & Webster, 1982). These deficits do not appear to be simple artifacts of wider deficits in mental speed and motor functioning (Boller et al., 1984). Levin et al. (1991) demonstrated that there is a complex relationship between Parkinson's disease and deficits in visual perception. The decline in some perceptual tasks appears to be primarily related to the presence of dementia, with the decline in other tasks related to disease duration. Interactions between disease duration and dementia are also present for some tasks.

Delays in the visual evoked potential occur in many patients with Parkinson's disease (Bodis-Wollner, Yahr, Mylin, & Thornton, 1982). Also, such patients may also have deficits in color discrimination despite normal visual acuity (Price, Feldman, Adelberg, & Kayne, 1992). In Parkinson's disease there is a depletion of central dopaminergic neurons. As some retinal neurons are dopaminergic, it is possible that the source of some visual deficits in patients with Parkinson's disease may be retinal.

NEUROLOGICAL AND COGNITIVE CORRELATES OF PERCEPTUAL DISORDERS

Relation to Visual Field Defects

A number of investigations have observed a relationship between visuoperceptual and visuospatial deficits and the presence of left visual field defects (Benton et al., 1978; De Renzi, Faglioni, & Spinnler, 1968; Newcombe, 1969). However, the association between right-sided visual field defects and perceptual impairments is not significant. Thus, the relationship between left-sided visual field defects and perceptual impairments appears to be more correlative than causative in nature, in that both may result from the presence of lesions situated in the posterior right hemisphere.

Relation to Aphasia

Complex perceptual deficits are rarely present in patients sustaining focal lesions of the left hemisphere, unless the patient suffers from an accompanying aphasia with a language comprehension deficit (Hamsher, 1991). Among patients with language comprehension deficits, a substantial minority will perform defectively on tests of visuoperceptual and visuoconstructional ability, with a higher rate of defective performance observed among those with the more severe comprehension deficits (Benton, 1973; Benton et al., 1983; Hamsher et al., 1979). This phenomenon defies simple explanation. It is not that the patients are simply incapable of comprehending task demands, because for some of the tasks, such as Three-Dimensional Block Construction, the demands are self-evident, and because many aphasic patients perform well above chance levels on perceptual tasks.

Two traditional explanations, reviewed by Hamsher (1991), have been invoked to explain defective perceptual performances in aphasics with language comprehension deficits. The "anatomical hypothesis" proposes that the perceptual impairments sometimes observed in aphasic patients are caused by encroachment of an aphasia-causing lesion on a cortical area in the left hemisphere that also mediates extralinguistic performances. However, the anatomical hypothesis fails to account for the association of visuoperceptual impairment with language comprehension deficits regardless of the anterior versus posterior locus of lesion (Hamsher et al., 1979). Also, there has been a failure to identify a consistent locus of lesion associated with impairments in extralinguistic performances (Varney & Damasio, 1986, 1987).

The "psychological hypothesis" proposes that language plays an overarching role in cognition such that even tasks that appear to be completely nonverbal may nevertheless make vital demands on some aspects of language functioning. However, the psychological explanation fails to account for the substantial proportion of patients with severe language comprehension impairments who do perform adequately on perceptual and constructional tasks (Benton, 1973; Hamsher et al., 1979).

Hamsher (1991) has suggested that nonverbal deficits in aphasic patients with language comprehension deficits may not reflect simple losses in specific perceptual abilities, but rather the onset of new error tendencies, such as semantic slippage coupled with pervasive difficulties in self-monitoring. In this way, the defective perceptual and visuoconstructive performances of some aphasic patients may represent "positive" symptoms of brain dysfunction, rather than "negative" symptoms.

CROSS-CULTURAL ISSUES

Increasingly, the relevance and accuracy of neuropsychological tests for individuals from various ethnic and cultural groups are being questioned (Matthews, 1992). As a rational assumption, tests of visual perception should be relatively resistant to confounding by cultural factors or minority status. Also, valid interpretation of neuropsychological tests for nonwhite individuals demands that the right-hemisphere specialization for visuoperceptual, visuospatial, and visuoconstructive performances should also be observed in different racial groups. Two studies are described below that empirically examined these assumptions.

Roberts and Hamsher (1984) tested a sample of 94 neurologically normal urban African-Americans on the Visual Naming subtest of the Multilingual Aphasia Examination (MAE; Benton & Hamsher, 1989) and on the Facial Recognition Test to determine whether a significant proportion of minority patients would be misclassified as impaired using the Iowa control groups (composed almost exclusively of white rural and urban Americans). All the stimuli in the Facial Recognition Test are of white Americans. Although a significant proportion (22%) of African-American patients would have been misclassified as impaired on the basis of the confrontation naming test using the conventional norms, a very small proportion (2%) of black patients would have been misclassified as impaired on the Facial Recognition Test.

Lee, Sasanuma, Hamsher, and Benton (1991) found that Japanese (n = 100) and American (n = 120) neurologically normal controls performed at equivalent levels on Three-Dimensional Block Construction. The relationship of defective performance to the presence of right-hemisphere disease and aphasia with language comprehension deficits was also equivalent for Japanese and American patients with unilateral cerebral lesions. These investigators concluded that the right hemisphere appears to be specialized for visuoconstructional performance for both Japanese patients and occidental Americans.

METHODS OF ASSESSMENT

General Considerations

A wide variety of techniques may be employed to determine the presence, nature, and severity of higher visual deficits. Readers desiring a comprehensive guide to neuropsychological tests of visuoperceptual, visuospatial, and visuoconstructive abilities are referred to Lezak (1983) and to Spreen and Strauss (1991). The selection of techniques used is likely to vary depending on the background and preference of the clinician, and the clinical questions raised by the individual patient who has been referred for evaluation. This section will illustrate the application of a limited number of tests and techniques that have been found to be useful in our respective laboratories. The advantage of using these particular tests include their brevity, sound normative basis, and most important, the fact that they were specifically designed to answer the question of whether a certain type of perceptual deficit common in neurological disease is present in a given patient (Benton et al., 1983). A select summary of published research on these tests, indicating the relationship of performance to hemispheric locus of lesion and the presence of aphasic deficit, is presented in Table 6.2.

Visual Acuity

Before embarking on a neuropsychological investigation of deficits in visual perception, the examiner should perform a brief screening of visual acuity under the condition of good ambient lighting. One of the variety of pocket screening charts available will serve adequately for this purpose. As a convention, near-point visual acuity of 20/70 or better (with corrective lenses) is considered adequate for most neuropsychological tasks. As previously stated, visual acuity is generally resistant to the effects of focal cerebral disease (Bisiach et al., 1976; Taylor & Warrington, 1973) and is relatively unaffected by Alzheimer's disease until very late in the disorder (Cronin-Golumb et al., 1991).

Visual Field Defects

Gross evaluation of visual fields may be performed by having the patient stare straight ahead while an object is brought gradually into his or her field of vision from the periphery. This procedure should be performed for all four quadrants of the visual field in each eye. Formal mapping of hemianopic and quadrantic visual field defects may be performed using perimetry. The presence of visual field defects does not necessarily invalidate performance on visually mediated tasks if the examiner properly positions the test materials and ensures that the patient has adequately scanned them (see below).

TABLE 6.2. Rates of Defective Performance on Tests of Visuoperceptual, Visuospatial, and Visuoconstructional Ability in Patients with Brain Disease

	Hemispheric locus of lesion						
	Left				Right		
	LH	LHNA	LHA	LHAC	RH	RHA	RHP
	Facial Recognition Test						
Benton & Van Allen (1968)	14%	–	–	–	67%	–	–
Hamsher et al. (1979)	20%	0%	30%	39%	42%	26%	53%
Lee & Hamsher (1988)	–	–	–	–	70%	–	–
Capruso & Risser (1992)	22%	9%	43%	–	52%	–	–
	LH	LHNA	LHA	LHAC	RH	RHA	RHP
	Judgment of Line Orientation						
Benton et al. (1978)	10%	–	–	–	40%	0%	75%
Levick (1982)	4%	–	–	–	44%	–	–
Lee & Hamsher (1988)	–	–	–	–	67%	–	–
Trahan (1991)	26%	–	–	–	56%	–	–
Hamsher et al. (1992)	17%	0%	24%	–	63%	–	–
	LH	LHNA	LHA	LHAC	RH	RHA	RHP
	Three-Dimensional Block Construction						
Benton & Fogel (1962)	14%	–	–	–	32%	–	–
Benton (1967)	23%	–	–	–	54%	–	–
Benton (1973)	32%	13%	38%	50%	36%	–	–
Lee & Hamsher (1988)	–	–	–	–	44%	–	–

LH, left-hemisphere lesion; LHNA, left-hemisphere lesion, nonaphasic; LHA, left-hemisphere lesion, aphasic; LHAC, left-hemisphere lesion, aphasic with comprehension deficit; RH, right-hemisphere lesion; RHA, right-hemisphere anterior lesion; RHP, right-hemisphere posterior lesion.

WAIS-R Performance Subtests

The WAIS-R Performance scale subtests are multifactorial and performed under speeded conditions. For these reasons they are sensitive to lesions of either hemisphere and are impure measures for the assessment of perceptual ability. The Digit Symbol subtest, in particular, represents a measure of psychomotor (more specifically, graphomotor) speed and does not load with the other Performance subtests in many factor-analytic solutions (Matarazzo, 1972). Yet, a significant depression in the Performance IQ, when compared to the Verbal IQ, is typically seen in the context of unilateral right-hemisphere disease (Matarazzo, 1972; McFie, 1975; Walsh, 1978; Zillmer, Waechtler, Harris, Khan, & Fowler, 1992). A Verbal–Performance discrepancy of 15 points is conventionally regarded as significant, although a discrepancy of this magnitude may be found in many normal subjects, $p = .15$ (Matarazzo & Herman, 1984). Thus, the finding of a significant Verbal–Performance IQ discrepancy is consistent with, but not diagnostic of, visuospatial and/or visuoperceptual dysfunction, and must be carefully interpreted in light of the patient's history and the clinical reason for the evaluation. In some respects, the WAIS-R Verbal–Performance discrepancies tend to raise more questions than they answer.

Relative deficits on the Performance scale or its constituent subtests can be further understood by both qualitative and quantitative analysis of performance. For example, some patients working productively toward achieving correct solutions may be unduly penalized by the time constraints imposed by the WAIS-R standardization (Hamsher, 1984), whereas other patients may be unable to perform any complex visual tasks due to a visual neglect syndrome. In our respective laboratories, poor performance on WAIS-R Performance subtests is also considered with respect to performance on specific tests of visuoperceptual, visuospatial, and visuoconstructional ability using the relatively pure measures of these abilities devised by Benton and his colleagues (1983; see Table 6.2). Thus, empirical conclusions about the level of the patient's perceptual abilities may be made on a precise actuarial basis, without excessive reliance on subjective qualitative analysis of the Performance subtests.

Assessment of Visuoperceptual Disorders

Visual Object Agnosia

Despite the attention that has been paid to agnosia in the clinical and experimental literature, this disorder is rare, and few clinicians are likely to encounter a "pure" visual associative agnosia uncomplicated by the presence of dementia or severe visuoperceptual deficits. Despite the extremely low base rate of visual associative agnosia, techniques for its assessment will be reviewed in the event that the clinician is called on to evaluate such a case. These techniques have not fundamentally changed since the days of Lissauer (cited in Benton, 1982).

To satisfy the definition of associative visual object agnosia, the patient must have a deficit in recognition restricted to the visual mode, with relative preservation of visuoperceptual functioning. First, the presence of a specific anomia should be ruled out by determining if the patient can describe the ways in which various common objects are used (e.g., the Description of Use subtest of the Neurosensory Center Comprehensive Examination for Aphasia; Spreen & Benton, 1969), or by testing the ability to name objects when their uses are described (e.g., the Responsive Naming subtest of the Boston Diagnostic Aphasia Examination; Goodglass & Kaplan, 1983). Since visual associative agnosia is considered to be a modality-specific disorder of recognition, the patient's naming ability should be tested in both visual and tactile modes. The Neurosensory Center Comprehensive Examination for Aphasia (Spreen & Benton, 1969) is especially suitable for testing naming abilities through a variety of modalities. The role of visuoperceptive deficits may be investigated by having patients draw common objects that they have failed to recognize. In prosopagnosic patients, the Facial Recognition Test (Benton et al., 1983) may be used to determine the possible contribution of visuoperceptive deficits to the syndrome. Patients are considered to have an apperceptive agnosia if their inability to recognize common objects is part of a severe visuoperceptive syndrome and they are unable to describe or draw the objects.

Patients are considered to have an associative agnosia if their inability to recognize common objects takes place in the context of intact visuoperceptual ability.

Visuoperceptual Deficit

Deficits in visual perception that are not severe enough to warrant the diagnosis of agnosia may be elicited through some of the techniques previously described such as closure tasks, overlapping or embedded figures, or the discrimination of unfamiliar faces.

Clinicians should critically examine the actual task demands and validity data of the techniques they are using to investigate visuoperceptual ability. For example, the Visual Form Discrimination test developed by Benton et al. (1983), although most sensitive to lesions of the posterior right hemisphere, has proven vulnerable to lesions in other areas of the brain. As illustrated in Figure 6.8, the test calls for the patient to

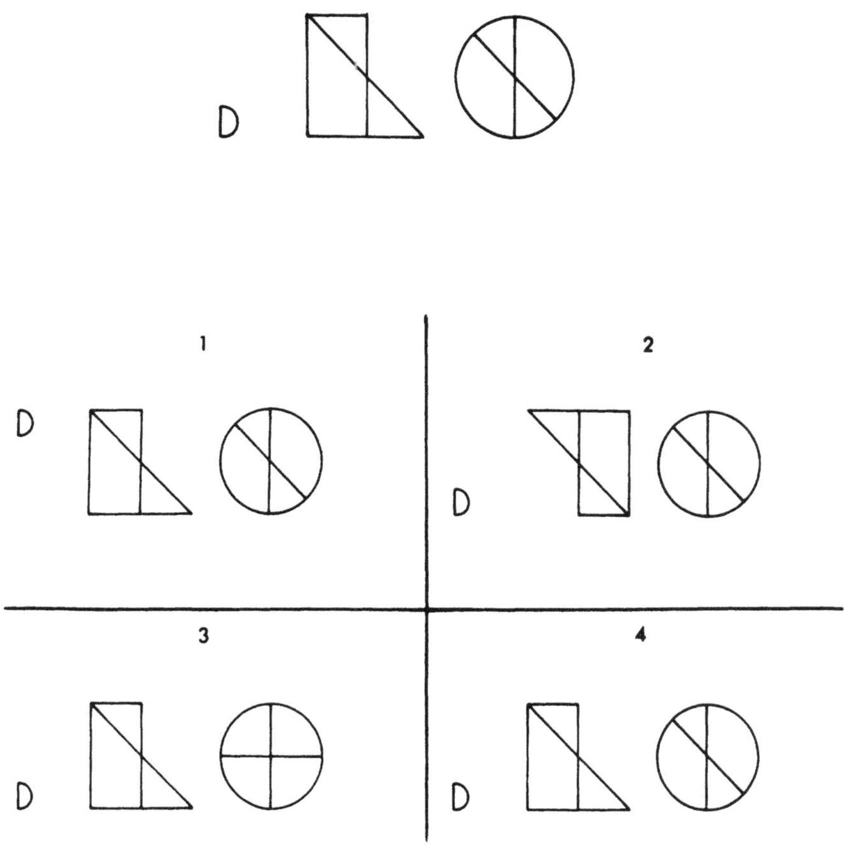

FIGURE 6.8. Item from the Visual Form Discrimination test. The task is to match the design at top with the correct choice from the four designs at bottom. From Benton, A. L., Hamsher, K. deS., Varney, N. R., & Spreen, O. (1983). *Contributions to neuropsychological assessment: A clinical manual.* New York: Oxford University Press. Copyright © 1983 by Oxford University Press, Inc. Reprinted by permission.

match a stimulus consisting of a group of three figures with an identical group of figures accompanied by three incorrect foils. If the patient carefully examines the stimulus figures and response choices, then 15 figures must be examined for each item of the test. The demands on sustained attention are obvious and probably account for the test's lack of specificity, since some disturbance in attentional processing is a frequent and generic clinical finding in patients with acute neurological and acute or chronic psychiatric disease (Hamsher & Lee, 1986).

Assessment of Visuospatial and Visuoconstructive Disorders

Visual Neglect

The presence of visual neglect is easily assessed by cancellation tasks such as that of Albert (1973) or Hamsher (1976). An example of severe visual neglect on such a task is illustrated in Figure 6.9. Line bisection tasks are also useful measures of neglect (Benton, 1969; Schenkenberg, Bradford, & Ajax, 1980). Patients are asked to draw an "X" or a vertical line through the middle of a horizontal line on a piece of paper. Patients with hemispatial neglect may show gross deviation in their placement of the center of the line. In many cases, neglect will appear as a pervasive factor across tests that require, but do not intend to measure, visual skills. For example, the patient may show such obvious errors as reading only one side of words or sentences (e.g., reading "ball" for baseball). In such cases, the examiner may attempt to compensate for the patient's neglect by placing stimuli eccentrically in the intact hemiattentional space, with frequent demonstrations to the patient of the necessity of scanning the entire stimulus field. Admittedly, this approach may be of limited value in some cases. Yet, to place all stimuli directly to the center of the patient will convert every test into a test of visual neglect. For example, the WAIS-R manual indicates that the model for the Block Designs should be placed slightly to the left side of right-handed subjects. When this is done with a patient suffering from a right-hemisphere lesion, the patient may respond to the instruction that he or she reproduce the design by asking, "What design?" Patients may then be able to attempt the design when the model is moved into their intact right hemiattentional space.

Visuospatial and Visuoconstructional Deficit

Two- and Three-Dimensional Block Designs. The Wechsler Block Design task is sensitive to disease of either hemisphere (Benton, 1973). This result likely derives from the fact that a patient may perform poorly on Block Design because of visual neglect, visuospatial impairment, visuoconstructional impairment, motor slowing, poor planning ability, or intellectual impairment. Of course, poor performance on any specific subtest may also represent a normal variant in a patient's WAIS-R profile (Matarazzo, 1990).

Patients who demonstrate impairment on Block Design should receive further visuospatial and visuoconstructional testing to clarify the nature of the deficit. A nonmotoric test of visuospatial ability (e.g., Judgment of Line Orientation) and a nonintellectual

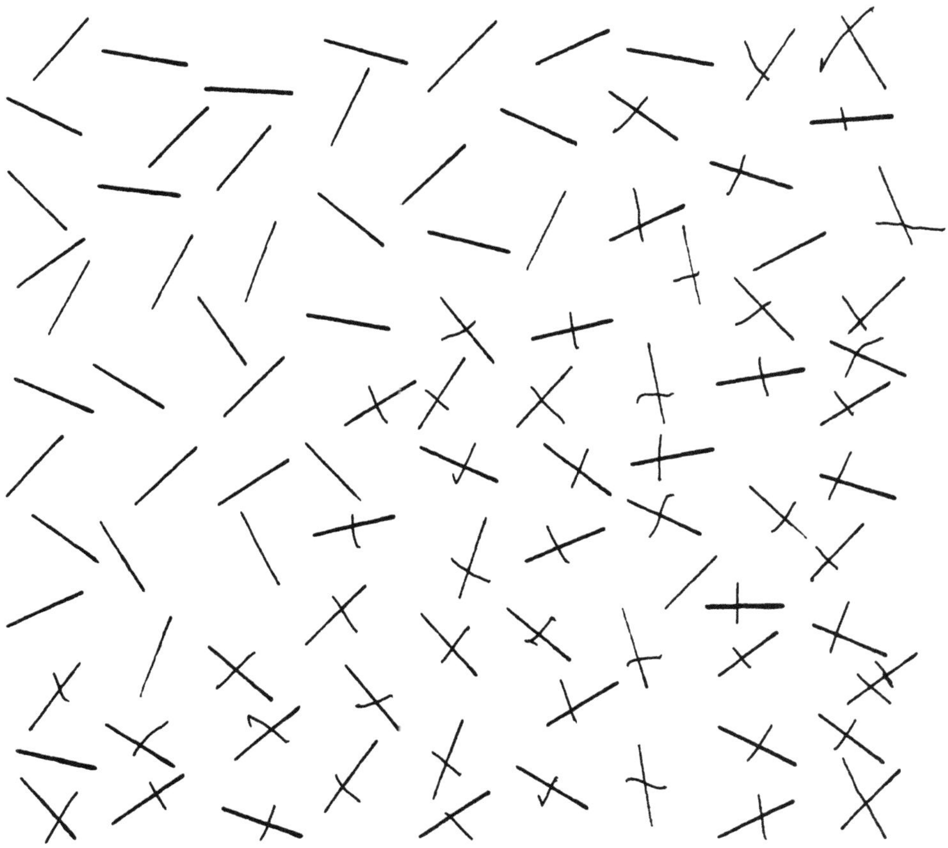

FIGURE 6.9. Severe left hemispatial neglect on a Line Cancellation task shown by a 65-year-old female with areas of infarction in the region of right anterior basal ganglia and right anterior parietal lobe. Stimulus item from Hamsher, K. deS. (1976). *Line Cancellation Test.* Iowa City: University of Iowa. Reprinted by permission.

test of visuoconstructive ability (e.g., Three-Dimensional Block Construction) are suitable for this exploration of performance. Careful qualitative analysis of Block Design performance is also useful in this regard (Kaplan, 1990; Milberg, Hebben, & Kaplan, 1986). Walsh (1985) has called attention to the fact that some of the WAIS-R Block Designs are much more difficult than others, regardless of the number of blocks necessary to complete the task. Patients often perform well when assembling designs where each block corresponds to a specific feature of the stimulus model. However, when specific features of the designs transcend individual blocks and must be assesmbled from combinations of blocks (as in the four-block "chevron" design of the WAIS-R), patients often demonstrate disproportionate difficulty.

Patients suffering from left-hemisphere lesions tend to construct Block Designs with the correct 2 × 2 or 3 × 3 configuration, but they often make errors concerning the internal details of the design. Patients with right-hemisphere lesions often construct designs that may preserve the pattern of internal detatil but grossly deviate from the square 2 × 2 or 3 × 3 configuration (Critchley, 1953; Kaplan, 1990; Paterson & Zangwill, 1944). In many instances, errors in 2 × 2 or 3 × 3 configuration can be an artifact of the neglect syndrome. An analgous pattern of performance may be observed on the Three-Dimensional Block Construction test, in which a patient may construct half the design, leaving some blocks balanced precariously on the edge of hemiattentional space (Benton et al., 1983). Patients in our respective laboratories have even been observed to have blocks repeatedly fall from the apex of a pyramidal three-dimensional construction because they fail to place a block underneath it on the left side.

Delis, Kiefner, and Fridlund (1988) have suggested that the tendency of patients with left-hemisphere lesions to make internal detail errors, while patients with right-hemisphere lesions make errors in 2 × 2 or 3 × 3 configuration, is related to a wider tendency for the left hemisphere to mediate processing of "local" stimulus features and for the right hemisphere to mediate processing of "global" stimulus features (e.g., van Kleeck, 1989). In support of this contention, Kramer, Kaplan, Blusewicz, and Preston (1991) found that the tendency to produce configural errors on WAIS-R Block Designs was related to the tendency to selectively process local, as opposed to global, stimulus features on a graphomotor copying task.

Patients with right-hemisphere disease often produce grossly inaccurate WAIS-R Block Designs. When asked whether their product matches the stimulus model, the patient will frequently answer in the affirmative. In contrast, patients with left-hemisphere lesions are usually aware that their designs are inaccurate. This phenomenon may be an aspect of the larger tendency of patients with right-hemisphere disease to be unaware of the extent of their deficits (McGlynn & Schacter, 1989). Patients with right-hemisphere disease may also commit the "closing-in" phenomenon of Mayer-Gross (1935). In this remarkable error type, patients may attempt to build a design by adjoining their block constructions directly onto the stimulus model.

Graphomotor Designs. Qualitative aspects of performance on the copy trial of the Rey-Osterrieth complex figure and other graphomotor drawing tasks also differ depending on the presence of diffuse or focal disease of either hemisphere (a full-scale copy of the complex figure may be found in Lezak, 1983). Patients with left-hemisphere lesions typically reproduce the spatial elements of drawings successfully, but may produce oversimplified reproductions with significant omission of details (Gainotti, 1985; Kirk & Kertesz, 1989; McFie & Zangwill, 1960). Kirk and Kertesz have questioned whether performance by some patients with left-hemisphere lesions will be affected by poor motor control in the preferred right hand, or by forced use of the nonpreferred left hand. Some patients with right-hemisphere lesions tend to neglect the left side of drawings. They may reproduce individual details accurately, but often with gross distortion and misplacement of spatial features of stimuli. An example of a spatially distorted complex figure is illustrated in Figure 6.10. Patients with dementia may show increased perseveration of elements on graphomotor designs (Ober, Jagust, Koss, Delis, & Friedland, 1991), and may display an increased tendency toward the closing-in phenomenon (Critchley, 1953; Gainotti, 1972; Gainotti, Parlato, Monteleone, & Carlomagno, 1992).

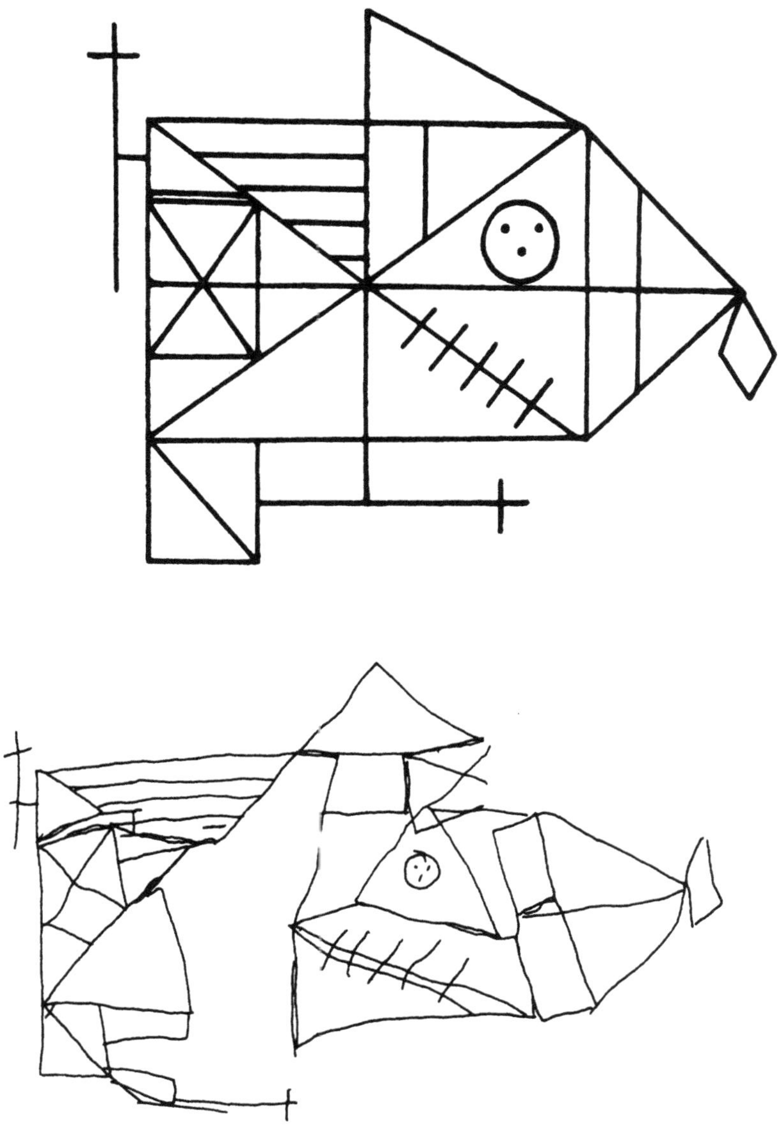

FIGURE 6.10. Rey-Osterrieth Complex Figure stimulus (at top), with copy (at bottom) produced by a 20-year-old white female with chronic seizure disorder. Note the preservation of many details from the stimulus, but with significant spatial distortions, particularly in the left hemifield. This patient had a Performance IQ of 83, but performed defectively on the Facial Recognition Test, Judgment of Line Orientation, and Three-Dimensional Block Construction.

CLINICAL CASE EXAMPLES

Described below are two clinical cases that illustrate the visuoperceptual, visuospatial, and visuoconstructional disorders that have been discussed. The general strategy represented in these cases reflects a traditional or "flexible" assessment approach.

There are two basic components. The first part of the assessment consists of more or less routine measures used to identify the presence of, and differentially diagnose, the major neurobehavioral disorders (Hamsher, 1984). These include measures of orientation and recent memory, attention, verbal and nonverbal intelligence, and naming. The results from these measures help to determine the presence or absence of an attentional disorder, aphasia, amnesia, confusional state, and dementia. These disorders have overarching diagnostic significance. For example, if a patient had dementia, but this had not been assessed or identified, then with a small collection of tests, one could seem to demonstrate almost any focal syndrome merely because the patient with dementia is likely to fail most cognitive tasks. Likewise, there are known deficit patterns associated with each of these major neurobehavioral syndromes, some of which could simulate focal disorders if not adequately assessed (e.g., Lee & Hamsher, 1988). The results of this initial core battery can also point to possible focal syndromes that can be investigated in the second part of the evaluation. The second part of the evaluation is then tailored to questions that arise from the reason for referral, presenting problems or patient complaints, lesion information such as that from neuroimaging studies, observations derived from the patient's behavior during the first part of the assessment, including a qualitative analysis of test performances, or the pattern of obtained results. Since behavior has multiple determinants, it is necessary to consider different reasons for failure on any particular task. For example, defects on a complex task such as Block Design could occur due to psychomotor retardation, general intellectual decline, or a specific defect in spatial or constructional ability because of neglect, or defects could be due to a visuoperceptive disorder (assuming poor visual acuity has been excluded as a factor). Likewise, a defect in visual naming could represent an aphasia, general intellectual decline, or a visual agnosia. Thus multiple hypotheses must be considered and systematically tested in the second portion of the examination.

Case 1

The patient was a 65-year-old white male. He was predominately right-handed, but was capable of using either hand for a variety of skilled activities. He had a family background that included mixed-handedness and sinistrality. The patient had 11 years of formal education and had worked for 30 years as a carpenter. The patient was admitted to the hospital after suffering a massive stroke in the territory of the right middle cerebral artery with left-sided hemiplegia. CT scan of the brain is presented in Figure 6.11. Past medical history was significant for five-vessel bypass surgery, left carotid endarterectomy, low back surgery, gallbladder removal, and a significant heart failure 1 year before the current stroke.

Perceptual examination of this patient was indicated because of the location of the lesions. A selection of tasks was included in the examination to measure the patient's recognition of familiar objects (MAE Visual Naming), scanning of visual space (Line Cancellation), constructional performance (WAIS-R Block Design), visuoperceptual performance (Facial Recognition Test), and visuospatial performance (Judgment of Line Orientation).

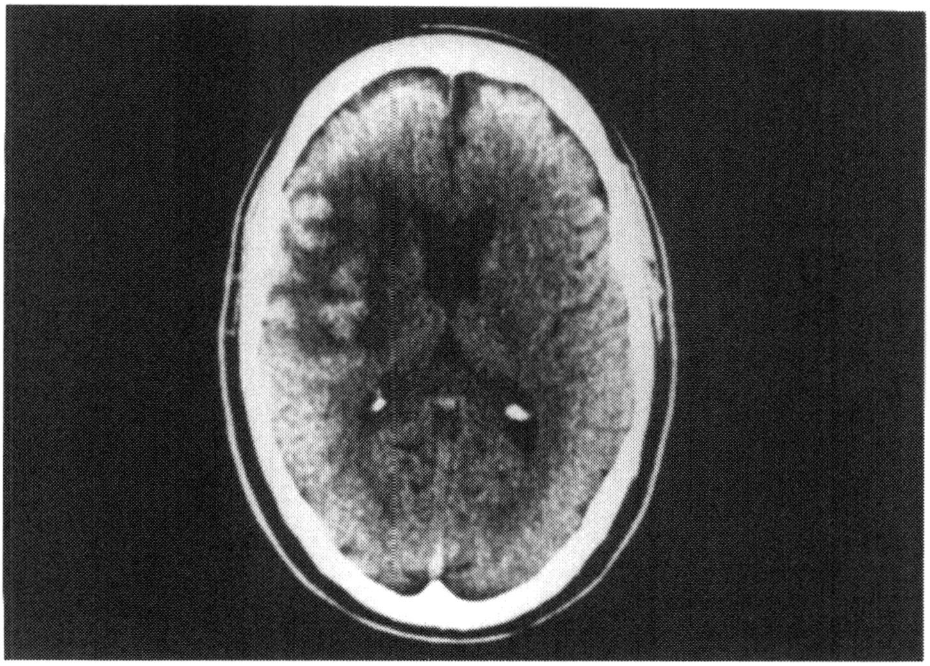

FIGURE 6.11. CT scan of the brain of the patient in Case 1. Areas of hemorrhage and infarction are apparent in the distribution of the right-hemisphere middle cerebral artery. Courtesy of Freeport Memorial Hospital, Freeport, IL.

A summary of the patient's formal psychometric performance is contained in Table 6.3. The patient showed very minimal left-sided inattention on a line cancellation task. Recent memory, verbal intellect, and recognition of common objects were normal. On the WAIS-R Block Design subtest, despite obtaining a score in the low average range, the patient made the gross configural errors that are often seen in the context of right-hemisphere disease. An example of this error type is illustrated in Figure 6.12. Visuoperceptual performance (Facial Recognition Test) and visuospatial performance (Judgment of Line Orientation) were both defective. The diagnostic impression was of visuoperceptual and visuospatial deficits in the context of otherwise essentially normal cognitive performances. This patient's deficits were judged to be consistent with, and typical of, the known cognitive effects of the lesion documented by CT scan.

Case 2

The patient was a 51-year-old, right-handed, white male with a dextral family background. He had 12 years of formal education and had been employed as a foreman. He was referred for neuropsychological evaluation of complaints of progressive memory loss and depression. Medical history was significant for long-standing hypertension. Angioplasty and cardiac revascularization were performed 10 years previous

TABLE 6.3. Psychometric Results for Case 1

	Raw score	Percentile rank	Interpretation
Recent memory			
Orientation			
Temporal (errors)	−3	5th	Borderline
Presidents Test			
Verbal Naming	6/6	65th	Normal
Verbal Sequencing	Rho = 1.0	64th	Normal
Photo Naming	6/6	51st	Normal
Photo Sequencing	Rho = 1.0	65th	Normal
New learning			
Verbal			
Serial Digit Learning (8)	18/24	63rd	Normal
	Standard/age scale score	**Percentile rank**	**Performance level**
WAIS-R			
Verbal IQ	94	34th	Average
Performance IQ	86	18th	Low average
Full Scale IQ	90	25th	Average
Information	9	37th	Average
Similarities	10	50th	Average
Verbal–Conceptual DQ	97	42nd	Average
Digit Span [5F/4B]	8	25th	Average
Arithmetic	9	37th	Average
Attention–Concentration DQ	92	30th	Average
Picture Arrangement	8	25th	Average
Block Design	7	16th	Low average
Perceptual–Constructional DQ	86	18th	Low average
	Raw score	**Percentile rank**	**Interpretation**
Language			
Multilingual Aphasia Examination (MAE)			
Visual Naming	52/60	75th	Normal
Visuoperceptual/spatial			
Line Cancellation	86/90	4th	Mild defect
Right Visual Field	29/30	12th	Low normal
Left Visual Field	27/30	<1st	Defective
Facial Recognition Test	32/54	<1st	Defective
Judgment of Line Orientation	10/30	<1st	Defective

to the neuropsychological examination, and were complicated by a small myocardial infarction during the procedure. MRI of the brain performed 1 month previous to the neuropsychological examination suggested a mildly prominent ventricular system, especially at the occipital horns, with high-intensity signals in the central occipital lobes and posterior parietal lobes, especially on the left, and extending superiorly toward the vertex. Focal cortical atrophy was seen in adjacent areas, particularly in the left posterior parietal region. Small foci of increased signal intensity were noted in the right

A

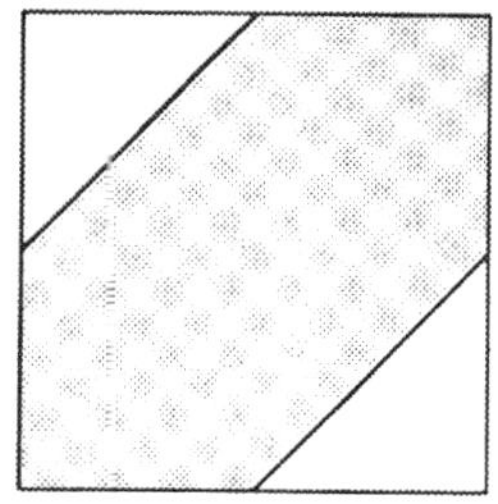

B

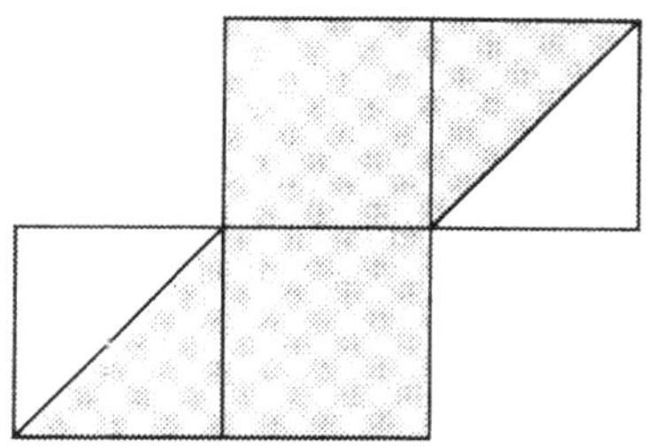

FIGURE 6.12. (A) WAIS-R Block Design stimulus model and (B) finished construction by the patient in Case 1. This is an example of a "configuration error" with retention of the internal features of the model. The patient was not aware that he had made an error, and after a redemonstration of the correct solution by the examiner, he produced exactly the same error. Block Design stimulus model from Wechsler, D. (1981). *Wechsler Adult Intelligence Scale-Revised.* San Antonio: Psychological Corporation. Copyright © 1981, 1955 by the Psychological Corporation. Reprinted by permission.

cerebellum and right frontal lobe. The general impression was that of diffuse white matter changes with adjacent extensive cortical atrophy, consistent with a combination of demyelinating disease and cortical ischemia.

A summary of the patient's formal psychometric performance is contained in Table 6.4. The range and severity of the patient's deficits warranted a diagnosis of dementia. However, the configuration of the test results also indicated especially severe impairments of perceptual functions, in the context of relative preservation of verbal functions. For example, examination of the WAIS-R profile indicated a 20-point discrepancy between verbal–conceptual and perceptual–constructional factor scores. The patient had performed particularly poorly on WAIS-R Block Design, so the Three-Dimensional Block Construction task was administered to determine whether the patient's deficits reflected a loss of nonverbal intelligence, or were a component of a more basic constructional apraxia that would be seen even on a constructional task with minimal demands on problem-solving skills or motor speed. The patient was able to construct the first and simplest of the designs (see Figure 6.7, upper stimulus item),

TABLE 6.4. Psychometric Results for Case 2

	Raw score	Percentile rank	Interpretation
Recent memory			
Orientation			
Temporal (errors)	−11	<1st	Defective
Personal Information and Place	12/12	52nd	Normal
Presidents Test			
Verbal Naming	3/6	65th	Normal
Verbal Sequencing	Rho = .83	9th	Low normal
Photo Naming	6/6	51st	Normal
Photo Sequencing	Rho = .88	14th	Low normal
New learning			
Verbal			
Serial Digit Learning (9)	4/24	8th	Low normal
Nonverbal			
Form Sequence Learning (4)	6/20	1st	Defective
Discrimination Score	28/40	1st	Defective
Sequence Score	25/40	2nd	Defective
	Standard/age scale score	**Percentile rank**	**Performance level**
WAIS-R			
Verbal IQ	80	9th	Low average
Performance IQ	66	1st	Defective
Full Scale IQ	72	3rd	Borderline
Information	8	25th	Average
Similarities	7	16th	Low average
Verbal–Conceptual DQ	86	18th	Low average
Digit Span [5F/3B]	6	9th	Low average
Arithmetic	6	9th	Low average
Attention–Concentration DQ	77	6th	Borderline
Picture Completion	6	9th	Low average
Picture Arrangement	5	5th	Borderline
Block Design	2	<1st	Defective
Perceptual–Constructional DQ	66	1st	Defective
	Raw score	**Percentile rank**	**Interpretation**
Language			
Multilingual Aphasia Examination (MAE)			
Visual Naming	46/60	27th	Normal
Controlled Oral Word Association	22	11th	Low normal
Token Test	40/44	24th	Low normal
Visuoperceptual/visuospatial			
Visual Acuity OU (Corrected)	20/25	–	Adequate
Line Cancellation	87/90	5th	Borderline
Right Visual Field	28/30	3rd	Defective
Left Visual Field	29/30	12th	Low normal
Facial Recognition Test	34/54	<1st	Defective
Judgment of Line Orientation	16/30	4th	Defective
3-D Block Construction	10/29	<1st	Defective

TABLE 6.4. (Continued)

	Raw score	Percentile rank	Interpretation
Somatoperceptual			
Right–Left Orientation	15/20	3rd	Defective
Own Body	10/12	–	–
Confrontation	5/8	–	–
Finger Localization	41/60	<1st	Defective
Right Hand	19/30	<1st	Defective
Left Hand	22/30	1st	Defective

but his constructions of the more complex designs (see Figure 6.7, middle and lower stimulus items) were severely distorted, with omitted and displaced blocks. Further investigation of the patient's perceptual ability with tests from the Benton Laboratory revealed deficits in both visuoperceptual (Facial Recognition Test) and visuospatial ability (Judgment of Line Orientation), despite adequate near-point acuity (20/25) and no evidence of lateralized visual neglect. In view of the left parietal lesions, tests of Finger Localization and Right–Left Orientation were administered, with impairments on these tasks indicating somatoperceptual deficits in addition to the higher visual impairments already documented. In contrast to the patient's perceptual deficits, language testing proved normal using selected subtests of the MAE.

The diagnostic impression was of dementia with prominent perceptual deficits. This case illustrates that testing of visual perception is not solely of relevance to patients with unilateral right-hemisphere lesions. Perceptual deficits may appear as prominent manifestations of a wider dementia syndrome in patients suffering from progressive neurodegenerative disorders.

SUMMARY

Visuoperceptual and visuopspatial functioning are mediated by two anatomically and functionally segregated systems within the brain. The visuoperceptual system processes the form and color of objects and is represented in the inferior temporal cortex. The visuospatial system processes the movement and location of objects, regardless of their form or color, and is represented in the posterior parietal cortex. Dissociation of these two systems may be seen following focal lesions of the brain.

High rates of defective performance in visuoperceptual, visuospatial, and visuoconstructional functioning are typically observed following right-hemisphere lesions. A minority of patients with left-hemisphere lesions perform defectively on these tasks, and the severity of deficit is usually less than that observed following right-hemisphere lesions. Substantial rates of defective performance on complex visual tasks are typically observed following left-hemisphere lesions when aphasic language comprehension deficits are present. Impairments in visuoperceptual, visuospatial, and visuoconstructive functioning are also prominent features of a variety of diffuse and degenerative brain diseases.

REFERENCES

Albert, M. C. (1973). A simple test of visual neglect. *Neurology, 23*, 658–664.

Arena, R., & Gainotti, G. (1978). Constructional apraxia and visuoperceptive disabilities in relation to laterality of cerebral lesions. *Cortex, 14*, 463–473.

Arrigoni, G., & De Renzi, E. (1964). Constructional apraxia and hemispheric locus of lesion. *Cortex, 1*, 170–197.

Ayres, A. J. (1972). *Sensory integration and praxis tests.* Los Angeles: Western Psychological Services.

Benton, A. L. (1967). Constructional apraxia and the minor hemisphere. *Confinia Neurologica, 29*, 1–16.

Benton, A. L. (1968). Differential behavioral effects of frontal lobe disease. *Neuropsychologia, 6*, 53–60.

Benton, A. L. (1969). Disorders of spatial orientation. In P. J. Vinken & G. W. Bruyn (Eds.), *Handbook of clinical neurology, Vol. 3. Disorders of higher nervous activity* (pp. 212–218). New York: Wiley.

Benton, A. L. (1973). Visuoconstructive disability in patients with cerebral disease: Its relationship to side of lesion and aphasic disorder. *Documenta Ophthalmologica, 34*, 67–76.

Benton, A. L. (1978). The interplay of experimental and brain lesion approaches in brain lesion research. In S. Finger (Ed.), *Recovery from brain damage: Research and theory* (pp. 49–68). New York: Plenum Press.

Benton, A. L. (1979). Visuoperceptive, visuospatial, and visuoconstructional disorders. In K. M. Heilman & E. Valenstein (Eds.), *Clinical neuropsychology* (pp. 186–232). New York: Oxford University Press.

Benton, A. L. (1980). The neuropsychology of facial recognition. *American Psychologist, 35*, 176–186.

Benton, A. L. (1982). Spatial thinking in neurological patients: Historical aspects. In M. Potegal (Ed.), *Spatial abilities: Development and physiological foundations* (pp. 253–271). New York: Academic Press.

Benton, A. L. (1985a). Facial recognition 1984. In L. Costa & O. Spreen (Eds.), *Studies of neuropsychology: Selected papers of Arthur Benton* (pp. 224–235). New York: Oxford University Press.

Benton, A. L. (1985b). Visuoperceptive, visuospatial, and visuoconstructional disorders. In K. M. Heilman & E. Valenstein (Eds.), *Clinical neuropsychology* (2nd ed., pp. 151–185). New York: Oxford University Press.

Benton, A. L. (1990). Facial recognition 1990. *Cortex, 26*, 491–499.

Benton, A. L., & Fogel, M. L. (1962). Three-dimensional constructional praxis: A clinical test. *Archives of Neurology, 7*, 347–354.

Benton, A. L., & Hamsher, K. deS. (1989). *Multilingual Aphasia Examination* (2nd ed.). Iowa City, IA: AJA Associates.

Benton, A. L., Hamsher, K. deS., Varney, N. R., & Spreen, O. (1983). *Contributions to neuropsychological assessment: A clinical manual.* New York: Oxford University Press.

Benton, A. L., Hannay, H. J., & Varney, N. R. (1975). Visual perception of line direction in patients with unilateral brain disease. *Neurology, 25*, 907–910.

Benton, A. L., & Hécaen, H. (1970). Stereoscopic vision in patients with unilateral cerebral disease. *Neurology, 20*, 1084–1088.

Benton, A. L., & Van Allen, M. W. (1968). Impairment in facial recognition in patients with cerebral disease. *Cortex, 4*, 344–358.

Benton, A. L., & Van Allen, M. W. (1972). Prosopagnosia and facial recognition. *Journal of Neurological Sciences, 15*, 167–172.

Benton, A. L., Varney, N. R., & Hamsher, K. deS. (1978). Visuospatial judgment: A clinical test. *Archives of Neurology, 35*, 364–367.

Bisiach, E., & Luzzatti, C. (1978). Unilateral neglect of representational space. *Cortex, 14*, 129–133.

Bisiach, E., Nichelli, P., & Spinnler, H. (1976).. Hemispheric functional asymmetry in visual discrimination between univariate stimuli: An analysis of sensitivity and response criterion. *Neuropsychologia, 14*, 335–342.

Bodamer, J. (1947). Die Prosop-Agnosie. *Archive für und Nervenkrankheiten, 179,* 6–54.
Bodis-Wollner, I., Yahr, M. D., Mylin, L., & Thornton, J. (1982). Dopaminergic deficiency and delayed visual evoked potentials in humans. *Annals of Neurology, 11,* 478–483.
Boller, F., Passafiume, D., Keefe, N. C., Rogerse, K., Morrow, L., & Kim, Y. (1984). Visuospatial impairment in Parkinson's disease: Role of perceptual and motor factors. *Archives of Neurology, 41,* 485–490.
Brain, W. R. (1941). Visual disorientation with special reference to lesions of the right cerebral hemisphere. *Brain, 64,* 224–272.
Brun, A., & Englund, E. (1981). Regional pattern of degeneration in Alzheimer's disease: Neuronal loss and histopathological grading. *Histopathology, 5,* 549–564.
Capruso, D. X., Hamsher, K. deS., Levin, H. S., & Barr, W. B. (1993). Retrograde memory in patients with unilateral CVA vs. patients with amnesia. *Neurology, 43*(Suppl. 2), A298–299.
Capruso, D. X., & Risser, A. H. (1992) Facial Recognition Test: Identical stimulus matching and transformed stimulus matching. *Journal of Clinical and Experimental Neuropsychology, 14,* 41.
Carmon, A., & Bechtoldt, H. P. (1969). Dominance of the right cerebral hemisphere for stereopsis. *Neuropsychologia, 7,* 29–39.
Chagas, C., Gattass, R., & Gross, C. (1985). *Pattern recognition mechanisms.* New York: Springer-Verlag.
Corkin, S. (1979). Hidden-Figures-Test performance: Lasting effects of unilateral penetrating head injury and transient effects of bilateral cingulotomy. *Neuropsychologia, 17,* 585–605.
Costa, L. D., & Vaughan, H. G. (1962). Performance of patients with lateralized cerebral lesions. I: Verbal and perceptual tests. *Journal of Nervous and Mental Disease, 134,* 162–168.
Cowey, A., & Gross, C. G. (1970). Effects of foveal prestriate and inferotemporal lesions on visual discrimination by rhesus monkeys. *Experimental Brain Research, 11,* 128–144.
Cowey, A., & Wilkinson, F. (1991). The role of the corpus callosum and extra striate visual areas in stereoacuity in the macaque monkeys. *Neuropsychologia, 29,* 465–479.
Critchley, M. (1953). *The parietal lobes.* New York: Hafner.
Cronin-Golumb, A., Corkin, S., Rizzo, J. F., Cohen, J., Growdon, J. H., & Banks, K. S. (1991). Visual dysfunction in Alzheimer's disease: Relation to normal aging. *Annals of Neurology, 29,* 41–52.
Damasio, A. R., & Benton, A. L. (1979). Impairment of hand movements under visual guidance. *Neurology, 29,* 170–178.
Damasio, A. R., & Damasio, H. (1983). Localization of lesions in achromatopsia and prosopagnosia. In A. Kertesz (Ed.), *Localization in neuropsychology* (pp. 417–428). New York: Academic Press.
Damasio, A. R., Damasio, H., & Chui, H. C. (1980). Neglect following damage to frontal lobe or basal ganglia. *Neuropsychologia, 18,* 123–132.
Damasio, A. R., Damasio, H., & Van Hoesen, G. W. (1982). Prosopagnosia: Anatomic basis and behavioral mechanisms. *Neurology, 32,* 331–341.
Dee, H. L. (1970). Visuoconstructive and visuoperceptive deficit in patients with unilateral cerebral lesions. *Neuropsychologia, 8,* 305–314.
Delis, D. C., Kiefner, M. G., & Fridlund, A. J. (1988). Visuospatial dysfunction following unilateral brain damage: Dissociations in hierarchical and hemispatial analysis. *Journal of Clinical and Experimental Neuropsychology, 10,* 421–431.
De Renzi, E. (1982). *Disorders of space exploration and cognition.* Chichester, England: Wiley.
De Renzi, E. (1985). Disorders of spatial orientation. In J. A. M. Frederiks (Ed.), *Handbook of clinical neurology, Vol. 1(45). Clinical neuropsychology* (pp. 405–422). North Holland: Elsevier.
De Renzi, E. (1986). Current issues on prosopagnosia. In H. D. Ellis, M. A. Jeeves, F. Newcombe, & A. Young (Eds.), *Aspects of face processing* (pp. 243–252). Dordrecht: Martinus Nijhoff.
De Renzi, E., Faglioni, P., & Scotti, G. (1970). Hemispheric contribution to the exploration of space through the visual and tactile modality. *Cortex, 6,* 191–203.
De Renzi, E. Faglioni, P., & Scotti, G. (1971). Judgment of spatial orientation in patients with focal brain damage. *Journal of Neurology, Neurosurgery, and Psychiatry, 34,* 489–495.
De Renzi, R., Faglioni, P., Scotti, G., & Spinnler, H. (1972). Impairment of color sorting behavior after hemispheric damage: An experimental investigation with the Holmgren skein test. *Cortex, 8,* 147–163.

De Renzi, E., Faglioni, P., & Spinnler, H. (1968). The performance of patients with unilateral damage on facial recognition tests. *Cortex, 4,* 17–34.

De Renzi, E., & Spinnler, H. (1966). Visual recognition in patients with unilateral cerebral disease. *Journal of Nervous and Mental Disease, 142,* 515–525.

De Renzi, E., & Spinnler, H. (1967). Impaired performance on color tasks in patients with hemispheric damage. *Cortex, 3,* 194–216.

Desimone, R., Schein, S. J., Moran, J., & Ungerleider, L. G. (1985). Contour, color, and shape analysis beyond the striate cortex. *Vision Research, 25,* 441–452.

Deutsch, G., Bourbon, W. T., Papanicolaou, A. C., & Eisenberg, H. M. (1988). Visuospatial tasks compared via regional cerebral blood flow. *Neuropsychologia, 26*(3), 445–452.

Duensing, F. (1953). Raumagnostiche und Ideatorisch-Apraktische Störung des gestaltenden Handelns. *Deutsche Zeitschrift für Nervenheilkunde, 170,* 72–94.

Eslinger, P. J., & Benton, A. L. (1983). Visuoperceptual performances in aging and dementia: Clinical and theoretical implications. *Journal of Clinical Neuropsychology, 5,* 213–220.

Eslinger, P. J., Damasio, A. R., Benton, A. L., & Van Allen, M. (1985). Neuropsychological detection of abnormal mental decline in older persons. *Journal of the Americn Medical Association, 253,* 670–674.

Ettlinger, G. (1990). "Object vision" and "spatial vision": The neuropsychological evidence for the distinction. *Cortex, 26,* 319–341.

Ettlinger, G., Warrington, E., & Zangwill, O. L. (1957). A further study of visuo-spatial agnosia. *Brain, 80,* 335–361.

Farah, M. J. (1990). *Visual agnosia: Disorders of object recognition and what they tell us about normal vision.* Cambridge, MA: MIT Press.

Farah, M. J., Wong, A. B., Monheit, M. A., & Morrow, L. A. (1989). Parietal lobe mechanisms of spatial attention: Modality-specific or supramodal? *Neuropsychologia, 27*(94), 461–470.

Fontenot, D. J., & Benton, A. L. (1972). Perception of direction in the right and left visual fields. *Neuropsychologia, 10,* 447–452.

Freedman, L., & Dexter, L. E. (1991). Visuospatial ability in cortical dementia. *Journal of Clinical and Experimental Neuropsychology, 13,* 677–690.

Freud, S. (1953). *On aphasia.* New York: International Universities Press. (Original work published 1891)

Gainotti, G. (1972). A quantitative study of the "closing-in" symptom in normal children and in brain-damaged patients. *Neuropsychologia, 10,* 429–436.

Gainotti, G. (1985). Constructional apraxia. In J. A. M. Frederiks (Ed.), *Handbook of clinical neurology, Vol. 1(45). Clinical neuropsychology* (pp. 491–506). North Holland: Elsevier.

Gainotti, G., Messerli, P., & Tissot, R. (1972). Qualitative analysis of unilateral spatial neglect in relation to laterality of cerebral lesions. *Journal of Neurology, Neurosurgery, and Psychiatry, 35,* 545–550.

Gainotti, G., Parlato, V., Monteleone, D., & Carlomagno, S. (1992). Neuropsychological markers of dementia on visual-spatial tasks: A comparison between Alzheimer's type and vascular forms of dementia. *Journal of Clinical and Experimental Neuropsychology, 14,* 239–254.

Geschwind, N. (1965). Disconnexion syndromes in animals and man. *Brain, 88,* 237–294.

Geschwind, N., & Fusillo, M. (1964). Color-naming defects in association with alexia. *Transactions on the American Neurological Association, 89,* 172–176.

Geschwind, N., & Fusillo, M. (1966). Color-naming defects in association with alexia. *Archives of Neurology, 15,* 137–146.

Gloning, I., Gloning, K., & Hoff, H. (1968). *Neurological symptoms and syndromes in lesions of the occipital lobe and the adjacent areas.* Paris: Gauthier-Villars.

Goodglass, H., & Kaplan, E. (1983). *The assessment of aphasia and related disorders* (2nd ed.). Philadelphia, PA: Lea & Febiger.

Gross, C. G., Desimone, R., Albright, T. D., & Schwartz, E. L. (1985). Inferior temporal cortex and pattern recognition. In Chagas, C., Gattass, R., & Gross, C. (Eds.), *Pattern recognition mechanisms* (pp. 179–201). New York: Springer-Verlag.

Hamsher, K. deS. (1976). Line Cancellation Test. Iowa City: University of Iowa.

Hamsher, K. deS. (1978a). Stereopsis and unilateral brain disease. *Investigative Ophthalmology and Visual Science, 4,* 336–343.
Hamsher, K. deS. (1978b). Stereopsis and the perception of anomalous contours. *Neuropsychologia, 16,* 453–459.
Hamsher, K. deS. (1984). Specialized neuropsychological assessment methods. In G. Goldstein & M. Hersen (Eds.), *Handbook of psychological assessment* (pp. 235–256). New York: Pergamon Press.
Hamsher, K. deS. (1991). Intelligence and aphasia. In M. T. Sarno (Ed.), *Acquired aphasia* (2nd ed., pp. 339–372). New York: Academic Press.
Hamsher, K. deS., Capruso, D. X., & Benton, A. L. (1992). Visuospatial judgment and right hemisphere disease. *Cortex, 28,* 493–495.
Hamsher, K. deS., & Lee, G. P. (1986). *Aprosexia: An actuarial study of a nomen nudem.* Paper presented at the meeting of the International Neuropsychological Society, Veldhoven, The Netherlands.
Hamsher, K. deS., Levin, H. S., & Benton, A. L. (1979). Facial recognition in patients with focal brain lesions. *Archives of Neurology, 36,* 837–839.
Hécaen, H., Ajuriaguerra, J., & Massonet, J. (1951). Les troubles visuoconstructive par lésion pariéto-occipitale droite. *Encéphale, 40,* 122–179.
Hécaen, H., & Angelergues, R. (1962). Agnosia for faces (prosopagnosia). *Archives of Neurology, 7,* 92–100.
Hécaen, H., Penfield, W., Bertrand, C., & Malmo, R. (1956). The syndrome of apractognosia due to lesions of the minor cerebral hemisphere. *Archives of Neurology and Psychiatry, 75,* 400–434.
Heilman, K. M., Bowers, D., Coslett, H. B., & Watson, R. T. (1983). Directional hypokinesia in neglect. *Neurology, 33*(Suppl. 2), 104.
Heilman, K. M., & Valenstein, E. (1972). Frontal lobe neglect in man. *Neurology, 22,* 660–664.
Heilman, K. M., Watson, R. T., & Valenstein, E. (1985). Neglect and related disorders. In K. M. Heilman & E. Valenstein (Eds.), *Clinical neuropsychology* (2nd ed., pp. 243–294). New York: Oxford University Press.
Heilman, K. M., Watson, R. T., Valenstein, E., & Damasio, A. R. (1983). Localization of lesions in neglect. In A. Kertesz (Ed.), *Localization in neuropsychology* (pp. 471–492). New York: Academic Press.
Hooper, H. E. (1983). Hooper Visual Organization Test. Los Angeles: Western Psychological Services.
Huber, S. J., Shuttleworth, E. C., & Paulson, G. W. (1986). Dementia in Parkinson's diseae. *Archives of Neurology, 43,* 987–990.
Iwai, E., & Mishkin, M. (1968). Two visual foci in the temporal lobe of monkeys. In N. Yoshii & N. A. Buchwald (Eds.), *Neurophysiological basis of learning and behavior.* Osaka, Japan: Osaka University Press.
Jackson, J. H. (1875/1958). On the anatomical and physiological localization of movements in the brain. In J. Taylor (Ed.), *Selected writings of John Hughlings Jackson, Vol. 1. On epilepsy and epileptiform convulsion* (pp. 37–76). London: Staples Press.
Jackson, J. H. (1876/1958). Case of large cerebral tumor without optic neuritis and with left hemiplegia and imperception. In J. Taylor (Ed.), *Selected writings of John Hughlings Jackson, Vol. 2. Evolution and dissolution of the nervous system, speech, various papers, addresses, and lectures* (pp. 146–152). London: Staples Press.
Jones, B. M. (1971). Verbal and spatial intelligence in short- and long-term alcoholics. *Journal of Nervous and Mental Disease, 153,* 292–297.
Jones, B. M., & Parsons, O. A. (1972). Specific vs. generalized deficits of abstracting ability in chronic alcoholics. *Archives of General Psychiatry, 26,* 380–384.
Julesz, B. (1971). *Foundations of cyclopean perception.* Chicago: University of Chicago Press.
Kanizsa, G. (1986). Subjective contours. In J. M. Wolfe (Ed.), *The mind's eye.* New York: W. H. Freeman.
Kaplan, E. (1990). The process approach to neuropsychological assessment of psychiatric patients. *Journal of Neuropsychiatry and Clinical Neurosciences, 2*(1), 72–87.
Kertesz, A., & Dobrowlski, S. (1981). Right hemisphere deficits: Lesion size and location. *Journal of Clinical Neuropsychology, 3*(4), 283–299.

Kinsbourne, M., & Warrington, E. K. (1962). A disorder of simultaneous form perception. *Brain, 85*, 461–486.
Kinsbourne, M., & Warrington, E. K. (1963). The localizing significance of simultaneous form perception. *Brain, 85*, 697–702.
Kirk, A., & Kertesz, A. (1989). Hemispheric contributions to drawing. *Neuropsychologia, 27*(6), 881–886.
Kleist, K. (1912). Der Gang und der gegenwärtige Strand der Apraxieforschung. *Ergebnisse der Neurologie und Psychiatrie, 1*, 342–452.
Kleist, K. (1922). Kriegsverletungen des Gehims in ihrer Bedeutung für die Hirnlokalisation und Hirnpathologie. In O. von Schjerning (Ed.), *Handbuch der ärtzlichen Erfahrung im Weltkrieg*, Bd. 4. Leipzig: Barth.
Kleist, K. (1934). *Gehirnpathologie*. Leipzig: Barth.
Kramer, J. H., Kaplan, E., Blusewicz, M. J., & Preston, K. A. (1991). Visual hierarchical analysis of Block Design configural errors. *Journal of Clinical and Experimental Neuropsychology, 13*, 455–465.
Lansdell, H. (1970). Relation of extent of temporal removals to closure and visuomotor factors. *Perceptual and Motor Skills, 31*, 491–498.
Lawler, K. A., & Cowey, A. (1986). The effects of pretectal and superior colliculus lesions on binocular vision. *Experimental Brain Research, 63*, 402–408.
Lee, G. P., & Hamsher, G. P. (1988). Neuropsychological findings in toxicometabolic confusional states. *Journal of Clinical and Experimental Neuropsychology, 10*, 769–778.
Lee, G. P., Sasanuma, S., Hamsher, K. deS., & Benton, A. L. (1991). Constructional praxis performance of Japanese and American normal and brain-damaged patients. *Archives of Clinical Neuropsychology, 6*, 15–25.
Levick, W. (1982). *The Judgment of Line Orientation test—A clinical validation*. Unpublished master's thesis, University of Newcastle, Australia.
Levin, B. E., Llabre, M. M., Reisman, S., Weiner, W. J., Sanchez-Ramos, J., Singer, C., & Brown, M. C. (1991). Visuospatial impairment in Parkinson's disease. *Neurology, 41*, 365–369.
Levin, B. E., Llabre, M. M., & Weiner, W. J. (1989). Cognitive impairments associated with early Parkinson's disease. *Neurology, 39*, 557–561.
Levin, H. S., Grossman, R. G., & Kelly, P. J. (1977). Impairment of facial recognition after closed head injury of varying severity. *Cortex, 13*, 119–130.
Lewis, D. A., Campbell, M. J., Terry, R. D., & Morrison, J. H. (1987). Laminar and regional distributions of neurofibrillary tangles and neuritic plaques in Alzheimer's disease: A quantitative study of visual and auditory cortices. *Journal of Neuroscience, 7*, 1799–1808.
Lezak, M. D. (1983). *Neuropsychological assessment* (2nd ed.). New York: Oxford University Press.
Livingstone, M., & Hubel, D. (1987). Psychophysical evidence for separate channels for the perception of form, color, movement, and depth. *Journal of Neuroscience, 7*, 3416–3468.
Livingstone, M., & Hubel, D. (1988). Segregation of form, color, movement, and depth: Anatomy, physiology, and perception. *Science, 240*, 740–749.
Luria, A. R., & Tsvetkova, L. D. (1964). The programming of constructive activity in local brain injuries. *Neuropsychologia, 2*, 95–108.
Masure, M. C., & Benton, A. L. (1983). Visuospatial performance in left-handed patients with unilateral brain lesions. *Neuropsychologia, 21*, 179–181.
Masure, M. C., & Tzavaras, A. (1976). Perception de figures entrécroisees par des sujets atteints de lésions corticales unilatérales. *Neuropsychologoia, 14*, 371–374.
Matarazzo, J. D. (1972). *Wechsler's measurement and appraisal of adult intelligence* (5th ed.). Baltimore: Williams & Wilkins.
Matarazzo, J. D. (1990). Psychological assessment versus psychological testing: Validation from Binet to the school, clinic, and classroom. *American Psychologist, 45*, 999–1017.
Matarazzo, J. D., & Herman, D. O. (1984). Base-rate data for the WAIS-R: Test-retest reliability and VIQ-PIQ differences. *Journal of Clinical Neuropsychology, 6*, 351–366.
Matthews, C. G. (1992). Truth in labeling: Are we really an international society? *Journal of Clinical and Experimental Neuropsychology, 14*, 418–426.

Maunsell, J. H. R. (1987). Psychological evidence for two visual subsystems. In L. M. Vaina (Ed.), *Matters of intelligence: Conceptual structures in cognitive neuroscience* (pp. 59–87). Boston: Reidel.

Mayer-Gross, W. (1935). Some observations on apraxia. *Proceedings of the Royal Society of Medicine, 28,* 1203–1212.

McFie, J. (1975). *Assessment of organic intellectual impairment.* New York: Academic Press.

McFie, J., Piercy, M. F., & Zangwill, O. L. (1950). Visual spatial agnosia associated with lesions of the right hemisphere. *Brain, 73,* 167–190.

McFie, J., & Zangwill, O. A. (1960). Visual constructive disabilities associated with lesions of the left cerebral hemisphere. *Brain, 83,* 243–260.

McGlynn, S. M., & Schacter, D. L. (1989). Unawareness of deficits in neuropsychological syndromes. *Journal of Clinical and Experimental Neuropsychology, 11,* 143–205.

Meadows, J. C. (1974). The anatomical basis of prosopagnosia. *Journal of Neurology, Neurosurgery, and Psychiatry, 37,* 615–632.

Mehta, Z., Newcombe, F., & Damasio, H. (1987). A left hemisphere contribution to visuospatial processing. *Cortex, 23,* 447–461.

Mendez, M. F., Mendez, M. A., Martin, R., Smyth, K. A., & Whitehouse, P. J. (1990). Complex visual disturbances in Alzheimer's disease. *Neurology, 40,* 439–443.

Milberg, W. P., Hebben, N., & Kaplan, E. (1986). The Boston process approach to neuropsychological assessment. In I. Grant & K. M. Adams (Eds.), *Neuropsychological assessment of neuropsychiatric disorders* (pp. 65–86). New York: Oxford University Press.

Mohr, E., Litvan, I., Williams, J., Fedio, P., & Chase, T. N. (1990). Selective deficits in Alzheimer and Parkinsonian dementia: Visuospatial function. *Canadian Journal of Neurological Sciences, 17*(3), 292–297.

Mooney, C. M. (1956). Closure with negative after-images under flickering light. *Canadian Journal of Psychology, 10,* 191–199.

Mortimer, J. A., Pirozzolo, F. J., Hansch, E. C., & Webster, D. D. (1982). Relationship of motor symptoms to intellectual deficits in Parkinson's disease. *Neurology, 32,* 133–137.

Mountcastle, V. B., Lynch, J. C., Georgopoulos, A., Sakata, H., & Acuna, C. (1975). Posterior parietal association cortex of the monkey: Command functions for operations within extrapersonal space. *Journal of Neurophysiology, 38,* 871–908.

Newcombe, F. (1969). *Missile wounds of the brain: A study of psychological deficits.* London: Oxford University Press.

Newcombe, F. (1985). Neuropsychology *qua* interface. *Journal of Clinical and Neuropsychology, 7,* 663–681.

Newcombe, F., & Ratcliff, G. (1989). Disorders of visuospatial analysis. In F. Boller & J. Grafman (Eds.), *Handbook of neuropsychology* (Vol. 2, pp. 333–356). Amsterdam: Elsevier.

Newcombe, F., Ratcliff, G., & Damasio, H. (1987). Dissociable visual and spatial impairments following right posterior cerebral lesions: Clinical, neuropsychological, and anatomic evidence. *Neuropsychologia, 25,* 149–161.

Newcombe, F., & Russell, W. R. (1969). Dissociated visual perceptual and spatial deficits in focal lesions of the right hemisphere. *Journal of Neurology, Neurosurgery, and Psychiatry, 32,* 73–81.

Ober, B. A., Jagust, W. J., Koss, E., Delis, D. C., & Friedland, R. P. (1991). Visuoconstructive performance and regional cerebral glucose metabolism in Alzheimer's disease. *Journal of Clinical and Experimental Neuropsychology, 13,* 752–772.

Parsons, O. A., & Farr, S. P. (1981). The neuropsychology of alcohol and drug use. In S. B. Filskov & T. J. Boll (Eds.), *Handbook of clinical neuropsychology* (pp. 320–365). New York: Wiley-Interscience.

Parsons, O. A., & Leber, W. R. (1981). The relationship between cognitive dysfunction and brain damage in alcoholics: Causal, interactive, or epiphenomenal? *Alcoholism: Clinical and Experimental Research, 5,* 326–343.

Paterson, A., & Zangwill, O. L. (1944). Disorders of visual space perception associated with lesions of the right hemisphere. *Brain, 67,* 331–358.

Paterson, A., & Zangwill, O. A. (1945). A case of topographical disorientation associated with unilateral cerebral lesion. *Brain, 68,* 188–211.

Piercy, M. F., & Smyth, V. (1962). Right hemisphere dominance for certain nonverbal intellectual skills. *Brain, 85,* 775–790.

Poggio, G. F. (1984). The analysis of stereopsis. *Annual Review of Neuroscience, 7,* 379–412.

Pohl, W. (1973). Dissociation of spatial discrimination deficits following frontal and parietal lesions in monkeys. *Journal of Comparative and Physiological Psychology, 82,* 227–239.

Poppelreuter, W. (1990). Disturbances of lower and higher visual capacities caused by occipital damage. Oxford: Clarendon Press. (Original work published 1917)

Price, M. J., Feldman, R. G., Adelberg, D., & Kayne, H. (1992). Abnormalities in color vision and contrast sensitivity in Parkinson's disease. *Neurology, 42,* 887–890.

Ptito, A., Zatorre, R. J., Larson, W. L., & Tosoni, C. (1991). Stereopsis after unilateral temporal lobectomy. *Brain, 114,* 1323–1333.

Quaglino, A., & Borelli, G. (1867). Emiplegia sinistra con amaurosi—guarigione—perdita totale della percezione dei colori e della memoria della configurazione degli oggetti. *Giornale d'Oftalmologia Italiano, 10,* 106–117.

Rizzo, M., & Damasio, H. (1985). Impairment of stereopsis with focal brain lesions. *Annals of Neurology, 18,* 112.

Roberts, R. J., & Hamsher, K. deS. (1984). Effects of minority status on facial recognition and naming performance. *Journal of Clinical Psychology, 40,* 539–545.

Rosenberger, P. (1974). Discriminative aspects of visual hemi-inattention. *Neurology, 24,* 17–23.

Russo, M., & Vignolo, L. A. (1967). Visual figure-ground discrimination in patients with unilateral cerebral disease. *Cortex, 3,* 118–127.

Ryan, C. J., & Butters, N. (1982). Cognitive effects in alcohol abuse. In B. Kissin & H. Begleiter (Eds.), *Biology of alcoholism, Vol. VI. Biological pathogenesis of alcoholism* (pp. 485–538). New York: Plenum Press.

Schenkenberg, T., Bradford, D. C., & Ajax, E. T. (1980). Line bisection and unilateral visual neglect in patients with neurologic impairment. *Neurology, 30,* 509–517.

Scotti, G., & Spinnler, H. (1970). Colour imperception in unilateral hemisphere-damaged patients. *Journal of Neurology, Neurosurgery, and Psychiatry, 33,* 23–28.

Selemon, L. D., & Goldman-Rakic, P. S. (1988). Common cortical and subcortical targets of the prefrontal and posterior parietal cortices in the rhesus monkey: Relation between intraparietal and principal sulcal cortex. *Journal of Neuroscience, 8,* 4049–4068.

Semmes, J., Weinstein, S., Ghent, L., & Teuber, H. L. (1955). Spatial orientation in man after cerebral injury—I: Analyses by locus of lesion. *Journal of Psychology, 39,* 227–244.

Sergent, J., Ohta, S., & McDonald, B. (1992). Functional neuroanatomy of face and object processing: A positron emission tomography study. *Brain, 115,* 15–36.

Sergent, J., & Signoret, J. L. (1992). Functional and anatomical decomposition of face processing: Evidence from prosopagnosia and PET study of normal subjects. *Philosophical Transactions of the Royal Society of London, B355,* 55–62.

Ska, B., Poissant, A., & Joanette, Y. (1990). Line orientation judgment in normal elderly and subjects with dementia of Alzheimer's type. *Journal of Clinical and Experimental Neuropsychology, 12,* 695–702.

Spreen, O., & Benton, A. L. (1969). *Neurosensory Center Comprehensive Examination for Aphasia.* Victoria, B.C.: University of Victoria, Neuropsychology Laboratory.

Spreen, O., & Strauss, E. (1991). *A compendium of neuropsychological tests.* New York: Oxford University Press.

Street, R. F. (1931). *A gestalt completion test* (Contributions to education, No. 481). New York: Bureau of Publications, Teacher's College, Columbia University.

Talland, G. A. (1965). *Deranged memory.* New York: Academic Press.

Tarter, R., & Edwards, K. (1985). Neuropsychology of alcoholism. In R. Tarter & D. Van Thiel (Eds.), *Alcohol and the brain: Chronic effects* (pp. 217–242). New York: Plenum Press.

Taylor, A. M., & Warrington, E. K. (1973). Visual discrimination in patients with localized brain lesions. *Cortex, 9,* 82–83.

Teuber, H. L. (1965). Disorders of higher tactile and visual functions. *Neuropsychologia, 3,* 287–294.
Teuber, H. L., Battersby, W. S., & Bender, M. B. (1951). Performance of complex visual tasks after cerebral lesions. *Journal of Nervous and Mental Disease, 114,* 413–429.
Teuber, H. L., Battersby, W. S., & Bender, M. B. (1960). *Visual field defects after penetrating missile wounds of the brain.* Cambridge, MA: Harvard University Press.
Thurstone, L. L. (1944). *Primary mental abilities.* Chicago: University of Chicago Press.
Trahan, D. E. (1991). Judgment of line orientation in patients with unilateral vascular lesions or severe head trauma. *Journal of Clinical and Experimental Neuropsychology, 13,* 23–24.
Ungerleider, L. G., & Mishkin, M. (1982). Two cortical visual systems. In D. J. Ingle, M. A. Goodale, & R. J. W. Mansfield (Eds.), *Analysis of visual behavior* (pp. 549–585). Cambridge, MA: MIT Press.
van Kleeck, M. H. (1989). Hemispheric differences in global versus local processing of hierarchical visual stimuli in normal subjects: New data and a meta-analysis of previous studies. *Neuropsychologia, 27,* 1165–1178.
Varney, N. R. (1982). Colour association and "colour amnesia" in aphasia. *Journal of Neurology, Neurosurgery, and Psychiatry, 45,* 248–252.
Varney, N. R., & Damasio, H. (1986). CT scan correlates of sound recognition defect in aphasia. *Cortex, 22,* 483–486.
Varney, N. R., & Damasio, H. (1987). Locus of lesion in impaired pantomime recognition. *Cortex, 23,* 699–703.
Walsh, K. W. (1978). *Neuropsychology: A clinical approach.* New York: Churchill Livingstone.
Walsh, K. W. (1985). *Understanding brain damage: A primer of neuropsychological evaluation.* Edinburgh: Churchill Livingstone.
Warrington, E. K. (1982). Neuropsychological studies of object recognition. *Philosophical Transactions of the Royal Society of London, B298,* 15–33.
Warrington, E. K., & James, M. (1967). An experimental investigation of facial recognition in patients with unilateral lesions. *Cortex, 3,* 317–326.
Warrington, E. K., & Rabin, P. (1970). Perceptual matching in patients with cerebral lesions. *Neuropsychologia, 8,* 475–487.
Wasserstein, J., Zappulla, R., Rosen, J., Gerstman, L., & Rock, D. (1987). In search of closure: Subjective contour illusions, gestalt completion tests, and implications. *Brain and Cognition, 6,* 1–14.
Watson, R. T., & Heilman, K. M. (1979). Thalamic neglect. *Neurology, 29,* 690–694.
Watson, R. T., Heilman, K. M., Cauthen, J. C., & King, F. A. (1973). Neglect after cingulectomy. *Neurology, 23,* 1003–1007.
Wechsler, D. (1981). *WAIS-R manual.* New York: Psychological Corporation.
Whitely, A. M., & Warrington, E. K. (1977). Prosopagnosia: A clinical, psychological, and anatomical study of three patients. *Journal of Neurology, Neurosurgery, and Psychiatry, 40,* 395–403.
Wise, S. P., & Desimone, R. (1988). Behavioral neurophysiology: Insights into seeing and grasping. *Science, 242,* 736–741.
Zeki, S. M. (1973). Colour coding in the rhesus monkey prestriate cortex. *Brain Research, 53,* 422–427.
Zeki, S. M. (1983). Colour coding in the cerebral cortex: The responses of wavelength-selective and colour-coded cells in monkey visual cortex to changes in wavelength composition. *Neuroscience, 9,* 767–781.
Zillmer, E. A., Waechtler, C., Harris, B., Khan, F., & Fowler, P. C. (1992). The effects of unilateral and multifocal lesions on the WAIS-R: A factor analytic study of stroke patients. *Archives of Clinical Neuropsychology, 7,* 29–40.

7

Assessment of Learning and Memory

GLENN J. LARRABEE and THOMAS H. CROOK III

Assessment of learning and memory is a critical component of neuropsychological evaluation, since impaired learning and memory are among the most common symptoms and neuropsychological deficits in neurological and psychiatric patients (Kapur, 1988; Spreen & Strauss, 1991). Learning and memory can be impaired in the context of relatively normal intellectual functions in the organic amnesias; alternatively, learning and memory can be impaired in the context of general intellectual decline in the dementias. Disordered learning and memory can also result from traumatic brain injury (TBI), brain tumors, and cerebrovascular disease, presenting as generalized or material-specific (verbal or visual nonverbal) impairment (Kapur, 1988). Finally, a variety of nonneurological, psychiatric factors—in particular, depression—can also affect learning and memory (Weingartner, 1986).

In addition to diagnostic assessment, there has been an increasing emphasis on accurate and relevant measurement of learning and memory functions in clinical trials of drugs intended to enhance memory (Crook, Johnson, & Larrabee, 1990; Larrabee & Crook, 1988). Such investigations have been conducted on persons suffering amnestic disorders and Alzheimer-type dementia (AD; McEntee & Crook, 1989). Additionally, there has been a rapid increase in clinical drug trials directed at modifying the changes seen in age-associated memory impairment (AAMI; Crook et al., 1991).

AAMI is a new descriptive category for persons aged 50 or over, who have subjectively noticed a decline in memory function relative to their young adult years, perform at least one standard deviation below the mean level of performance for young adults on measures of secondary memory, are not depressed or demented, and do not have any other condition that can account for performance decline (Crook, 1989; Crook et al., 1986). AAMI, referenced to young adult levels of performance, is a

GLENN J. LARRABEE • 630 South Orange, Suite 202, Sarasota, Florida 34236. THOMAS H. CROOK III • Memory Assessment Clinics, Inc., 8311 Wisconsin Avenue, Suite B8, Bethesda, Maryland 20814.

Clinical Neuropsychological Assessment: A Cognitive Approach, edited by Robert L. Mapou and Jack Spector. Plenum Press, New York, 1995.

broader descriptive category than "benign senescent forgetfulness" (Kral, 1962), which is referenced to age peer levels of performance.

The development of the new descriptive category AAMI and the fact that many clinical memory disorders occur in aged individuals also underscore the need for comprehensive, age-based normative data on measures of learning, memory, and related functions. Indeed, age-associated decline in memory test performance can be quite dramatic, with healthy, normal 70- and 80-year-old persons performing at half the level of young adults on measures of verbal and visual learning and memory (Larrabee, Trahan, Curtiss, & Levin, 1988; Trahan, Larrabee, & Levin, 1986).

Thus, learning and memory assessment is an integral part of any neuropsychological evluation. In this chapter, we will describe the components necessary for memory evaluation. Instruments available to assess each component will be critically reviewed. We will conclude with an illustration of clinical memory assessment.

ESSENTIAL COMPONENTS OF THE MEMORY EXAMINATION

In their seminal review, Erickson and Scott (1977) trace the origins of clinical memory testing to informal mental status testing. Following their review of the Wechsler Memory Scale (WMS) and other existing measures for evaluation of memory functions, Erickson and Scott (1977) recommended that future efforts in the evaluation of learning and memory should include dimensions of orientation and remote memory, immediate memory, and new learning for both verbal and visual material. In particular, these authors emphasized the importance of assessing acquisition of material (learning), as well as measuring retention of acquired material over time (memory). Finally, they recommended that material for memory tasks should be meaningful and should have "face validity" for the patient.

Since this review, research on organic amnesia, dementia, and clinical conditions known to result in memory impairment, such as severe TBI, has grown substantially. Paralleling this rapid expansion, there has been a similar expansion in development of memory testing procedures, including a revised version of the WMS (the WMS-R; Wechsler, 1987). Over this period, there has also been an increasing impact of experimental psychology on memory research and memory testing procedures (cf. Butters & Cermak, 1980). This experimental influence has been twofold: (1) theoretical and (2) methodological (Larrabee & Crook, 1988).

Theoretically, there has been a major influence of information processing (Butters & Cermak, 1980; Kaszniak, Poon, & Riege, 1986). This influence has included structural information processing models of sensory memory; primary, secondary, and tertiary memory (Kaszniak et al., 1986); and information processing models focusing on the mental processes relevant to memory functioning, such as levels of processing (Craik & Lockhart, 1972) and release from proactive inhibition (Wickens, 1970).

Methodologically, tasks such as the consonant trigrams procedure, developed for research on decay/interference in short-term memory (Brown, 1958; Peterson & Peterson, 1959), have been applied to the investigation of impaired memory in organic amnesia (Butters & Cermak, 1980). Signal detection, which allows a differentiation between response bias and sensitivity (Hannay, 1986), has been applied to recognition memory paradigms for facial memory (Ferris, Crook, Clark, McCarthy, & Rae, 1980), familiar figures (Hannay, Levin, & Grossman, 1979), and abstract geometric forms (Trahan & Larrabee, 1988). The delayed nonmatching-to-sample paradigm used in primate research (Mishkin, 1978) has been extended to investigation of impaired memory processes in demented humans (Albert & Moss, 1984).

This rapid growth of memory research has demonstrated the complexity and multivariate nature of learning and memory processes. Although the unitary construct of the Memory Quotient was promoted by Wechsler (1945) in the original WMS, several subsequent factor analyses of the WMS have yielded multiple factors or dimensions, including General Memory, Attention/Concentration and Immediate Memory, and Orientation (Larrabee, Kane, & Schuck, 1983; Prigatano, 1978). Factor analyses of other memory and problem-solving tests have yielded factor structures that are remarkably similar to structural information processing models. Hence, factors have been reported for primary/immediate memory (and concentration), secondary/long-term/recent memory for verbal and visual material, and tertiary/very long-term/remote memory (Larrabee et al., 1983; Larrabee, Kane, Schuck, & Francis, 1985; Larrabee & Levin, 1986; Prigatano, 1978; Wechsler, 1987). Factor analyses have not typically yielded separate dimensions of material-specific (i.e., verbal versus visual nonverbal) dimensions. Only one report using a balanced set of verbal and visual memory and intellectual tests, with separate factor analyses for immediate and delayed scores, has yielded material-specific (verbal and visual) factors in a group of normal subjects (Larrabee, Trahan, & Curtiss, 1992).

In summary, the review by Erickson and Scott (1977), a more recent review by Kapur (1988), experimental and clinical research on amnesia, dementia, and TBI, and factor-analytic investigations suggest that there are five components for the clinical examination of learning and memory. These are (1) orientation, (2) a general category of attention/concentration, information processing and immediate memory, (3) verbal learning and memory, (4) visual learning and memory, and (5) recent and remote memory. Erickson and Scott's (1977) recommendation that testing include assessment of acquisition (learning) and retention over a period of time delay (memory) is underscored by the recent report by Welsh, Butters, Hughes, Mohs, and Heyman (1991), who found that delayed-recall measures provided better discrimination between patients with AD and normals than did scores based on acquisition.

In the remainder of this chapter, we selectively review measures falling under the five learning and memory components, as well as general (omnibus) memory batteries. Additionally, we will briefly review metamemory (self-report) scales, as well as measures of everyday memory function, in particular, a computerized everyday memory battery designed for use in clinical trials of memory-enhancing compounds. We will not cover recent work on implicit memory and procedural learning, since this is still restricted primarily to experimental investigations of memory disorders. However, it is possible that in the future, assessment of implicit learning and procedural learning processes may yield information predictive of those memory-disordered patients who will benefit from memory rehabilitation (cf. Glisky & Schacter, 1987).

STANDARDIZED ASSESSMENT OF LEARNING AND MEMORY

Orientation

Assessment of orientation is a common component of the mental status examination (Benton, Hamsher, Varney, & Spreen, 1983; Strub & Black, 1985). Orientation is typically evaluated in four spheres: time, place, person, and situation. Strub and Black (1985) observed that orientation to time and place are actually measures of recent memory, since they evaluate the patient's ability to learn and remember continuing changes in these spheres. Benton et al. (1983) observed that disorientation to time suggests the presence of some type of abnormal condition. Finally, disorientation to time is a cardinal feature of posttraumatic amnesia (PTA), or the period of gross confusion, disorientation, and amnesia for ongoing events after the TBI patient regains consciousness (Levin, Benton, & Grossman, 1982; Levin, O'Donnell, & Grossman, 1979).

Benton et al. (1983) have developed a brief, well-standardized measure of temporal orientation, the Temporal Orientation Test, with specific criteria for five scored responses: the stated day of the week, day of the month, month, year, and time of day. In nonaphasic patients, those with bilateral brain disease showed the highest frequency of disorientation (57%), whereas disorientation was less frequent in patients with right- (14%) and left- (17%) hemisphere lesions (Benton et al., 1983). A screening battery composed of the Temporal Orientation Test, the Benton Visual Retention Test (Benton, 1974), and Controlled Oral Word Association (Benton & Hamsher, 1983) correctly classified 89% of dementia patients and normal age- and sex-matched controls (Eslinger, Damasio, Benton, & Van Allen, 1985).

Varney and Shepherd (1991) advocated using the Temporal Orientation Test as a screening task to determine the need for further assessment of memory functions. They found that eight error points or greater on the Temporal Orientation Test was associated with failure on three memory tests (WMS Associate Learning, Benton Visual Retention Test, Serial Digit Learning). Additionally, these authors noted that since the Temporal Orientation Test has a lower "floor," it could be used to measure improvement in recent memory, when such improvement would not be measurable on standard tests of secondary memory function.

The Galveston Orientation and Amnesia Test (GOAT) was developed by Levin et al. (1979) to evaluate PTA. The GOAT contains a brief series of questions concerning orientation to time (the questions from the Temporal Orientation Test), place, and person, as well as questions related to retrograde (recall of events prior to trauma) and anterograde (recall of events subsequent to trauma) amnesia. Levin et al. (1979) demonstrated that GOAT scores were significantly related to both the Glasgow Coma Scale (Teasdale & Jennett, 1974) and the Glasgow Outcome Scale (Jennett & Bond, 1975). High, Levin, and Gary (1990) have analyzed the pattern of recovery of orientation on the GOAT, following TBI of varying severity. They found that the most common pattern of return of orientation was person, place, and time in 70% of those studied. In 13%, return of orientation to time preceded orientation to place, and in 7%, return of orientation to place or time preceded the return of orientation to person. When disoriented to time, 68% of patients' estimates of the date were displaced backward in time, specifying a date that was, on average, 7.3 years in the past.

Attention/Concentration, Information Processing, and Immediate Memory

Several different neuropsychological tests can be listed under this heading, since measures of attention, speed of processing, and immediate memory are fairly closely interrelated, as reflected by various factor analyses of tests of memory and concentration (Larrabee et al., 1983, 1985; Prigatano, 1978). The prototypic measure of immediate memory, digit span (cf. Miller, 1956), has been demonstrated to load with factors that are also defined by the Wechsler Adult Intelligence Scale (WAIS; Wechsler, 1955) Digit Symbol subtest (Matarazzo, 1972), as well as with factors that are defined by the WMS Mental Control subtest (Larrabee et al., 1983; Larrabee, Kane, Schuck, & Francis, 1985). Measures of attention, rapid information processing, and sensitivity of short-term memory to interference, such as the Paced Auditory Serial Addition Test (PASAT; Gronwall, 1977), the Trail Making Test (Army Individual Test Battery, 1944), and the Consonant Trigrams procedure (Brown, 1958; Peterson & Peterson, 1959), have been widely applied in investigations of TBI, Korsakoff's syndrome, and orbitofrontal brain damage (Butters & Cermak, 1980; Levin et al., 1982; Stuss et al., 1982; Stuss, Stethem, Hugenholtz, & Richard, 1989). All of these measures are also sensitive to nonneurological (psychiatric) conditions (Niederehe, 1986; Reisberg et al., 1986; Weingartner, 1986).

Tests of Immediate Memory Processes

Tasks of digit recall following a single presentation have a long history in clinical psychology and neuropsychology. Such tasks are found on both intelligence and memory test batteries (Wechsler, 1945, 1955, 1974, 1981, 1987; Williams, 1991). Forward digit span is minimally sensitive to normal aging effects, while reverse digit recall is more sensitive to aging (Craik, 1984). Moreover, some evidence suggests that performance on reverse digit recall may be related to visual scanning and visuospatial skill (Costa, 1975; Larrabee & Kane, 1986). Psychiatric patients may perform relatively better (*percentile-wise*) on reversed digit recall compared to forward recall, and malingering subjects may actually recall more digits in reverse than forward sequence (Larrabee, 1990). These observations suggest that separate normative data should be provided for digits forward and reversed (a practice followed in the WMS-R; Wechsler, 1987), in addition to existing normative data that base scoring on the combined total.

Stuss and colleagues have used the Consonant Trigrams procedure (Brown, 1958; Peterson & Peterson, 1959) to evaluate short-term memory in frontal-leukotomized schizophrenics (Stuss et al., 1982). In this procedure, subjects are provided with three consonants, then must engage in an interfering activity (e.g., counting) for 3, 9, and 18 seconds. Consonant Trigrams was the only test out of several measures of learning and memory that was sensitive to orbitofrontal leukotomy. Subsequently, Stuss et al. (1989) analyzed recovery patterns on the Trail Making Test, the PASAT, and the Consonant Trigrams procedure in patients with mild and severe TBI. All three tests significantly discriminated control subjects from severe TBI patients, whereas only Consonant Trigrams discriminated mild TBI patients from controls. Stuss, Stethem, and Poirer (1987) provided normative data for a 9-, 18-, and 36-second version of the test.

Measures of Attentional Tracking and Information Processing Rate

Both the Trail Making Test and the PASAT have been considered as information processing tasks (Lezak, 1983; Spreen & Strauss, 1991; Stuss et al., 1987). However, a recent factor analysis of memory and information processing tasks showed that the PASAT loaded on an attention/information processing factor, whereas Trail Making B loaded on a visual intellectual/visuospatial factor defined by WAIS-R Block Design and Object Assembly (Larrabee & Curtiss, 1991). This calls for caution in interpreting Trail Making Test performance solely as a basic measure of attention and information processing rate.

The reader is referred to Chapter 2 by Mirsky, Fantie, and Tatman (this volume), for more detailed discussion of the various types of attention and information processing tasks. Normative data for Gronwall's (1977) original version of the PASAT are provided by Stuss et al. (1987). This version differs from the PASAT used in the study by Levin et al. (1987) of recovery from mild TBI (the version by Levin et al. uses 50 rather than 61 numbers per trial block). Normative data for the version by Levin et al. (1987) are available in two sources (Brittain, La Marche, Reeder, Roth, & Boll, 1991; Roman, Edwall, Buchanan, & Patton, 1991). Several sets of normative data exist for Trail Making, including Stuss et al. (1987), a composite set of data in Spreen and Strauss (1991), and new data published by Heaton, Grant, and Matthews (1991).

Verbal Learning and Memory

A variety of tasks have been developed for evaluation of verbal learning and memory, including recall of prose (WMS Logical Memory Subtest; Wechsler, 1945), and multiple-trial supraspan (i.e., beyond immediate memory span) learning tests including Serial Digit Learning (Benton et al., 1983), the Expanded Paired Associates Test (EPAT; Trahan, Larrabee, Quintana, Goethe, & Willingham, 1989), the California Verbal Learning Test (CVLT; Delis, Kramer, Kaplan, & Ober, 1987), the Verbal Selective Reminding Test (VSRT; Buschke, 1973; Larrabee et al., 1988), and the Rey Auditory Verbal Learning Test (RAVLT; Lezak, 1983; Rey, 1964).

It is important to note that learning (acquisition) and retention (memory) are confounded during the learning/presentation trials of these tests. Hence, delayed recall should also be examined to test for retention (memory). Delayed-recall trials are included in the RAVLT, CVLT, and VSRT. Serial Digit Learning does not include a delayed trial, and a recent factor analysis (Larrabee & Curtiss, 1991) demonstrated that this test had equivalent loadings on memory and attentional factors. Moreover, recall of text or prose after a single presentation, such as for the WMS Logical Memory Procedure, may be adversely affected by attentional fluctuation, thereby creating a confound of attention, learning, and retention. In view of these considerations, Russell (1975) developed a delayed-recall trial for WMS Logical Memory, a modification that has been carried over to the WMS-R (Wechsler, 1987).

The remainder of this section will consider, in greater detail, the EPAT, RAVLT, CVLT, and VSRT. The reader interested in Serial Digit Learning is referred to the chapter concerning this test in Benton et al. (1983). Those interested in WMS Logical Memory specifically, and prose/text recall in general, are referred to the critical discussion of WMS Logical Memory by Loring and Papanicolaou (1987).

Expanded Paired Associates Test

The EPAT (Trahan et al., 1989) is a modification of the Associate Learning subtest from Form I of the WMS, and was designed to address the two limitations of the original version: (1) there was no delayed-recall trial, and (2) the test was too easy for some subjects, with "ceiling effects" for normal subjects and relatively intact patients. The EPAT contains an additional four "hard" pairs: lampshade–sidewalk, crossroad–pillow, lawnmower–envelope, and automobile–scissors. These and the original four "hard" and six "easy" paired associates are administered over three learning trials, with a fourth recall trial conducted following 30 minutes of other nonverbal testing.

Normative data are provided for 306 adults, ages 18 to 91, screened for psychiatric or neurological factors (Trahan et al., 1989). Trahan et al. (1989) also presented performance data on patients with left and right cerebrovascular accident (CVA), severe TBI, and presumptive AD. With failure defined as performance below the fifth percentile, approximately half of left-CVA patients (aphasics excluded) failed either the EPAT acquisition or delay, whereas approximately 60% of severe TBI and 75% of presumptive AD patients failed either the acquisition or the delay trial. By contrast, only 25% of right-CVA patients failed either EPAT condition. Of particular interest, those right-CVA patients failing the test had poorer attention (measured by WAIS-R Digit Span) than those right-CVA patients passing the test. A similar association of Digit Span with EPAT performance was *not* demonstrated in the left-CVA group.

Factorial validity has been demonstrated in two separate samples. In the first, the EPAT and the VSRT loaded on a verbal memory factor in a sample of normal subjects (Larrabee et al., 1992). In the second, the EPAT loaded on a general (verbal and visual) memory factor along with the VSRT, Continuous Recognition Memory (Hannay et al., 1979; Trahan et al., 1986), and Continuous Visual Memory Test (Trahan & Larrabee, 1988), in a sample of psychiatric and neurological patients (Larrabee & Curtiss, 1991).

The Rey Auditory Verbal Learning Test

The RAVLT (Rey, 1964) has gained popularity through the writings of Taylor (1959) and Lezak (1983). The subject is presented with 15 unrelated words (A List) over five trials, with recall assessed after each trial. This is followed by a single trial of a new 15-word list (B List), to serve as interference, subsequent short delay recall of the original list, and a delayed-recall trial (20 to 30 minutes later, varying by specific laboratory; Lezak, 1983; Spreen & Strauss, 1991). Lezak (1983) also provided a 50-word list (containing A List, B List, and 20 novel words) for recognition testing following the delayed-recall trial. Scrutiny of the pattern of performance across the various trials of the RAVLT can yield data on serial position effects (particularly on the first trial of the A List and single trial of the B List), proactive interference (of A List on B List recall), retroactive interference (of B List on A List short delay recall), forgetting over delay, and consistency of performance in suspected nonneurological contributions to performance (e.g., better B List than first trial of A List recall; better A List short delay than on the fifth or final trial of A List acquisition; better recall on long delay A List testing than on short delay recall). Bernard (1991) has reported that malingerers suppressed recall from the first third of the RAVLT list, compared to controls and to patients with TBI.

The RAVLT is sensitive to a variety of disorders of brain function (Lezak, 1983). Ogden (1986) has reported reduced RAVLT performance in young adults with hydrocephalus. Ponsford, Donnan, and Walsh (1980) have reported lowered RAVLT scores in patients suffering vertebrobasilar insufficiency. Factor analysis of RAVLT scores and other neuropsychological measures yielded a factor on which the RAVLT and WMS verbal memory scores loaded (Ryan, Rosenberg, & Mittenberg, 1984). Macartney-Filgate and Vriezen (1988) reported a moderate degree of intercorrelation among the RAVLT, the VSRT, and the WMS "hard" associates.

RAVLT normative data are provided by Ivnik et al. (1990); Geffen, Moar, O'Hanlon, Clark, and Geffen (1990); and Wiens, McMinn, and Crossen (1988). Ryan, Geisser, Randall, and Georgemiller (1986) compared the alternate-form reliability and equivalency of List A and List C (see Lezak, 1983, p. 423). With approximately a 2-hour test–retest interval, forms A and C intercorrelated .60 to .77 and yielded comparable mean levels of performance. Crawford, Stewart, and Moore (1989) developed alternate, parallel forms for the original List A and List B.

The California Verbal Learning Test

The CVLT was designed to evaluate the process of verbal learning and the amount of material acquired and retained, using an everyday verbal memory task (Delis et al., 1987). The subject is presented with a "Monday" list of 16 items (four each, in the categories of clothing, spices/herbs, tools, and fruits) over five trials, followed by a second "Tuesday" list to serve as intereference. Short delay (immediately following interference) with free and category-cued recall, long delay (20 minutes) with free and cued recall, and yes–no recognition of the original list items among distractors are assessed. Multiple dimensions of performance can be evaluated, including semantic versus serial learning strategies, vulnerability to proactive and retroactive interference, retention of information over time, and free versus cued recall versus recognition memory. Normative data are available across the age range of 17 to 80. The CVLT has good split-half reliability (.92). Test–retest values are somewhat lower (e.g., List A total recall = .59); however, the retest interval was 1 year. The CVLT correlates significantly with various WMS subtests (Delis, Cullum, Butters, & Cairns, 1988). The test manual summarizes CVLT data on a variety of clinical populations.

Additional research further supports the construct and criterion-related validity of the CVLT. Delis, Freeland, Kramer, and Kaplan (1988) reported a factor structure representing multiple underlying memory processing components, including general verbal learning, response discrimination, proactive effect, and serial position effect, among others. Crosson, Novack, Trenerry, and Craig (1988) reported data comparing the performance of severe TBI patients with neurologically normal adult males. These subject groups differed on the CVLT in both level and process of verbal learning (e.g., TBI subjects as a group did not typically use semantic grouping strategies). Kramer, Levin, Brandt, and Delis (1989) used discriminant function analysis in demonstrating correct classification of over 76% of cases of Huntington's disease (HD), AD, and Parkinson's disease (PD) on the basis of CVLT performance. Schear and Craft (1989) reported significant correlations among CVLT, WMS, and VSRT scores (Levin et al., 1982). Delis et al. (1991) recently developed an alternate form of the CVLT.

Verbal Selective Reminding Test

The VSRT was originally developed by Buschke (1973). This procedure differs from the CVLT and the RAVLT in that the only time the subject hears the entire supraspan list is on the first trial; thereafter, the examiner presents only those items not recalled on the immediately preceding trial, yet the subject is still expected to provide all of the words (reminded and not-reminded) on the list. Several different versions of the test exist (Spreen & Strauss, 1991). Perhaps the most widely used version is that developed by Levin and colleagues (Hannay & Levin, 1985; Levin et al., 1982). Spreen and Strauss (1991) and Larrabee et al. (1988) provide the test stimuli (12 unrelated words presented over 12 trials) and instructions for administration. Normative data cover the adult age range of 18 to 91 (Larrabee et al., 1988; Ruff, Light, & Quayhagen, 1989). Data are also available for 13- to 18-year-old adolescents (Levin & Grossman, 1976). There are children's versions consisting of 12 unrelated words presented for eight trials (for ages 9 to 12 years; see Spreen & Strauss, 1991) and eight animal names presented for eight trials (see Spreen & Strauss, 1991).

On the VSRT, it is assumed that if a word is recalled at least once, without reminding, it is in long-term storage (LTS). If it is then recalled to criterion (correct recall of the entire list for three consecutive trials or to the final trial of the test), the word is considered to be in consistent long-term retrieval (CLTR). Some have questioned the validity of these assumptions (Loring & Papanicolaou, 1987). Indeed, Larrabee et al. (1988) found that the various VSRT scores (CLTR, LTS, Short-Term Storage, Short-Term Recall, Random Long-Term Retrieval) defined only one factor. However, Larrabee and Levin (1986) found separate verbal learning and retrieval dimensions when a subset of VSRT scores was factored with other memory test measures. These data suggest that caution should be exercised in literal interpretations of CLTR, LTS, and other VSRT scores.

The adult version of the Levin VSRT exists in four forms; however, only three are equivalent (forms 2, 3, and 4; Hannay & Levin, 1985). This is unfortunate, since normative data are based on form 1. Larrabee et al. (1988) have suggested that on repeat testing using one of forms 2, 3, or 4, the raw scores should be reduced by 10%, prior to calculating percentiles, since Hannay and Levin (1985) found form 1 to be approximately 10% more difficult.

The Levin form of the VSRT has been used extensively in research on TBI and AD (Larrabee, Largen, & Levin, 1985; Levin et al., 1982; Masur, Fuld, Blau, Crystal, & Aronson, 1990; Masur et al., 1989). In patients with TBI, more pronounced deficits are more likely to be seen in VSRT performance with left-hemisphere mass lesion, bilateral mass lesions, or severe diffuse injury, than with right-hemisphere mass lesion or mild TBI (Levin et al., 1982). VSRT scores most sensitive to AD tend to be CLTR, sum of recall, and delayed recall (Larrabee, Largen, & Levin, 1985; Masur et al., 1989; Masur et al., 1990). Variable data have been reported for reliability, ranging from .414 (Hannay & Levin, 1985) to .92 (Masur et al., 1989).

Visual Learning and Memory

Two major methodologies have been used in evaluating visual learning and memory: (1) design reproduction from memory and (2) visual recognition memory. Lesser used methodologies have included recall of object placement, such as abstract symbols (Malec, Ivnik, & Hinkeldey, 1991) or marbles (Levin & Larrabee, 1983) in a spatial array, or learning a supraspan spatial sequence (Milner, 1971, describing a task developed by P. Corsi).

Various time delays have been incorporated in measures of design reproduction. The popular Revised Visual Retention Test (Benton, 1974; commonly referred to as the Benton Visual Retention Test, or BVRT) can be administered using two different delay periods: immediate reproduction (following either 5 or 10 seconds of exposure) and reproduction following a delay of 15 seconds (after an initial exposure of 10 seconds). The Complex Figure Test (Lezak, 1983; Osterrieth, 1944; Rey, 1941; Spreen & Strauss, 1991) has been administered (following a copy trial) using immediate recall from memory, and anywhere from 20- to 45-minute delayed-recall trials. Spreen and Strauss (1991) noted that a 30-minute delay is one of the most widely used delay periods. These authors provide normative data from Kolb and Whishaw (1985) and from their own laboratory, for both the copy and 30-minute delay conditions. The original Visual Reproduction (VR) subtest of the WMS (Wechsler, 1945) required immediate design reproduction following a 10-second exposure. Russell (1975) modified the administraton to include a 30-minute delayed trial.

A variety of visual recognition memory tests are available. Kimura (1963) devised a test containing geometric nonsense figures, some of which recur and others that appear only once in a deck of 140 cards. The subject must discriminate recurring from nonrecurring stimuli. This same format has been employed by Hannay et al. (1979) using line drawings of familiar objects (Continuous Recognition Memory; CRM) and by Trahan and Larrabee (1988) using complex ambiguous stimuli (Continuous Visual Memory Test; CVMT). Additionally, Trahan and Larrabee (1988) have incorporated a 30-minute delayed-recognition trial. Warrington (1984) has developed a two-alternative forced-choice test of facial recognition memory.

As with verbal learning and memory, learning (acquisition) and memory (retention) are confounded during visual memory acquisition trials. Of greater importance, however, is the confound of visual memory testing procedures with general visuospatial processing ability. Factor-analytic studies of memory tests that have employed a balanced set of WAIS or WAIS-R marker variables for verbal intelligence and visuospatial intellectual ability, and that have analyzed memory test acquisition scores independently of retention scores (to avoid a method variance confound), have routinely demonstrated that for measures of verbal learning and memory (e.g., WMS Logical Memory), these tests load on a memory factor that is independent of verbal and visuospatial intellectual skills (Larrabee & Curtiss, 1991; Larrabee, Kane, Schuck, & Francis, 1985; Larrabee et al., 1992). The same has not been demonstrated, however, for measures of visual memory. Tests requiring immediate design reproduction show primary loadings with visuospatial intellectual skills and weaker or minimal loadings on a memory factor (Larrabee & Curtiss, 1991; Larrabee, Kane, Schuck, & Francis, 1985; Larrabee et al., 1992; Leonberger, Nicks, Goldfader, & Larrabee, 1990; Leonberger, Nicks, Larrabee, & Goldfader, 1992). When delayed-reproduction scores are factored, there is a shift in factor loadings, demonstrating a stronger relationship with a memory factor. This is depicted in Table 7.1, which shows the results from four independent samples using WMS Immediate and Delayed VR (Larrabee & Curtiss, 1991; Larrabee, Kane, Schuck, & Francis, 1985) and WMS-R Immediate and Delayed VR (Leonberger et al., 1990; Leonberger et al., 1992). For the WMS, Immediate VR shows stronger loadings on a spatial intellectual factor than on a general memory factor, whereas the reverse pattern is obtained for delayed VR. For the WMS-R, the Immediate VR condition shows an even stronger loading on a spatial intellectual factor and weaker loading on general memory than that demonstrated by the WMS Immediate VR test. For WMS-R Delayed VR, the loading increases on the memory factor, but

TABLE 7.1. Factor Loadings of WMS and WMS-R Immediate and Delayed Visual Reproduction

	Factor	
Test	General memory	Spatial intellectual
WMS Visual Reproduction		
Immediate Recall		
Larrabee et al., 1985[a]	.41	.66
Larrabee & Curtiss, 1991[b]	.42	.59
Delayed Recall		
Larrabee et al., 1985	.59	.51
Larrabee & Curtiss, 1991	.68	.33
WMS-R Visual Reproduction		
Immediate Recall		
Leonberger et al., 1990[c]	.21	.72
Leonberger et al., 1992[d]	.17	.64
Delayed Recall		
Leonberger et al., 1990	.44	.66
Leonberger et al., 1992	.49	.55

[a]Larrabee, Kane, Schuck, & Francis, 1985; $n = 102$.
[b]Larrabee & Curtiss, 1991; $n = 112$.
[c]Leonberger, Nicks, Goldfader, & Larrabee, 1990; $n = 99$.
[d]Leonberger, Nicks, Larrabee, & Goldfader, 1992; $n = 237$.

the Delayed VR subtest still shows a primary association with spatial intellectual ability. These data demonstrate two important points: (1) it is critical to include delayed-recall or -recognition trials in visual memory testing to reduce the confound of visual memory with spatial intellectual ability, and (2) the WMS VR appears, factorially, to be a better measure of visual memory than the WMS-R VR subtest.

Wechsler Memory Scale Immediate and Delayed Visual Reproduction

Over 15 years have passed since Russell (1975) first published data on a 30-minute delayed-recall trial for WMS Logical Memory and VR. This modification greatly enhanced the clinical utility of these two subtests and was one of the major factors influencing the development of delayed-recall trials for various subtests of the new WMS-R (Wechsler, 1987). Since the original paper, other papers have appeared that have expanded the normative base for the procedure, including data for children and adolescents (Curry, Logue, & Butler, 1986) and for the elderly (Haaland, Linn, Hunt, & Goodwin, 1983). More recently, Russell (1988) has published expanded normative data for 188 normal adults ranging in age from 30 to over 80.

Trahan, Quintana, Willingham, and Goethe (1988) have published normative data for 255 neurologically normal adults, covering the age range of 18 to 91. As expected, there was a significant association of age with performance on both the Immediate and Delayed VR scores. Data were also presented for patients with left and right CVA, severe TBI, and presumptive AD. In all cases, the clinical groups performed more poorly than the normal control subjects. The percentage of impairment (i.e., in the bottom 5% of control group performance) ranged from 46% (Immediate VR in the left-CVA group) to 92% (Delayed VR in the group with presumptive AD). The Delayed VR score was the most sensitive score in terms of detecting impairment in the clinical groups.

As depicted in Table 7.1, the Delayed VR score shows a stronger association with memory than Immediate VR. More recently, Larrabee et al. (1992) have demonstrated separate verbal and visual memory factors in a group of normal subjects, where the visual memory factor was defined by the Delayed Recognition CVMT score and Delayed VR.

Although the factor-analytic data indicate greater construct validity for WMS Delayed VR as a measure of visual memory, caution should be exercised in using this procedure with patients with dominant hand motor impairment, severe visuospatial or visuoperceptual problems, or neglect. These same cautions apply to other visual memory tests using a design-reproduction format. Alternative visual memory assessment procedures for patients with motor impairment but normal spatial/perceptual abilities would include visual recognition memory tests, such as the CRM or the CVMT.

Continuous Recognition Memory

The CRM was originally developed for evaluation of the effects of TBI on visual recognition memory (Hannay et al., 1979). The CRM employs 120 line drawings of living things and objects (e.g., flowers, sea shells, birds) as stimuli. There are several different categories of stimuli. Eight categories contain six perceptually similar yet different exemplars, one of which recurs, the others that occur only once in the 120 cards. The subject's task is to identify the recurring stimuli as "old," and the nonrecurring stimuli as "new." Signal detection procedures are used to score CRM performance.

In the original investigation, Hannay et al. (1979) found that excessive false alarms (misidentification of a "new" stimulus as "old" or previously seen) differentiated persons with moderate TBI from those with mild TBI and from performance of nonneurological medical control patients. Levin et al. (1982) report a dissociation in the memory performance of patients with mass lesion in the left temporal lobe. These patients performed defectively on the VSRT but normally on the CRM. No dissociation was found in patients with right-hemisphere mass lesions.

More recently, Hannay and Levin (1989) evaluated CRM performance in normal adolescents and adolescents with TBI of varying degrees of severity. Adolescents with mild TBI (Glasgow Coma Scale or GCS, 13–15) did not perform differently from normal adolescents. Adolescents with moderate TBI (GCS 9–12) had significantly lower CRM d prime values, fewer hits, and fewer total correct than normal adolescents, but did not differ in terms of test age, false alarms, or c (criterion). Adolescents with severe TBI (GCS of 8 or less) differed from normal adolescents on all CRM variables. Overall, 42% of adolescents surviving TBI that resulted in coma exhibited residual impairment on the CRM, whereas defective CRM scores were found for 30% of teens who had sustained moderate TBI, and for 9% of those with mild TBI. Patients with diffuse injury and left-hemisphere mass lesions differed the most from normal controls, but the different lesion groups (left, right, bilateral, and diffuse hemispheric injury) did not differ significantly from one another.

In addition to being sensitive to the effects of TBI, the CRM is also sensitive to normal age-related changes in visual recognition memory. Trahan et al. (1986), in an investigation of 299 normal persons ages 10 to 89, found age-associated differences for CRM false alarms, d prime, and hits. The most pronounced effects of aging were on false alarms and d prime, where age accounted for over four times the variance that it accounted for in association with hits.

Continuous Visual Memory Test

Trahan and Larrabee (1988) developed the CVMT to incorporate five basic features: (1) a recognition memory format; (2) use of complex ambiguous designs not easily susceptible to verbal labeling; (3) a large number of stimuli, including classes of perceptually similar stimuli; (4) limited exposure time to each stimulus; and (5) a delayed-recognition test. The CVMT has 112 designs, seven of which are repeated six times. Each of the repeated stimuli are from categories containing six perceptually similar stimuli that do not recur. The subject must identify the recurring stimuli as "old" and the nonrecurring stimuli as "new" in a signal detection format similar to the CRM. Indeed, Drake and Hannay (1992) found that both the CRM and the CVMT met the assumptions of signal detection theory.

The CVMT manual contains normative data for d prime (d′), total correct, and delayed multiple-choice recognition for 310 adults ages 18 to 91, in addition to CVMT data on failure rates for patients with amnestic disorder, AD, and severe TBI. One hundred percent of the amnestics, 92% of the AD subjects, and 68% of the TBI subjects were impaired on at least two CVMT scores (Trahan & Larrabee, 1988).

Larrabee et al. (1992), in a factor analysis of CVMT performance in normal subjects, found that CVMT d′ loaded on attentional, verbal intellectual, and visual intellectual factors. By contrast, CVMT delayed recognition loaded on a visual memory factor that was independent of verbal and visual intellectual factors and a verbal memory factor. Larrabee and Curtiss (1991), in a factor analysis of CVMT performance in a mixed group of psychiatric and neurological patients, found that CVMT total correct and CVMT delayed multiple-choice recognition memory loaded on a general (verbal and nonverbal) memory factor in separate factor analyses of acquisition and delayed scores. Trahan and Larrabee (1990) have developed an alternate form of the CVMT. Test–retest reliability over a 1-week period ranges from .80 to .98 in normal and TBI patients (Trahan & Larrabee, 1988). Trahan, Larrabee, and Quintana (1990) demonstrated significantly poorer CVMT performance for patients with right-CVA lesions than for those with left-CVA lesions.

Forgetting Scores

Analysis of forgetting rates for verbal and visual memory tasks has become an important consideration in the differentiation of various amnestic and dementing conditions (Butters, 1992). Butters et al. (1988) demonstrated discrimination of patients with HD, AD, and amnestic syndrome from both young and old normal controls, based on savings scores (Delayed Recall/Immediate Recall × 100) for WMS-R Logical Memory, VR, Visual Paired Associates, and Verbal Paired Associates. Additionally, HD patients showed greater saving than AD and amnestic patients. Martin, Loring, Meador, and Lee (1988) found more rapid forgetting in patients with temporal lobe epilepsy, compared to normal controls, matched on a pairwise basis for initial learning on the VSRT. AD and PD patients forgot at a faster rate than HD patients on the CVLT (Kramer et al., 1989).

Recently, normative data for evaluation of forgetting rates for several memory procedures have become available. Forgetting data have been published for the RAVLT (Geffen et al., 1990; Ivnik et al., 1990), the WMS-R (Ivnik et al., 1992), the EPAT (Trahan & Larrabee, 1992), the original (form 1) WMS VR with delayed recall (Trahan, 1992), and the VSRT (Trahan & Larrabee, 1993). Table A3 of the CVLT manual also provides normative data relevant to analysis of forgetting (Delis et al., 1987).

Recent and Remote Memory Functions

Although combining the terms *recent* and *remote* in one section may seem counterintuitive, it is difficult to assess the point at which recent memory crosses over into remote memory. Basically, the material being assessed is material that the subject "brings with" him or her to the evaluation. Moreover, one is interested in evaluating *episodic* or context-dependent material as opposed to *semantic* memory. Consider an information item on an intelligence test requesting that the patient identify who or what the Enola Gay was. For a 65-year-old person who recalls the precise context of seeing a newspaper headline concerning the dropping of the atomic bomb, this is in episodic memory. For the 14-year-old history and trivia buff, this material is more likely to be in semantic memory. The distinction is important, as demonstrated by the normal performance of Korsakoff's patients on the WAIS Information subtest (Butters & Cermak, 1980) contrasted with the marked retrograde amnesia apparent on the Albert, Butters, and Levin (1979) Remote Memory Battery assessing memory for famous faces and famous events from the 1920s through the 1970s. These examples point out the difficulty in evaluating remote, episodic memory. The ideal test would ensure that once a newsworthy event occurs in a given time frame, say, 1963, it would never be highlighted by the media again. Unfortunately, famous persons and newsworthy events are frequently repeated across several different temporal contexts.

Memory for Famous Faces and Famous Events

Development of tests assessing remote episodic memory for famous faces and/or events dates to work by Warrington and Silberstein (1970), Seltzer and Benson (1974), and Marslen-Wilson and Teuber (1975). Perhaps the best-known example of this type of examination is the Remote Memory Battery (RMB) developed by Albert et al. (1979).

In describing the rationale for their investigation, the authors noted that Ribot (1881) and Talland (1965) had observed a temporal gradient of impairment for patients with Korsakoff's syndrome, in which memories acquired in the remote past were typically better preserved than those acquired during the more recent past (10 or 15 years prior to the current evaluation of the patient). Despite these clinical observations, Albert et al. (1979) observed that experimental investigations into the temporal gradient in organic amnestic patients had produced conflicting results, with Marslen-Wilson and Teuber (1975) and Seltzer and Benson (1974) demonstrating the gradient, in contrast to Sanders and Warrington (1971), who found generalized impairment in remote memory with no evidence to support relative preservation of remote relative to recent episodic memories. To further address this issue, Albert et al. (1979) carefully constructed a remote-memory battery composed of famous faces and public events covering the period 1920 to 1975, employing both recall and recognition testing. This battery was administered to 11 patients with alcoholic Korsakoff's syndrome and 15 control subjects. The data strongly confirmed the presence of a gradient of impairment, with greater impairment for both recall and recognition of both faces and events for more recent as opposed to more remote memoranda.

Subsequently, Albert, Butters, and Brandt (1981) employed the RMB to contrast the remote-memory performance of patients with alcoholic Korsakoff's syndrome, HD, and normal control subjects. Albert et al. (1981) replicated the previous finding of a temporal gradient of impairment in remote memory for the Korsakoff's patients. By contrast, patients with HD exhibited a global impairment in remote memory, equivalent across all decades examined, with no evidence for a temporal gradient. In this respect, it is noteworthy that when Wilson, Kaszniak, and Fox (1981) administered the RMB to a group of patients with presumptive AD, AD performance also reflected a global impairment in remote memory, equivalent across all decades examined.

Thus, the RMB has yielded important empirical data on the differential impairment of remote memory in Korsakoff's amnestic disturbance and in dementing conditions, with the temporal gradient being confirmed in the former. By contrast, dementing conditions apparently result in global, equivalent impairment across all decades examined. As mentioned earlier in the general discussion concerning problems related to measuring remote episodic memory, the problem arising from recurring news and entertainment media exposure of previously famous persons and events remains. Also, the complete RMB is lengthy (although a short form does exist; see White, 1987).

Recognition Memory for Canceled Television Shows

One alternative to the problem of information recurring across several different temporal contexts was devised by Squire and Slater (1975). These investigators assessed recognition memory for television shows that had been on for only one season, then canceled. This results in a definite restriction of material to a specific time period of 1 year, but may result in other psychometric problems, since previous research demonstrating temporal gradients in amnestics has covered much larger time spans (decades). Indeed, Levin et al. (1985) were unable to demonstrate a retrograde gradient for TBI patients in PTA, using a variant of the Squire and Slater (1975) TV Memory test, contrasted with the classic gradient found when remote memory was assessed using autobiographical information drawn from four developmental periods (primary school, junior high school, high school, and young adult life).

The Presidents Test

Hamsher (1982) has developed a novel, brief measure of recent and remote memory: the Presidents Test. This is a standardized test procedure, derived from common mental status examination questions concerning memory for recent U.S. presidents. Hamsher and Roberts (1985) presented detailed discussion of the development of the Presidents Test, as well as normative data, and test data obtained on patients with cerebral disease.

The test has four parts: (1) Verbal Naming, requiring free recall of the current and five previous U.S. presidents; (2) Verbal Sequencing, requiring sequencing of six cards imprinted with the names of the presidents (presented in quasi-random order) in the order of office; (3) Photo Naming, requiring confrontation naming of photographs (presented in the same quasi-random order as Verbal Sequencing); and (4) Photo Sequencing, requiring sequencing of the photographs in the order of office. Verbal Naming and Photo Naming are scored in terms of number correct. Verbal and Photo Sequencing are scored by computing the Spearman rho between the actual sequence of office and the patient's sequence. Of particular interest, the initial development of the test used the six presidents between Eisenhower and Carter, inclusive. When Reagan came into office, subsequent normative data collection was conducted on the six presidents between Kennedy and Reagan, inclusive. Comparison between both sets of normative data did not disclose significantly different patterns of performance. This suggests that future restandardizations, as presidents change office, do not require extensive restandardization (a potentially significant problem with other measures of recent and remote memory). The original normative data are based on 250 hospitalized nonneurological, nonpsychiatric medical patients.

Hamsher and Roberts (1985) reported that the Verbal Naming test was the most difficult, whereas Photo Naming was the easiest. Additionally, patients with diffuse cerebral disease and/or general intellectual decline performed the poorest on the various Presidents Test subtests. In a subsequent investigation, Roberts, Hamsher, Bayless, and Lee (1990) found that 88% of control subjects and patients with diffuse cerebral disease were correctly classified on the basis of their Presidents Test performance. Moreover, a selective impairment in temporal sequencing was found in patients with right-hemisphere disease, whereas patients with left-sided lesions demonstrated verbal deficit patterns (i.e., poor Verbal Naming and Photo Naming). Generalized memory impairment for recent presidents was rare for patients with unilateral lesions. Finally, the factorial validity of the Presidents Test is supported by an investigation concerning memory self-report and actual performance in normal elderly, conducted by Larrabee and Levin (1986). These authors found a factor that was defined by self-rated change in remote memory, the Presidents Test, and the Levin version of Squire and Slater's (1975) Recognition Memory Test for canceled television shows.

The advantages of the Presidents Test include good standardization and brief administration time. The major disadvantage is that performance cannot be analyzed for a temporal gradient of impairment.

OTHER DEVELOPMENTS IN THE ASSESSMENT OF LEARNING AND MEMORY

There have been two basic approaches to the development of tests of learning and memory. One approach focuses on the development of a specific measure of one aspect of learning and memory, such as verbal memory (e.g., RAVLT, CVLT, VSRT) or visual memory (e.g., CRM, CVMT). The other approach focuses on development of omnibus memory batteries, where subtests are designed and standardized as a battery, exemplified by the WMS-R and the newly published Memory Assessment Scales (MAS; Williams, 1991). Each approach has advantages and disadvantages. Individual tests designed to measure specific memory functions benefit from attention to the nature of the test stimuli and other psychometric issues, a focus that may be considerably diluted in development of an omnibus battery. Additionally, batteries such as the WMS-R and MAS may omit certain areas such as remote memory (WMS-R and MAS) or orientation (MAS). By contrast, standardization of test batteries allows calculation of base rates of difference scores between different subtests, which cannot be done if one employs an evaluation based on individually developed tests (e.g., combining the CVLT and the CVMT to assess verbal and visual memory).

The reader interested in test batteries such as the WMS-R or MAS is referred to other sources. An entire issue of *The Clinical Neuropsychologist* (1988, Volume 2, number 2) was devoted to the WMS-R. It is important to note that although this special issue presents the WMS-R in positive terms, subsequent reviews have criticized the psychometric properties of the battery and have called for caution prior to widespread implementation (Loring, 1989). Indeed, information in the current chapter questions the psychometric properties of the WMS-R VR and Paired Associate Learning subtests.

The newly published MAS is just beginning to undergo independent peer review. Larrabee (1991) noted that strengths of this battery include an extensive normative base (843 adult subjects), test design emphasizing research from cognitive psychology (e.g., semantic clustering, Brown-Peterson-type interference), and incorporation of an everyday memory task (Name Face Learning). One potential weakness is an apparent ceiling effect in the normative data (age-associated differences do not appear until the 70-plus group). This may not pose significant problems when using the scale in patient groups with significant neurological abnormalities, since the MAS summary scores for the clinical groups reported in the test manual are quite close to related scores reported for similar clinical groups in the WMS-R manual. This does suggest that additional research is needed on the sensitivity of the MAS to subtle neuropsychological deficit. The reader is referred to the MAS review by Larrabee (1991) for more details concerning this instrument.

Other memory batteries appeared during the 1980s but are not in widespread use. These include the Denman Neuropsychology Memory Scale (Denman, 1984) and the NYU Memory Battery (Randt, Brown, & Osborne, 1980). The NYU Memory Battery has been used as a validation measure for the Memory Function Questionnaire (Gilewski, Zelinski, & Schaie, 1990; Zelinski, Gilewski, & Anthony-Bergstone, 1990). Franzen, Tishelman, Smith, Sharp, and Friedman (1989) reported on the equivalence of Form A and Form B of the NYU Memory Battery. Larrabee and Curtiss (1985) reported that the factor structure of the Denman does not support the recommended scoring of performance (Denman, 1984) by computing Verbal and Nonverbal memory quotients.

There has been an increasing interest in developing memory assessment techniques that encompass the demands of everyday life (Crook, Ferris, & McCarthy, 1979; Crook, Ferris, McCarthy, & Rae, 1980). The Rivermead Behavioural Memory Test (RBMT; Wilson, Cockburn, & Baddeley, 1985; Wilson, Cockburn, Baddeley, & Hiorns, 1989) was developed to evaluate memory in the context of the environment of the physician's office. It includes tasks requiring remembering a first and last name, the location of a hidden belonging, an appointment, a new route traced out in the office, and prospective memory for delivering a message at a later date, among others. Wilson et al. (1989) present extensive psychometric data on the RBMT, which is currently seeing growing application in rehabilitation settings.

Crook and colleagues have an extensive everyday memory test development program using advanced computer imaging and laser disk technology for simulation of everyday memory tasks (Crook et al., 1990; Crook & Larrabee, 1988; Larrabee & Crook, 1991). These procedures combine realistic simulations (e.g., using laser disk recordings of actors introducing themselves) with current memory measurement paradigms such as paired associate learning, delayed nonmatching-to-sample, and selective reminding. Tasks include grocery list acquisition, first and last name paired associate learning, object location recall in a computer simulation of the interior of a house, dialing telephone numbers from memory, prose recall for television and radio broadcasts, reaction time for a simulated driving task, and facial recognition memory. The tests, designed for evaluation of everyday memory in clinical trials of memory-enhancing compounds, are available in six or more equivalent forms (Crook, Youngjohn, & Larrabee, 1992); discriminate persons with AAMI from those with mild AD (Youngjohn, Larrabee, & Crook, 1992); demonstrate factors of everyday verbal memory, visual memory, attention, vigilance, and psychomotor speed (Crook & Larrabee, 1988; Larrabee & Crook, 1989); and reflect a significant association between self-report and actual performance (Larrabee, West, & Crook, 1991). Normative data average approximately 2,000 adult subjects per test. The procedures, currently employed in clinical research in the United States and Europe, are available in American English, British English, Danish, Finnish, Flemish, French, German (Austrian and German versions), Italian, Spanish, and Swedish.

Finally, a significant amount of research has been conducted evaluating the association between memory self-ratings and actual memory performance. This is comprehensively reviewed in two sources: Hermann (1982) and Gilewski and Zelinski (1986). As noted in these reviews, although self-rating scales can yield useful information about memory beliefs, they should not be used as the sole means of evaluating memory, due to the weak associations between memory self-report and actual performance. Moreover, as compared to *actual* impairment, self-report may result in underestimation of memory difficulties by patients with AD (Reisberg et al., 1986, Figure 12.1), but overestimation by depressed patients (Williams, Little, Scates, & Blockman, 1987). Consequently, it is advisable to analyze self-report data in the context of actual memory test performance, as well as ratings of the patient's memory completed by significant others.

Two new self-rating scales have appeared subsequent to the reviews by Hermann (1982) and Gilewski and Zelinski (1986): the Memory Function Questionnaire (MFQ; Gilewski et al., 1990; Zelinski et al., 1990) and the Memory Assessment Clinic Self-Rating of Everyday Memory Scale (MAC-S; Crook & Larrabee, 1990, 1992). The MFQ has a stable factor structure, reflects modest associations with standardized memory test performance and diaries of actual failures (Zelinski et al., 1990), and is also available in a relative/family-rating format. The MAC-S has a stable factor structure (Crook & Larrabee, 1990) and demonstrates a significant association with computer-simulated everyday memory performance after statistically removing the shared variance between depression and self-ratings in normal adult subjects (Larrabee et al., 1991). Table 7.2 displays the results of a canonical correlation between MAC-S scores, correlated with factor scores from the computer-simulated everyday memory battery (cf. Crook et al., 1990). The first canonical variate represents the overlap between the MAC-S and depression, while the second canonical variate represents the overlap between the MAC-S and a general everyday memory factor. The MAC-S is available in a relative-rating format, the MAC-F. Feher, Mahurin, Inbody, Crook, and

TABLE 7.2. Canonical Correlation of MAC-S Factors with the GDS and Computer-Simulated Everyday Memory Factors

Variables	Correlation with first canonical variate	Correlation with second canonical variate
MAC-S Ability[a]		
Remote	−.498	.353
Numeric	−.511	.072
Everyday	−.769	−.310
Semantic	−.414	.321
Spatial	−.430	.211
MAC-S Frequency		
Semantic	−.818	.051
Concentration	−.560	.351
Everyday	−.783	−.081
Forgetful	−.534	−.568
Facial	−.466	.151
Global Speed of Recall	−.458	−.205
Global Concern and Distress	−.729	.134
GDS[b]	.992	.010
Computerized Tests[c]		
General	−.173	.961
Attention/Vigilance	.043	.160
Psychomotor Speed	.066	.075
Attention	.183	.093

[a]MAC-S = Memory Assessment Clinic Self-Report Memory Scale.
[b]GDS = Geriatric Depression Scale.
[c]Factors from the computer-simulated everyday memory battery.
Note. First canonical correlation = .630; second = .528.
From Larrabee, West, and Crook (1991).

Pirozzolo (1991) have reported a modest association of difference scores (MAC-S minus MAC-F) with dementia severity in an investigation of anosognosia in AD.

CASE EXAMPLE

The following case illustrates clinical assessment of learning and memory, using the framework and many of the techniques described.

A 49-year-old, single, female, right-handed, retired schoolteacher, with a Master's degree in education, was seen for neuropsychological evaluation 16 years after surgical resection of a third ventricle colloid cyst. She attempted to return to teaching following the surgery, but could no longer function effectively in the classroom. Since that time, she had held a variety of semiskilled positions and was working as a bagger in a supermarket at the time of the present neuropsychological evaluation. Her physician was concerned over change in personality (poor hygiene, difficulty getting along with others) and memory (poor compliance concerning medication). She had been taking Dilantin since the onset of a seizure disorder in 1982.

Review of medical records disclosed that the cyst was approached through a right frontal craniotomy. She experienced surgical complications, became obtunded, and developed a right hemiparesis on the second postoperative day. A ventriculostomy tube was inserted, followed by some improvement. She then underwent a second craniotomy, swelling was noted, and the septum pellucidum was opened, connecting both lateral ventricles.

On formal assessment, language and perceptual/spatial functions were well preserved. On motor function testing, there was no evidence of residual right hemiparesis. She did have a left-hand fine-motor impairment, which was thought to be correlated with the right frontal craniotomy. Manual tactile functions were preserved, bilaterally. On the WAIS-R, she obtained a Verbal IQ of 111 and a Performance IQ of 96. On the Wide Range Achievement Test-Revised, Reading was at the 79th percentile, Spelling was at the 77th percentile, and Arithmetic was at the 77th percentile. The Wisconsin Card Sorting Test was performed poorly, with 33 perseverative responses and 28 perseverative errors. The Minnesota Multiphasic Personality Inventory was valid; there were no clinical elevations.

On formal assessment, she was well oriented to time. She correctly stated the month, day of the month, year, and day of the week, and her estimated time of day was within 12 minutes of actual clock time. This is an errorless performance per normative standards (Benton et al., 1983).

Attentional and information processing scores were variable. WMS Mental Control was at the 90th percentile (Lezak, 1983, p. 464). Trail Making was administered twice. Initially, she took 34 seconds for Part A and 140 seconds (two errors) for Part B, performances at the 12th and below the 1st percentiles, respectively (cf. Heaton et al., 1991). When repeated later in the day, she took 32 seconds for Part A and 75 seconds for Part B, performances at the 12th and 14th percentiles, respectively. PASAT performance, scored for her age (Roman et al., 1991), was at the 11th, 15th, 33rd, and 19th percentiles for trials 1 through 4. Of particular interest, her Consonant Trigrams performance was above average for the 9-second and 18-second delay conditions (77th and 66th percentiles; cf. Stuss et al., 1987), but dropped significantly for the 36-second condition (15th percentile). This suggested an increased susceptibility of short-term memory traces to interference, consistent with the known third-ventricle location of her surgery.

In the area of verbal learning and memory, rote memorization was preserved for the nine-digit sequence on Serial Digit Learning (31st percentile; Benton et al., 1983). Performance deteriorated on more complex verbal learning and memory. On the EPAT, her acquisition score was at the 3rd percentile, while 30-minute delay was below the 2nd percentile (Trahan et al., 1989). Her forgetting score on this test fell at the 12th percentile (Trahan & Larrabee, 1992). Performance was severely impaired on the VSRT, with LTS, CLTR, and 30-minute delay all falling below the 1st percentile (Larrabee et al., 1988). Her forgetting score, based on the number of words in LTS on the 12th trial (the most stable estimate of acquisition for analysis of VSRT forgetting; Trahan & Larrabee, 1993), was at the 46th percentile.

Visual memory performance also reflected significant difficulties. WMS Immediate Visual Reproduction was at the 13th percentile, with 30-minute delay below the 4th percentile (Trahan et al., 1988). Her forgetting score for WMS Visual Reproduction was at the 3rd percentile. Performance on the CRM was at the 4th percentile

(Trahan et al., 1986). On the CVMT, memory sensitivity was at the 9th percentile, total correct fell at the 3rd percentile, and 30-minute delayed multiple-choice recognition memory was at chance level of performance.

On the Presidents Test, she recalled only four of the last six presidents (12th percentile), but when presented with cards imprinted with their names, she could sequence them in the exact order of office (63rd + percentile; Hamsher, 1982). Naming of photographs of the last six presidents was perfect (54th + percentile), and she could sequence them in the exact order of office (62nd + percentile).

Overall, this woman presented with impaired verbal and visual secondary memory, with impairment greater for acquisition than for forgetting. This pattern was seen in the context of basically normal intellectual functioning, with some indication for frontal lobe dysfunction (personality change, by history; reduced performance on Trail Making B and the Wisconsin Card Sorting Test). The neuropsychological pattern is consistent with a moderately severe amnestic syndrome. She definitely can process and retain information, given her normal Temporal Orientation Test performance and basically normal Presidents Test performance. This may well be due to the fact that her Consonant Trigrams performance was normal for the 9- and 18-second delay periods, with drop-off observed only at the 36-second condition. Had she developed a severe amnestic syndrome, impairment would also have been observed in her Temporal Orientation and Presidents Test performance, as well as for the shorter delay periods on Consonant Trigrams.

This woman's relatively better forgetting relative to acquisition performance is consistent with the diencephalic location of her tumor (Butters, 1992). Actually, if one compares her forgetting performance across the EPAT, VSRT, and WMS VR, there is an inverse relationship of level of performance with number of preceding acquisition trials, with her poorest performance on Visual Reproduction (1 trial), followed by better performance on the EPAT (3 trials), and her best performance on the VSRT (12 trials). This suggests that although the patient has a reduced amount of information that can be processed into secondary memory (i.e., impaired acquisition scores), with sufficient repetition of to-be-learned material, she can maintain information over time.

REFERENCES

Albert, M. S., Butters, N., & Brandt, J. (1981). Patterns of remote memory in amnesic and demented patients. *Archives of Neurology, 38*, 495–500.

Albert, M. S., Butters, N., & Levin, J. (1979). Temporal gradients in the retrograde amnesia of patients with alcoholic Korsakoff's disease. *Archives of Neurology, 36*, 211–216.

Albert, M. S., & Moss, M. (1984). The assessment of memory disorders in patients with Alzheimer's disease. In L. R. Squire & N. Butters (Eds.), *The neuropsychology of memory* (pp. 236–246). New York: Guilford Press.

Army Individual Test Battery. (1944). *Manual of directions and scoring*. U.S. Army, Washington, DC: War Department, Adjutant General's Office.

Benton, A. L. (1974). *The Revised Visual Retention Test* (4th ed.). New York: Psychological Corporation.

Benton, A. L., & Hamsher, K. deS. (1983). *Multilingual Aphasia Examination*. Iowa City, IA: AJA Associates.
Benton, A. L., Hamsher, K. deS., Varney, N. R., & Spreen, O. (1983). *Contributions to neuropsychological assessment: A clinical manual*. New York: Oxford University Press.
Bernard, L. C. (1991). The detection of faked deficits on the Rey Auditory Verbal Learning Test. *Archives of Clinical Neuropsychology, 6*, 81–88.
Brittain, J. L., La Marche, J. A., Reeder, K. P., Roth, D. L., & Boll, T. J. (1991). Effects of age and IQ on Paced Auditory Serial Addition Task (PASAT) Performance. *The Clinical Neuropsychologist, 5*, 163–175.
Brown, J. (1958). Some tests of the decay theory of immediate memory. *Quarterly Journal of Experimental Psychology, 10*, 12–21.
Buschke, H. (1973). Selective reminding for analysis of memory and learning. *Journal of Verbal Learning and Verbal Behavior, 12*, 543–550.
Butters, N. (1992). Memory remembered: 1970–1991. *Archives of Clinical Neuropsychology, 7*, 285–295.
Butters, N., & Cermak, L. S. (1980). *Alcoholic Korsakoff's syndrome: An information processing approach*. New York: Academic Press.
Butters, N., Salmon, D. P., Cullum, C. M., Cairns, P., Troster, A. I., Jacobs, D., Moss, M., & Cermak, L. S. (1988). Differentiation of amnestic and demented patients with the Wechsler Memory Scale-Revised. *The Clinical Neuropsychologist, 2*, 133–148.
Costa, L. D. (1975). The relation of visuospatial dysfunction to digit span performance in patients with cerebral lesions. *Cortex, 11*, 31–36.
Craik, F. I. M. (1984). Age differences in remembering. In L. R. Squire & N. Butters (Eds.), *Neuropsychology of memory* (pp. 3–12). New York: Guilford Press.
Craik, F. I. M., & Lockhart, R. S. (1972). Levels of processing: A framework for memory research. *Journal of Verbal Learning and Verbal Behavior, 11*, 671–684.
Crawford, J. R., Stewart, L. E., & Moore, J. W. (1989). Demonstration of savings on the AVLT and development of a parallel form. *Journal of Clinical and Experimental Neuropsychology, 11*, 975–981.
Crook, T. H. (1989). Diagnosis and treatment of normal and pathologic memory impairment in later life. *Seminars in Neurology, 9*, 20–30.
Crook, T., Bartus, R. T., Ferris, S. H., Whitehouse, P., Cohen, G. D., & Gershon, S. (1986). Age-associated memory impairment: Proposed diagnostic criteria and measures of clinical change—Report of a National Institute of Mental Health work group. *Developmental Neuropsychology, 2*, 261–276.
Crook, T. H., Ferris, S. H., & McCarthy, M. (1979). The misplaced objects task: A brief test for memory dysfunction in the aged. *Journal of the American Geriatric Society, 27*, 284–287.
Crook, T. H., Ferris, S. H., McCarthy, M., & Rae, D. (1980). The utility of digit recall tasks for assessing memory in the aged. *Journal of Consulting and Clinical Psychology, 48*, 228–233.
Crook, T. H., Johnson, B. A., & Larrabee, G. J. (1990). New methods for assessing drug effects in Alzheimer's disease and age-associated memory impairment. In O. Benkert, W. Maier, & K. Rickels (Eds.), *Methodology of the evaluation of psychotropic drugs* (pp. 37–55). New York: Springer.
Crook, T. H., & Larrabee, G. J. (1988). Interrelationships among everyday memory tests: Stability of factor structure with age. *Neuropsychology, 2*, 1–12.
Crook, T. H., & Larrabee, G. J. (1990). A self-rating scale for evaluating memory in everyday life. *Psychology and Aging, 5*, 48–57.
Crook, T. H., & Larrabee, G. J. (1992). Normative data on a self-rating scale for evaluating memory in everyday life. *Archives of Clinical Neuropsychology, 7*, 41–51.
Crook, T. H., Tinklenberg, J., Yesavage, J., Petrie, W., Nunzi, M. G., & Massari, D. C. (1991). Effects of phosphatidylserine in age-associated memory impairment. *Neurology, 41*, 644–649.
Crook, T. H., Youngjohn, J. R., & Larrabee, G. J. (1992). Multiple equivalent test forms in a computerized everyday memory battery. *Archives of Clinical Neuropsychology, 7*, 221–232.
Crosson, B., Novack, T. A., Trenerry, M. R., & Craig, P. L. (1988). California Verbal Learning Test

(CVLT) performance in severely head-injured and neurologically normal adult males. *Journal of Clinical and Experimental Neuropsychology, 10*, 754–768.
Curry, J. F., Logue, P. E., & Butler, B. (1986). Child and adolescent norms for Russell's revision of the Wechsler Memory Scale. *Journal of Clinical Child Psychology, 15*, 214–220.
Delis, D. C., Cullum, C. M., Butters, N., & Cairns, P. (1988). Wechsler Memory Scale-Revised and California Verbal Learning Test: Convergence and divergence. *The Clinical Neuropsychologist, 2*, 188–196.
Delis, D. C., Freeland, J., Kramer, J. H., & Kaplan, E. (1988). Integrating clinical assessment with cognitive neuroscience: Construct validation of a multivariate verbal learning test. *Journal of Consulting and Clinical Psychology, 56*, 123–130.
Delis, D. C., Kramer, J. H., Kaplan, E., & Ober, B. A. (1987). *California Verbal Learning Test. Research edition. Manual*. San Antonio: Psychological Corporation.
Delis, D. C., McKee, R., Massman, P. J., Kramer, J. H., Kaplan, E., & Gettman, D. (1991). Alternate form of the California Verbal Learning Test: Development and reliability. *The Clinical Neuropsychologist, 5*, 154–162.
Denman, S. B. (1984). *Denman Neuropsychology Memory Scale*. Charleston, SC: Author.
Drake, A. I., & Hannay, H. J. (1992). Continuous recognition memory tests: Are the assumptions of the theory of signal detection met? *Journal of Clinical and Experimental Neuropsychology, 14*, 539–544.
Erickson, R. C., & Scott, M. L. (1977). Clinical memory testing: A review. *Psychological Bulletin, 84*, 1130–1149.
Eslinger, P. J., Damasio, A. R., Benton A. L., & Van Allen, M. (1985). Neuropsychologic detection of abnormal mental decline in older persons. *Journal of the American Medical Association, 253*, 670–674.
Feher, E. P., Mahurin, R. K., Inbody, S. B., Crook, T. H., & Pirozzolo, F. J. (1991). Anosognosia in Alzheimer's disease. *Neuropsychiatry, Neuropsychology, and Behavioral Neurology, 4*, 136–146.
Ferris, S. H., Crook, T., Clark, E., McCarthy, M., & Rae, D. (1980). Facial recognition memory deficits in normal aging and senile dementia. *Journal of Gerontology, 35*, 707–714.
Franzen, M. D., Tishelman, A., Smith, S., Sharp, B., & Friedman, A. (1989). Preliminary data concerning the test–retest and parallel forms reliability of the Randt Memory Test. *The Clinical Neuropsychologist, 3*, 25–28.
Geffen, G., Moar, K. J., O'Hanlon, A. P., Clark, C. R., & Geffen, L. B. (1990). Performance measures of 16- to 86-year-old males and females on the Auditory Verbal Learning Test. *The Clinical Neuropsychologist, 4*, 45–63.
Gilewski, M. J., & Zelinski, E. M. (1986). Questionnaire assessment of memory complaints. In L. W. Poon, T. Crook, K. L. Davis, C. Eisdorfer, B. J. Gurland, A. W. Kaszniak, & L. W. Thompson (Eds.), *Handbook for clinical memory assessment of older adults* (pp. 93–107). Washington, DC: American Psychological Association.
Gilewski, M. J., Zelinski, E. M., & Schaie, K. W. (1990). The memory functioning questionnaire for assessment of memory complaints in adulthood and old age. *Psychology and Aging, 5*, 482–490.
Glisky, E., & Schacter, D. (1987). Acquisition of domain-specific knowledge in organic amnesia: Training for computer-related work. *Neuropsychologia, 25*, 893–906.
Gronwall, D. M. A. (1977). Paced auditory serial-addition task: A measure of recovery from concussion. *Perceptual and Motor Skills, 44*, 367–373.
Haaland, K. Y., Linn, R. T., Hunt, W. C., & Goodwin, J. S. (1983). A normative study of Russell's variant of the Wechsler Memory Scale in a healthy elderly population. *Journal of Consulting and Clinical Psychology, 51*, 878–881.
Hamsher, K. deS. (1982). *Presidents Test: Manual of instructions*. Milwaukee, WI: University of Wisconsin Medical School at Mt. Sinai Medical Center.
Hamsher, K. deS., & Roberts, R. J. (1985). Memory for recent U.S. presidents in patients with cerebral disease. *Journal of Clinical and Experimental Neuropsychology, 7*, 1–13.
Hannay, H. J. (1986). Psychophysical measurement techniques and their application to neuropsychology. In H. J. Hannay (Ed.), *Experimental techniques in human neuropsychology* (pp. 45–94). New York: Oxford University Press.

Hannay, H. J., & Levin, H. S. (1985). Selective Reminding Test: An examination of the equivalence of four forms. *Journal of Clinical and Experimental Neuropsychology, 7,* 251–263.

Hannay, H. J., & Levin, H. S. (1989). Visual continuous recognition memory in normal and closed-head-injured adolescents. *Journal of Clinical and Experimental Neuropsychology, 11,* 444–460.

Hannay, H. J., Levin, H. S., & Grossman, R. G. (1979). Impaired recognition memory after head injury. *Cortex, 15,* 269–283.

Heaton, R. K., Grant, I., & Matthews, C. G. (1991). *Comprehensive norms for an expanded Halstead-Reitan Battery.* Odessa, FL: Psychological Assessment Resources.

Hermann, D. J. (1982). Know thy memory: The use of questionnaires to assess and study memory. *Psychological Bulletin, 92,* 434–452.

High, W. M., Levin, H. S., & Gary, H. E. (1990). Recovery of orientation following closed-head injury. *Journal of Clinical and Experimental Neuropsychology, 12,* 703–714.

Ivnik, R. J., Malec, J. F., Smith, G. E., Tangalos, E. G., Petersen, R. C., Kokmen, E., Kurland, L. T. (1992). Mayo's older Americans normative studies: WMS-R norms for ages 56–94. *The Clinical Neuropsychologist, 6,*(Suppl.), 49–82.

Ivnik, R. J., Malec, J. F., Tangalos, E. G., Petersen, R. C., Kokmen, E., & Kurland, L. T. (1990). The Auditory-Verbal Learning Test (AVLT): Norms for ages 55 years and older. *Psychological Assessment: A Journal of Consulting and Clinical Psychology, 2,* 304–312.

Jennett, B., & Bond, M. (1975). Assessment of outcome after severe brain damange. *Lancet, 1,* 480–487.

Kapur, N. (1988). *Memory disorders in clinical practice.* London: Butterworths.

Kaszniak, A. W., Poon, L. W., & Riege, W. (1986). Assessing memory deficits: An information processing approach. In L. W. Poon, T. Crook, K. L. Davis, C. Eisdorfer, B. J. Gurland, A. W. Kaszniak, & L. W. Thompson (Eds.), *Handbook for clinical memory assessment of older adults* (pp. 168–188). Washington, DC: American Psychological Association.

Kimura, D. (1963). Right temporal lobe damage. *Archives of Neurology, 8,* 264–271.

Kolb, B., & Whishaw, I. (1985). *Fundamentals of human neuropsychology* (2nd ed.). New York: W. H. Freeman.

Kral, V. A. (1962). Senescent forgetfulness: Benign and malignant. *Journal of the Canadian Medical Association, 86,* 257–260.

Kramer, J. H., Levin, B. E., Brandt, J., & Delis, D. C. (1989). Differentiation of Alzheimer's, Huntington's, and Parkinson's disease patients on the basis of verbal learning characteristics. *Neuropsychology, 3,* 111–120.

Larrabee, G. J. (1990). Cautions in the use of neuropsychological evaluation in legal settings. *Neuropsychology, 4,* 239–247.

Larrabee, G. J. (1991). The Memory Assessment Scales. A review. *Bulletin of the National Academy of Neuropsychology, 8,* 12–15.

Larrabee, G. J., & Crook, T. H. (1988). Assessment of drug effects in age-related memory disorders: Clinical, theoretical and psychometric considerations. *Psychopharmacology Bulletin, 24,* 515–522.

Larrabee, G. J., & Crook, T. H. (1989). Dimensions of everyday memory in age-associated memory impairment. *Psychological Assessment: A Journal of Consulting and Clinical Psychology, 1,* 92–97.

Larrabee, G. J., & Crook, T. H. (1991). Computerized memory testing in clinical trials. In E. Mohr & P. Brouwers (Eds.), *Handbook of clinical trials: The neurobehavioral approach* (pp. 293–306). Amsterdam: Swets & Zeitlinger.

Larrabee, G. J., & Curtiss, G. (1985). Factor structure and construct validity of the Denman Neuropsychology Memory Scale. *International Journal of Neuroscience, 26,* 269–276.

Larrabee, G. J., & Curtis, G. (1991). Factorial validity of various memory testing procedures [Abstract]. *The Clinical Neuropsychologist, 5,* 261–262.

Larrabee, G. J., & Kane, R. L. (1986). Reversed digit repetition involves visual and verbal processes. *International Journal of Neuroscience, 30,* 11–15.

Larrabee, G. J., Kane, R. L., & Schuck, J. R. (1983). Factor analysis of the WAIS and Wechsler Memory Scale: An analysis of the construct validity of the Wechsler Memory Scale. *Journal of Clinical Neuropsychology, 5,* 159–168.

Larrabee, G. J., Kane, R. L., Schuck, J. R., & Francis, D. E. (1985). The construct validity of various memory testing procedures. *Journal of Clinical and Experimental Neuropsychology, 7*, 239–250.

Larrabee, G. J., Largen, J. W., & Levin, H. S. (1985). Sensitivity of age-decline resistant ("Hold") WAIS subtests to Alzheimer's disease. *Journal of Clinical and Experimental Neuropsychology, 7*, 497–504.

Larrabee, G. J., & Levin, H. S. (1986). Memory self-ratings and objective test performance in a normal elderly sample. *Journal of Clinical and Experimental Neuropsychology, 8*, 275–284.

Larrabee, G. J., Trahan, D. E., & Curtiss, G. (1992). Construct validity of the Continuous Visual Memory Test. *Archives of Clinical Neuropsychology, 7*, 395–405.

Larrabee, G. J., Trahan, D. E., Curtiss, G., & Levin, H. S. (1988). Normative data for the Verbal Selective Reminding Test. *Neuropsychology, 2*, 173–182.

Larrabee, G. J., West, R. L., & Crook, T. H. (1991). The association of memory complaint with computer-simulated everyday memory performance. *Journal of Clinical and Experimental Neuropsychology, 13*, 466–478.

Leonberger, F. T., Nicks, S. D., Goldfader, P. R., & Larrabee, G. J. (1990). Construct validity of the WMS-R indices [Abstract]. *The Clinical Neuropsychologist, 4*, 284.

Leonberger, F. T., Nicks, S. D., Larrabee, G. J., & Goldfader, P. (1992). Factor structure of the Wechsler Memory Scale-Revised within a comprehensive neuropsychological battery. *Neuropsychology, 6*, 239–249.

Levin, H. S., Benton, A. L., & Grossman, R. G. (1982). *Neurobehavioral consequences of closed head injury*. New York: Oxford University Press.

Levin, H. S., & Grossman, R. G. (1976). Storage and retrieval. *Journal of Pediatric Psychology, 1*, 38–42.

Levin, H. S., High, W. M., Jr., Meyers, C. A., Von Laufen, A., Hayden, M. E., & Eisenberg, H. M. (1985). Impairment of remote memory after closed head injury. *Journal of Neurology, Neurosurgery, & Psychiatry, 48*, 556–563.

Levin, H. S., & Larrabee, G. J. (1983). Disproportionate decline in visuospatial memory in human aging. *Society for Neurosciences Abstracts, 9*, 918.

Levin, H. S., Mattis, S., Ruff, R. M., Eisenberg, H. M., Marshall, L. F., Tabaddor, K., High, W. M., & Frankowski, R. F. (1987). Neurobehavioral outcome following minor head injury: A three-center study. *Journal of Neurosurgery, 66*, 234–243.

Levin, H. S., O'Donnell, V. M., & Grossman, R. G. (1979). The Galveston Orientation and Amnesia Test: A practical scale to assess cognition after head injury. *Journal of Nervous and Mental Disease, 167*, 675–684.

Lezak, M. D. (1983). *Neuropsychological assessment* (2nd ed.). New York: Oxford University Press.

Loring, D. W. (1989). The Wechsler Memory Scale-Revised, or the Wechsler Memory Scale-revisited? *The Clinical Neuropsychologist, 3*, 59–69.

Loring, D. W., & Papanicolaou, A. C. (1987). Memory assessment in neuropsychology: Theoretical considerations and practical utility. *Journal of Clinical and Experimental Neuropsychology, 9*, 340–358.

Macartney-Filgate, M. S., & Vriezen, E. R. (1988). Intercorrelation of clinical tests of verbal memory. *Archives of Clinical Neuropsychology, 3*, 121–126.

Malec, J. F., Ivnik, R. J., & Hinkeldey, N. S. (1991). Visual Spatial Learning Test. *Psychological Assessment: A Journal of Consulting and Clinical Psychology, 3*, 82–88.

Marslen-Wilson, W. D., & Teuber, H. L. (1975). Memory for remote events in anterograde amnesia: Recognition of public figures from news photographs. *Neuropsychologia, 13*, 353–364.

Martin, R. C., Loring, D. W., Meador, K. J., & Lee, G. P. (1988). Differential forgetting in patients with temporal lobe dysfunction. *Archives of Clinical Neuropsychology, 3*, 351–358.

Masur, D. M., Fuld, P. A., Blau, A. D., Crystal, H., & Aronson, M. K. (1990). Predicting development of dementia in the elderly with the Selective Reminding Test. *Journal of Clinical and Experimental Neuropsychology, 12*, 529–538.

Masur, M., Fuld, P. A., Blau, A. D., Thal, L. J., Levin, H. S., & Aronson, M. K. (1989). Distinguishing normal and demented elderly with the Selective Reminding Test. *Journal of Clinical and Experimental Neuropsychology, 11*, 615–630.

Matarazzo, J. D. (1972). *Wechsler's measurement and appraisal of adult intelligence* (5th ed.). Baltimore, MD: Williams & Wilkins.
McEntee, W. J., & Crook, T. H. (1989). Pharmacological treatments of age-related cognitive loss. *Current Opinion in Psychiatry, 2*, 543–547.
Miller, G. A. (1956). The magical number seven, plus or minus two. *Psychological Review, 63*, 81–97.
Milner, B. (1971). Interhemispheric differences in the localization of psychological processes in man. *British Medical Bulletin, 27*, 272–277.
Mishkin, M. (1978). Memory in monkeys severely impaired by combined but not by separate removal of amygdala and hippocampus. *Nature, 273*, 297–298.
Niederehe, G. (1986). Depression and memory impairment in the aged. In L. W. Poon, T. Crook, K. L. Davis, C. Eisdorfer, B. J. Gurland, A. W. Kaszniak, & L. W. Thompson (Eds.), *Handbook for clinical memory assessment of older adults* (pp. 226–237). Washington, DC: American Psychological Association.
Ogden, J. A. (1986). Neuropsychological and psychological sequelae of shunt surgery in young adults with hydrocephalus. *Journal of Clinical and Experimental Neuropsychology, 8*, 657–679.
Osterrieth, P. A. (1944). Le test de copie d'une figure complex: Contribution a l'etude de la perception et de la memoire. *Archives de Psychologie, 30*, 286–356.
Peterson, L. R., & Peterson, M. J. (1959). Short-term retention of individual verbal items. *Journal of Experimental Psychology, 58*, 193–198.
Ponsfsord, J. L., Donnan, G. A., & Walsh, K. W. (1980). Disorders of memory in vertebrobasilar disease. *Journal of Clinical Neuropsychology, 2*, 267–276.
Prigatano, G. P. (1978). Wechsler Memory Scale: A selective review of the literature. *Journal of Clinical Psychology, 34*(Spec. Monogr. Suppl.), 816–832.
Randt, C. T., Brown, E. R., & Osborne, D. P. (1980). A memory test for longitudinal measurement of mild to moderate deficits. *Clinical Neuropsychology, 2*, 184–194.
Reisberg, B., Ferris, S. H., Borenstein, J., Sinaiko, E., de Leon, M. J., & Buttinger, C. (1986). Assessment of presenting symptoms. In L. E. Poon, T. Crook, K. L. Davis, C. Eisdorfer, B. J. Gurland, A. W. Kaszniak, & L. W. Thompson (Eds.), *Handbook for clinical memory assessment of older adults* (pp. 108–128). Washington, DC: American Psychological Association.
Rey, A. (1941). L'examen psychologique dans le cas de'encephalopathie traumatique. *Archives de Psychologie, 28*, 286–340.
Rey, A. (1964). *L'examen clinique en psychologie*. Paris: Presses Universitaires de France.
Ribot, T. (1881). *Diseases of memory*. New York: Appleton.
Roberts, R. J., Hamsher, K. deS., Bayless J. D., & Lee, G. P. (1990). Presidents Test performance in varieties of diffuse and unilateral cerebral disease. *Journal of Clinical and Experimental Neuropsychology, 12*, 195–208.
Roman, D. C., Edwall, G. E., Buchanan, R. J., & Patton, J. H. (1991). Extended norms for the Paced Auditory Serial Addition Task. *The Clinical Neuropsychologist, 5*, 33–40.
Ruff, R. M., Light, R. H., & Quayhagen, M. (1989). Selective reminding tests: A normative study of verbal learning in adults. *Journal of Clinical and Experimental Neuropsychology, 11*, 539–550.
Russell, E. W. (1975). A multiple scoring method for the assessment of complex memory functions. *Journal of Consulting and Clinical Psychology, 43*, 800–809.
Russell, E. W. (1988). Renorming Russell's version of the Wechsler Memory Scale. *Journal of Clinical and Experimental Neuropsychology, 10*, 235–249.
Ryan, J. J., Geisser, M. E., Randall, D. M., & Georgemiller, R. J. (1986). Alternate form reliability and equivalency of the Rey Auditory Verbal Learning Test. *Journal of Clinical and Experimental Neuropsychology, 8*, 611–616.
Ryan, J. J., Rosenberg, S. J., & Mittenberg, W. (1984). Factor analysis of the Rey Auditory-Verbal Learning Test. *International Journal of Clinical Neuropsychology, 6*, 239–241.
Sanders, H. I., & Warrington, E. K. (1971). Memory for remote events in amnesic patients. *Brain, 94*, 661–668.
Schear, J. M., & Craft, R. B. (1989). Examination of the concurrent validity of the California Verbal Learning Test. *The Clinical Neuropsychologist, 2*, 162–168.

Seltzer, B., & Benson, D. F. (1974). The temporal pattern of retrograde amnesia in Korsakoff's disease. *Neurology, 24*, 527–530.

Spreen, O., & Strauss, E. (1991). *A compendium of neuropsychological tests: Administration, norms, and commentary.* New York: Oxford University Press.

Squire, L. R., & Slater, P. C. (1975). Forgetting in very long-term memory as assessed by an improved questionnaire technique. *Journal of Experimental Psychology: Human Learning and Memory, 104*, 50–54.

Strub, R. L., & Black, F. W. (1985). *The mental status examination in neurology* (2nd ed.). Philadelphia: F. A. Davis.

Stuss, D. T., Kaplan, E. F., Benson, D. F., Weir, W. S., Chirilli, S., & Sarazin, F. F. (1982). Evidence for the involvement of orbitofrontal cortex in memory functions: An interference effect. *Journal of Comparative and Physiological Psychology, 96*, 913–925.

Stuss, D. T., Stethem, L. L., Hugenholtz, H., & Richard, M. T. (1989). Traumatic brain injury: A comparison of three clinical tests, and analysis of recovery. *The Clinical Neuropsychologist, 3*, 145–156.

Stuss, D. T., Stethem, L. L., & Poirer, C. A. (1987). Comparison of three tests of attention and rapid information processing across six age groups. *The Clinical Neuropsychologist, 1*, 139–152.

Talland, G. (1965). *Deranged memory.* New York: Academic Press.

Taylor, E. M. (1959). *The appraisal of children with cerebral deficits.* Cambridge, MA: Harvard University Press.

Teasdale, G., & Jennett, B. (1974). Assessment of coma and impaired consciousness: A practical scale. *Lancet, 2*, 81–84.

Trahan, D. E. (1992). Analysis of learning and rate of forgetting in age-associated memory differences. *The Clinical Neuropsychologist, 6*, 241–246.

Trahan, D. E., & Larrabee, G. J. (1988). *Professional manual: Continuous Visual Memory Test.* Odessa, FL: Psychological Assessment Resources.

Trahan, D. E., & Larrabee, G. J. (1990). The Continuous Visual Memory Test: Development of an alternate form [Abstract]. *Journal of Clinical and Experimental Neuropsychology, 12*, 56.

Trahan, D. E., & Larrabee, G. J. (1992). Effect of normal aging on rate of forgetting. *Neuropsychology, 6*, 115–122.

Trahan, D. E., & Larrabee, G. J. (1993). Clinical and methodological issues in measuring rate of forgetting with the verbal selective reminding test. *Psychological Assessment: A Journal of Consulting and Clinical Psychology, 5*, 67–71.

Trahan, D. E., Larrabee, G. J., & Levin, H. S. (1986). Age-related differences in recognition memory for pictures. *Experimental Aging Research, 12*, 147–150.

Trahan, D. E., Larrabee, G. J., & Quintana, J. W. (1990). Visual recognition memory in normal adults and patients with unilateral vascular lesions. *Journal of Clinical and Experimental Neuropsychology, 12*, 857–872.

Trahan, D. E., Larrabee, G. J., Quintana, J. W., Goethe, K. E., & Willingham, A. C. (1989). Development and clinical validation of an Expanded Paired Associate Test with delayed recall. *The Clinical Neuropsychologist, 3*, 169–183.

Trahan, D. E., Quintana, J., Willingham, A. C., and Goethe, K. E. (1988). The Visual Reproduction Subtest: Standardization and clinical validation of a delayed recall procedure. *Neuropsychology, 2*, 29–39.

Varney, N. R., & Shepherd, J. S. (1991). Predicting short-term memory on the basis of temporal orientation. *Neuropsychology, 5*, 13–16.

Warrington, E. K. (1984). *Recognition Memory Test.* Windsor, Berkshire: NFER-Nelson Publishing Company.

Warrington, E. K., & Silberstein, M. (1970). A questionnaire technique for investigating very long-term memory. *Quarterly Journal of Experimental Psychology, 22*, 508–512.

Wechsler, D. (1945). A standardized memory scale for clinical use. *Journal of Psychology, 19*, 87–95.

Wechsler, D. (1955). *Manual for the Wechsler Adult Intelligence Scale.* New York: Psychological Corporation.

Wechsler, D. (1974). *WISC-R manual. Wechsler Intelligence Scale for Children-Revised.* New York: Psychological Corporation.

Wechsler, D. (1981). *WAIS-R manual.* New York: Psychological Corporation.

Wechsler, D. (1987). *Wechsler Memory Scale-Revised manual.* San Antonio: Psychological Corporation.

Weingartner, H. (1986). Automatic and effort-demanding cognitive processes in depression. In L. W. Poon, T. Crook, K. L. Davis, C. Eisdorfer, B. J. Gurland, A. W. Kaszniak, & L. W. Thompson (Eds.), *Handbook for clinical memory assessment of older adults* (pp. 218–225). Washington, DC: American Psychological Association.

Welsh, K., Butters, N., Hughes, J., Mohs, R., & Heyman, A. (1991). Detection of abnormal memory decline in mild cases of Alzheimer's disease using CERAD neuropsychological measures. *Archives of Neurology, 48,* 278–281.

White, R. F. (1987). Differential diagnosis of probable Alzheimer's disease and solvent encephalopathy in older workers. *The Clinical Neuropsychologist, 1,* 153–160.

Wickens, D. D. (1970). Encoding categories of words: An empirical approach to meaning. *Psychological Review, 77,* 1–15.

Wiens, A. N., McMinn, M. R., & Crossen, J. R. (1988). Rey Auditory-Verbal Learning Test: Development of norms for healthy young adults. *The Clinical Neuropsychologist, 2,* 67–87.

Williams, J. M. (1991). *Memory Assessment Scales.* Odessa, FL: Psychological Assessment Resources.

Williams, J. M., Little, M. M., Scates, S., & Blockman, N. (1987). Memory complaints and abilities among depressed older adults. *Journal of Consulting and Clinical Psychology, 55,* 595–598.

Wilson, B. A., Cockburn, J., & Baddeley, A. D. (1985). *The Rivermead Behavioural Memory Test.* Titchfield: Thames Valley Test Company.

Wilson, B. A., Cockburn, J., Baddeley, A., & Hiorns, R. (1989). The development and validation of a test battery for detecting and monitoring everyday memory problems. *Journal of Clinical and Experimental Neuropsychology, 11,* 855–870.

Wilson, R. S., Kaszniak, A. W., & Fox, J. H. (1981). Remote memory in senile dementia. *Cortex, 17,* 41–48.

Youngjohn, J. R., Larrabee, G. J., & Crook, T. H. (1992). Discriminating age-associated memory impairment from Alzheimer's disease. *Psychological Assessment: A Journal of Consulting and Clinical Psychology, 4,* 54–59.

Zelinski, E. M., Gilewski, M. J., & Anthony-Bergstone, C. R. (1990). Memory functioning questionnaire: Concurrent validity with memory performance and self-reported memory failure. *Psychology and Aging, 5,* 388–399.

II

Selected Approaches to Assessment

8

The Approach of A. R. Luria to Neuropsychological Assessment

KASPER JØRGENSEN and ANNE-LISE CHRISTENSEN

LURIA'S CONCEPT OF HIGHER CORTICAL FUNCTIONS

The Historico-Cultural Tradition in Psychology

Luria's neuropsychology is based on the historico-cultural tradition in psychology, developed by Vygotsky and Luria in the late 1920s and early 1930s. It is a psychology rooted in historical materialism, in accordance with the Marxist ideology that characterized the scientific climate of the Soviet Union at that time.[1] The thesis of the historico-cultural tradition is that complex or "higher" cognitive functions are, to a large extent, determined by cultural and social conditions and formed through internalization of external cultural representational systems and codes (Goldberg, 1992). In order to explain the genesis and development of mental processes, historico-cultural psychology emphasizes both anthropology and developmental psychology. During the years of growth, the child internalizes a number of preexisting, culturally determined representational systems, particularly through the acquisition of language; these systems are thought to have decisive importance for the structuring of cognitive functions.

An interest in anthropology and developmental psychology dominated Luria's work and research until the end of the 1930s, when he supplemented his education in psychology with a medical degree and shifted his focus to biological psychology and

[1]In spite of its historical and materialistic basis, the historico-cultural tradition nevertheless was denounced as "idealistic," that is, bourgeois and reactionary, by those in power in the Soviet Union, whereupon the tradition was virtually unheard of over the next three decades.

KASPER JØRGENSEN • Department of Neurology, Bispebjerg Hospital, 2400 Copenhagen NV, Denmark. ANNE-LISE CHRISTENSEN • Center for Rehabilitation of Brain Injury, University of Copenhagen, 2300 Copenhagen S, Denmark.

Clinical Neuropsychological Assessment: A Cognitive Approach, edited by Robert L. Mapou and Jack Spector. Plenum Press, New York, 1995.

neurology. Throughout the rest of his career as a neurologist and neuropsychologist, Luria maintained a developmental and anthropological view in his studies of cognition and tried to combine this perspective with the rapidly accumulating knowledge concerning brain anatomy and physiology. This was gained, in part, during World War II, via assessment of patients with circumscribed brain lesions secondary to penetrating missile wounds. The ability to synthesize elements from various traditions also characterizes Luria's approach to neuropsychological assessment, in which he combined elements from experimental psychology and the Western tradition of psychological testing with methods of the clinical neurological examination.

Luria's assessment procedure has been criticized for lack of systematization and methodological rigor, as it rejected dealing with basic issues of standardization, normative data, reliability, and validity. As pointed out by Luria's student and former colleague Elkhonon Goldberg, the chief value of Luria's approach to assessment lies not in the battery of tests itself, but in the unique way the neuropsychological assessment is performed in close accordance with a theory of the cerebral organization of cognitive processes:

> What his approach does contribute to applied neuropsychology is a matrix, a logic of examination which in spite of its methodological looseness, offers an extremely systematic internal organization and dimensionalization of cognition, because it is rooted in a cohesive brain-behavioral model. . . . His clinical approach in many ways foreshadowed and served as the basis for the currently popular "process approach" to neuropsychological diagnosis. (Goldberg, 1990, p. 8)

The Hierarchical Organization of the Brain

Luria's concept of the organization of the brain is hierarchical. In the light of hypotheses about the cerebral organization of mental processes, Luria advanced the distinction among three functional cerebral units:

- *Unit One,* constituted by the metencephalon, mesencephalon, diencephalon, and the medial zones of the hemispheres
- *Unit Two,* consisting of the cortex posterior to the central sulcus
- *Unit Three,* consisting of the cortex anterior to the central sulcus

The division of the brain into three units is determined primarily by the types of mental activity taking place within these functional units. The *first unit* is described as a system for regulating arousal ("cortical tone") or alertness and for maintaining functions such as orientation, learning, and memory. The *second unit* is described as a system specialized for receiving, processing, and storing of input from the sensory organs. The *third unit* is described as a system for planning, initiating, regulating, and monitoring behavior and mental activity.

Luria emphasized that this division of the cerebrum into three functinal units does not mean that each unit is an autonomous module, independent of the two other units. On the contrary, Luria saw any complex mental process, such as perception, voluntary movement, or memory, as resulting from the activity in a *functional system,* that is, from a network of cooperating cortical and subcortical structures in all three functional units. The concept of "the functional system" will be elaborated later.

The hierarchical view of the organization of the brain is manifested partly in the reciprocal relationship among the functional units and partly in the internal organization of each unit. Concerning the reciprocal relationship among the three functional units, Unit Three, which among other areas includes the prefrontal cortex, is regarded as possessing a regulating influence on the two other units. The prefrontal cortex has vast reciprocal connections both with the cortex posterior to the central sulcus, particularly with the association areas or tertiary zones of Unit Two, and with subcortical structures that Luria included in Unit One. For example, the orbitomedial zone of the prefrontal cortex has extensive ascending and descending connections to the medial thalamic nuclei and the reticular formation. The prefrontal cortex has been demonstrated to have a regulating influence on the reticular formation and, through this, on the level of activity in the cerebrum as a whole.

The internal organization of each of the three functional units of the brain is also hierarchical. In the case of Units Two and Three, Luria discriminated among primary, secondary, and tertiary zones and proposed a hierarchical relationship among these three zones (Kagan & Saling, 1988). The *primary zones* correspond to the projection areas of the cortex. In the posterior part of the cortex, the projection zones are specialized for reception of afferent impulses from the sensory organs. In the anterior part of the cortex the primary zones correspond to the motor (precentral) cortex that controls the motor system through the pyramidal tracts.

The *secondary zones* are adjacent to the primary zones. In Unit Two, the secondary zones are specialized for analysis and synthesis of the afferent impulses received by the primary zones from the sensory organs. The secondary zones of the second functional unit are therefore sometimes labeled "gnostic" cortical zones, in order to express the idea that these zones form an important neuronal basis for the recognition of sensory impressions. The primary and secondary zones are together labeled "analyzers," as they are modally specific functional modules for reception and processing of information. As a rule, Luria's system operates with three analyzers: visual, auditory, and the somatosensory, which process sensory input. In Unit Three, the role of the secondary zones is the generation and preparation of motor programs and sequences, for which the motor cortex serves as an output channel.

Luria used the name *tertiary zones* for the association areas both in the posterior part of the cortex and in the prefrontal cortex. In unit Two, the tertiary zones manage the intermodal or polymodal integration of information from the modally specific analyzers. As previously mentioned, the tertiary zones of Unit Three correspond to the prefrontal cortex and are thought to be involved in the direction and control of behavior on a superior level. Luria introduced the concept of the "executive functions" of the brain as characteristic for the prefrontal areas. This concept refers to activities such as planning, initiation and monitoring of behavior, controlling the results of actions, and inhibition of irrelevant impulses for actions, among others.

The dual application of the concepts of primary, secondary, and tertiary zones in both the anterior and the posterior parts of the cortex is due to the fact that Luria saw a parallel between the hierarchical organization of these cortical areas. In both Units Two and Three, there is a controlling and regulating influence from the tertiary zones through the secondary and primary zones. In Unit Two, the regulation mainly affects the process of perception and gnosis, whereas in Unit Three regulation of behavior occurs.

This hypothesis or "law of the hierarchical organizaton of the cortex" is derived from the earlier work of Vygotsky and Luria in developmental psychology (Vocate, 1987). Vygotsky and Luria presumed that adequate functioning of the primary zones in the posterior part of the cortex of the child is essential for the normal development of the secondary and tertiary zones. Vygotsky used the expression that in the child the main direction of interaction between the cortical zones runs "from bottom, up."[2] Vygotsky's evolutionary point of view proposed that the development of normal spatial concepts depends on the integrity of the visual and somatosensory analyzers during infancy. Correspondingly, the development of verbal abilities seems to be dependent on intact functioning of the auditory analyzer. As the association areas of Unit Two develop, they are thought to become increasingly important for the perceptual processing by the analyzers. Thus, in the adult, the main direction of interaction between the cortical zones runs "from top, down."

In the adult, fully developed individual, perception seems very much controlled by complex cognitive processes connected to the tertiary zones. Sensory impressions are organized according to previously internalized concepts, experiences, and expectations. This evolutionary perspective forms the basis for a differentiated understanding of the relationship between the time of onset of a brain injury and the consequences of the injury for cognitive functioning. Lesioning or defective development of one of the analyzers in infancy will, according to Luria, cause more serious disturbances than a similar lesion occurring after the brain is fully developed, and intact functioning of the tertiary zones is ensured. Luria took the point of view that processes in the tertiary zones can, to some extent, compensate for dysfunctioning of the analyzers occurring late in development. The hypothesis of the regulating influence of the tertiary zones on the analyzers and the hypothesis of the potential for compensation in case of limited dysfunction at a hierarchically lower level hold implications both for Luria's method of neuropsychological assessment and for his understanding of the possibilities for remediation of cognitive functions. These implications will be elaborated below.

The Functional System

The discussion of the localization of cognitive functions dates back to the origins of neuropsychology in the seventeenth and eighteenth centuries and the prevailing faculty psychology. The mind was conceived as constituted by a number of specific mental functions or "faculties," such as "parental love," "destructiveness," and so on. The eighteenth-century anatomist Franz Josef Gall thus operated with 27 different faculties, which he tried to localize in circumscribed cortical areas. In contrast to the

[2]This hypothesis is supported by the observation that during fetal development and childhood, myelination develops earlier and faster in the primary and secondary areas than in the tertiary zones.

classic adynamic models of localization, there was the holistic or equipotentialist point of view held by, among others, the nineteenth-century French physiologist Pierre Flourens. The equipotentialists argued that the brain worked as an undifferentiated whole, with no exact cortical localization of mental functions. Similarly, twentieth-century neuropsychologists like K. S. Lashley argued for an equipotentialist viewpoint.

With Paul Broca and Carl Wernicke's discovery of specific language zones in the left hemisphere, in the second half of the nineteenth century, the way was opened for a dynamic comprehension of the cerebrum as a system of specialized and cooperating modules. Wernicke was among the first to articulate a network theory for brain functioning, as he argued that speech must result from coordinated activity in both language zones of the brain. Wernicke hereby took up a position that opposed both faculty psychology and the holistic viewpoint.

According to Luria, the concept of the functional system was originally introduced and developed by the Russian neurophysiologist P. K. Anokhin in the 1930s. Luria's own concept of the functional system can be seen as a further elaboration and differentiation of the network theory. He referred to the way that autonomous processes, such as respiration and digestion, are organized. A complex activity such as respiration is not performed by a single, isolated organ but by a number of cooperating groups of muscles and organs of which the lungs, of course, are crucial. Because of its complexity, a functional system is characterized by a certain amount of flexibility and potential for restructuring, since the way in which the overall task of the system is performed can be varied without major consequences. For instance, where *respiration* represents a functional system, Luria noted that, in the event of paralysis of the diaphragm, other groups of muscles begin to work and try to maintain the system's primary activity.

Luria characterized the functional system as follows: a constant task is performed through variable mechanisms bringing the process to a constant result (Luria, 1973). In his paper "The Functional Organization of the Brain," Luria analyzed how complex neuropsychological functions, such as voluntary movement and the skill of writing, are organized in functional systems (Luria, 1970). In keeping with the historico-cultural position, Luria argued that the organization of cognitive processes in complex networks is, to a large extent, influenced by external conditions, such as verbal and social stimulation, school attendance, and so on. The organization of functional systems varies from individual to individual according to environmental influences, and where there are important changes in biological or social conditions, the systems can, to some extent, be *reorganized*. Spontaneous reorganization of functional systems is thought to take place several times during childhood and adolescence, for example, in connection with the transfer of acquired skills from a conscious and voluntary mode of performance to a more automatic performance.

As an illustration, consider that a skill such as writing is originally acquired through the child's learning the shape characteristics of every single letter and laboriously "drawing" the lines that together constitute the letter. Through continued practice, the motor impulses necessary for writing the letter are combined into brief automated series of consecutive impulses, or "kinetic melodies," that can be released without the child being conscious of every single component in the activity. Combinations of letters occurring frequently, such as one's signature, can achieve a similar degree of automation, meaning that they can be performed without awareness of the serial order of the letters.

The spontaneous reorganization of functional systems during ontogenesis alters not only the functional structure of cognitive processes but also their cerebral organization. At the early stages of the writing process, when the child learns the connection between the spatial and auditory characteristics of each letter, activation of the motor areas of the cortex takes place, along with widespread activation of the cortical zones supporting visuospatial and auditory analysis and synthesis. In addition, executive functions, which are thought to regulate voluntary action, are involved. At a later, more automated stage, when motor engrams have been established and when spelling has become a matter of routine, the activity of writing presumably can be performed with less widespread cortical activation. The cerebral organization has thus become altered. The potential for reorganization of functional systems can be used when remediating cognitive functions.

Symptom and Syndrome Analysis

The concept of the functional system has vital importance for Luria's understanding of the effect of brain lesions on cognitive functions and for the neuropsychological assessment of these effects. Luria was among the first neuropsychologists to state clearly that no simple, unequivocal relation between symptom and localization can be proved. On the basis of a neuropsychological symptom such as specific disturbances of gnosis or praxis, there is, as a rule, no direct way to determine which areas of the cortex could be affected.

> If mental activity is a complex functional system, involving the participation of a group of concertedly working areas of the cortex . . . a lesion of each of these zones or areas may lead to disintegration of the entire functional system, and in this way the symptom or "loss" of a particular function tells us nothing about its "localization." (Luria, 1973, p. 35)

In other words, the relation between symptom and localization of lesion can be highly complex. On the one hand, the same symptom can be the manifestation of a number of differently localized brain lesions. A symptom, such as disturbance of expressive speech, can result from lesions of both anterior and posterior cortical areas or from a disruption of the intrahemispheric connections between the language zones. On the other hand, a circumscribed cortical lesion can simultaneously affect several functional systems, and consequently can result in various manifestations of symptoms. For example, lesions of the association areas or tertiary zones in the posterior part of the cortex can give rise to various complex symptoms, as these cortical areas seem to be involved in numerous functional systems. Luria described patients suffering from circumscribed lesions of the parieto-occipital region of the left hemisphere who, apart from disturbances in spatial orientation, also had problems with arithmetical calculations and comprehension of grammatical structures involving local relations and the genitive. The common cognitive factor in these three different types of mental activity is, according to Luria, the ability to handle spatial or "quasi-spatial" relations.[3]

As can be seen, most functional systems can be affected by a lesion in a large number of cortical areas, but there will be some variation of disturbances depending on which components of the system are affected. Consequently, Luria structured the neuropsychological asessment on the basis of a *systemic* way of thinking. This approach is guided by two fundamental questions:

1. Which processes are involved in the cognitive functions in consideration?
2. What cerebral structures support the functional system and constitute the neuronal basis for the functions in consideration?

Through a combination of clinical observations, empirical research, and theoretical considerations, Luria worked at providing the basic knowledge necessary to perform clinical syndrome analysis. When this knowledge could not be produced, he operated with theoretical models. For instance, his hypothesis as to the crucial importance of "inner speech" for the functioning of all higher cortical processes must be regarded as a theoretical construct that has not been verified empirically.

On the basis of a systematic mapping of which symptoms emerge as a result of lesions in a circumscribed cerebral area, Luria formulated assumptions about the functional systems supported by a particular brain area. Through careful analysis of the ways in which a functional system is affected by a lesion in one of its cerebral components, he made further hypotheses on what specific task in that functional system the component supports. Thus, a close connection among clinical observation, systemic cognitive models, and methods of neuropsychological assessment characterizes Luria's work.

LURIA'S NEUROPSYCHOLOGICAL INVESTIGATION

The Qualitative Approach to Neuropsychological Assessment

Luria's approach to neuropsychological assessment has been developed according to his theory of the organization of cognitive processes in functional systems, with complex cortical distribution. Through the application of a number of relatively simple, nonstandardized tasks and tests, the function in every single component of the functional system in question is examined, along with the dynamic interaction among the components.

Luria's assessment approach is rooted partly in the tradition of experimental psychology, from which many of the items in his collection of tests have their origin, and partly in the neurological examination. In the neurological examination, a screening of the function of the nervous system is carried out through systematic application of

[3]Some have attempted to summarize complexes of symptoms like these under specific syndromes (such as "Gerstmann's syndrome"), but due to the complexity and the individual variability in the composition of symptoms, such attempts have not proven very adequate.

observations and simple tests. In the light of any functional deficits, hypotheses are formed about their origin.

Luria's method of neuropsychological assessment differs radically from the psychometric tradition employed by the majority of Western neuropsychologists, which emphasizes quantification, normative data, reliability, and validity. In *Higher Cortical Functions in Man,* Luria disassociated himself from the psychometric tradition exemplified by Halstead's battery of tests, stating dogmatically that "any attempt to apply standardized experimental techniques [to neuropsychological investigation] must be entirely disouraged" (Luria, 1980, p. 392).

Luria's criticism of the psychometric tradition is built on two arguments. First, he held that psychometric tests are often constructed according to a theoretically based categorizing of cognitive functions that does not correspond to the disturbances of function due to brain lesions. Batteries of tests, such as Wechsler's Intelligence Scales, contain tests like "Information" and "Comprehension" that do not match unambiguously any one specific cognitive function. Second, Luria held that the psychometric tradition's emphasis on quantification of test results is not suitable for the examination of the complicated types of functional deficits resulting from brain injury. He argued that when test results are summarized in scores, valuable information on the individual process that has led to a given result is neglected.

Alternatively, Luria proposed a qualitatively oriented procedure, in which the performances of the patient on every single item and observation of his or her method of working and behavior are combined in the analysis of the functions being examined. According to Luria, it is not sufficient to assess whether the functions in question are intact or affected. Instead, the neuropsychological assessment should lead to a "qualitative, structural analysis" of the symptoms discovered through the assessment, and as far as possible, result both in a description of the individual character of the functional deficits demonstrated and in a hypothesis of the cause of the disturbance.

To illustrate Luria's point of view, we will consider the issue of reduced learning ability after brain injury. A strictly psychometric assessment of learning ability would lead typically to establishing the patient's level of performance relative to the performance of a representative population of normal controls, taking into consideration age and level of education. Knowledge or assumptions regarding the premorbid level of intelligence are also taken into consideration. The relative performance of the patient can be indicated by reporting percentile scores or standard deviations from the mean of the normative group. On the basis of this, the performance can furthermore be described through adjectives such as *normal, slightly reduced, moderately reduced,* or *severely reduced.*

In contrast, a Lurian assessment of learning ability would emphasize a qualitative analysis of the functional disturbances. The process of learning is conceived of as being composed of several elements, such as reception, storage, and retrieval. Other factors that could influence the learning process are also involved in the analysis. These could be relatively basic cognitive functions with a low position in the hierarchy, such as alertness, arousal level, general orientation, attention, and concentration; or more complex, hierarchically higher mental capacities such as executive functions, that is, voluntary, goal-directed application of cognitive abilities. Consequently, such assess-

TABLE 8.1. Levels of Analysis in Relation to Evaluating Test Performances

1. Neurophysiological level	Primary defect
2. Systemic level	Disturbances in functional systems
3. Descriptive or classificatory level	Neuropsychological syndrome

ment would result in a clarification of which components of the learning process are affected and which are intact, whether the disturbances affect lower or higher levels of the hierarchy of cognitive functioning, whether the learning difficulties are of a general or modally specific nature, and eventually, which strategies of compensation the patient applies to cope with the difficulties.

When evaluating test performances, Luria operated with multiple levels of analysis (Table 8.1). The lowest level in the hierarchy is the *neurophysiological* level where the connection between the localization and type of brain injury and the functional deficit is conceived of as rather unambiguous. The next level, the *systemic* level, is the level of disruptions derived from the primary defect in one or more functional systems. The highest level is the *descriptive* or *classificatory* level, where the disturbances and deficits are summarized in the identification of a neuropsychological syndrome, if possible.

At the hierarchically lowest level, Luria enumerated various types of neurophysiological defects[4] that can cause disturbances of function: pathological weakening of the neural activity in the primary analyzers, disturbances in the integrating activity of the brain, lack of inhibition of neural activity, pathological inertia in neural processes, and defective feedback from afferent systems.

To illustrate the three levels of analysis, let us consider a patient with a lesion of the left superior temporal gyrus, resulting in difficulties in impressive speech. The primary (neurophysiological) defect is a disturbance in the phonemic analysis of speech sounds. On the systemic level, these primary disturbances cause a disruption in the functional system that supports language, mainly in the form of difficulties in understanding the speech of others and oneself. Thus, the primary impressive difficulties can also cause difficulties in expressive speech, since the unreliable auditory feedback results in occasional lack of agreement between what the patient thinks he or she expresses and what is actually expressed. Other functional systems, such as reading and writing, also may be affected by such a disruption of phonemic analysis. Finally, on the classificatory level, the described pattern of symptoms characterized by a combination of impressive and expressive difficulties, plus possible disruption of reading and writing, can be summarized under the term *sensory aphasia, fluent aphasia,* or *Wernicke's aphasia,* depending on the system of classification being applied.

In addition to criticizing the psychometric tradition's quantification of test results, Luria also called into question the application of the concept of reliability to neuropsychological assessment. The performance level of the individual patient will, particularly during the postacute phase, often vary significantly. Even though highly reliable

[4]Luria, as a rule, used the Russian inspired term *neurodynamic defect,* which is synonymous with *neurophysiological defect.*

and repeatable tests are being used, according to Luria, test performance of a brain-injured patient on different occasions can vary considerably. He therefore refused to deal further with the issue of reliability and, alternatively, recommended that the reliability of the single test performances be evaluated in the light of the total pattern of test results. Luria thus cautioned against putting too much emphasis on single test performances and isolated occurrences of functional deficits. A specific type of functional deficit associated with a particular syndrome should be considered "reliable" only when it manifests itself consistently on different tests assessing similar functions.[5]

The psychometric and the qualitative approaches to assessment thus differ widely and can appear completely incompatible, regarding both the assessment procedure and the interpretation of test results. The psychometric approach applies standardized, carefully described guidelines for administration of tests (items, instruction, scoring), whereas the qualitative approach is characterized by a highly flexible and individualized procedure, in which the selection and succession of tests and the administration of these tests vary from one assessment to the next. The selection and ordering of tests are, in general, determined by the patient's performances and results during the assessment and the hypotheses being formed by the examiner.

In spite of the very different theoretical and methodological basis, some degree of reciprocal approximation and inspiration in the clinical application of the two approaches seems to have occurred over the years, perhaps as a consequence of the fact that both approaches in their pure forms might seem incomplete. On the one hand, a predominantly psychometric approach does not necessarily rule out the use of qualitative features. On the other hand, Luria's own presentation of the approach, as well as Anne-Lise Christensen's (1984) revision and adaptation of his procedures, has resulted in an incipient "standardization" of the approach. Both Luria's and Christensen's presentations hold tentative guidelines for administration and instructions, numerous examples of tests, and suggestions for variation and modification of the procedures.[6]

To be able to apply Luria's approach to neuropsychological assessment in a meaningful way, it is very important that the examiner have a comprehensive and thorough knowledge of clinical neurology and neuropsychology, based on several years of practical experience. As a consequence of the fact that the selection of tests and their order of administration are not decided in advance, but depend on the judgment of the examiner on a case-by-case basis and on the individual course of each testing, the utility of the approach stands or falls with matters such as the ability of the neuropsychologist to select relevant tests, the ability to discriminate between normal and pathologically deviant behavior and test performances, and the ability to generate meaningful hypotheses on latent causes for clinically manifested functional deficits.

[5]Luria's discussion does not seem to imply a proper critique of the concept of reliability as such but rather questions the relevance of emphasizing the issue of test–retest reliability in relation to neuropsychological assessment.

[6]Luria (1980) pointed out that only a limited number of the most useful tests and tasks that he applied in his clinical work are described.

The Course of the Investigation

The Preliminary Conversation

Like most other neuropsychologists, Luria recommended that the neuropsychological assessment begin with a clinical interview, the length of which is adjusted in consideration of the referral problems and the present condition of the patient. Luria mentioned a number of general objectives for the clinical interview. In addition to providing the patient with an occasion to account for his or her symptoms, the interview also provides an opportunity for a clinical estimate of the patient's state of consciousness and orientation. The examiner might also obtain a preliminary impression of the patient's personality and awareness of his or her present condition and situation. Finally, the psychologist must pay attention to occurrence of symptoms that can reflect the localization of any brain lesion and form the basis for hypotheses on pathology.

The First, General Stage of the Investigation

The first stage in the neuropsychological assessment proper is carrying out a broad-spectrum, preliminary estimate of the patient's general level of cognitive functioning. In this context, Luria discriminated among three levels of mental activity: direct sensorimotor reactions, mnestic organization of acts, and complex, volitional acts. Again, this is a hierarchical model, with the sensorimotor reactions at the lowest end of the hierarchy.

The assessment of sensorimotor reactions is carried out through a systematic screening of the functioning of the individual analyzers, that is, the visual, auditory, and somatosensory modalities plus the motor system. In current clinical practice, the sensory and motor systems of the patient usually have been examined by a neurologist or other medical specialist before the patient is referred for neuropsychological assessment. Consequently, it might seem superfluous for the neuropsychologist to undertake an additional assessment of these functions. However, considering the tests applied by Luria to assessment of sensorimotor functions, it appears that neuropsychologists are not merely repeating the neurological examination. The difference lies mainly in the scope and complexity of the approaches, as the neurological examination is concerned primarily with assessment of function on a more "fundamental" physiological level, whereas Luria's assessment approach involves basic and more complex gnostic and psychological aspects of sensory modalities and motor function.

The assessment of motor functions thus includes very simple motor tests, for the purpose of assessing muscle strength and tone, as is also the case in the neurological examination. Subsequently, tests of hand and finger positions are presented for the purpose of assessing kinesthetic and proprioceptive aspects of the functional system of voluntary movement. This section includes tests where the patient, sitting face to face with the examiner, is asked to reproduce the examiner's positioning of his or her hands (Head's test). The purpose of this is to assess the ability for visuospatial organization of movement. Finally, tests are administered to assess performance of complex sequences of movements, including the capacity for voluntary regulation and control of the motor system on a higher (executive) level.

It was Luria's hypothesis that the capacity for volitional regulation and control of acts is connected closely to the phenomenon "inner speech," conceived of as thinking mediated by linguistic symbols. In the case of disorders in the ability to regulate behavior, the patient is asked during the testing to accompany his or her behavior with verbalization. Through this, it is clarified whether the patient's "thinking aloud" and instructing himself or herself can compensate for the disruption of the executive functioning.

At this general stage of the assessment, Luria recommended the use of brief tests with a relatively "standardized" administration (not standardized in the psychometric meaning of the term), which are so easy that noninjured persons with limited schooling also can solve them without difficulty. However, he also recommended that the level of difficulty of the tests be adjusted according to the estimated premorbid level of intelligence (Luria, 1980). Thus, it is the examiner's duty to maintain a satisfactory balance between homogeneity of the tests and individualization.

Table 8.2 summarizes the areas of cognitive functioning that are assessed in Luria's neuropsychological investigation. Within each group of functions, a hierarchical assessment approach is applied, starting with very simple tests designed to examine basic aspects of the function and continuing with increasingly more complex tests, in order to examine the function in question in interaction with other groups of functions.[7]

The Second, Selective Stage of the Investigation

In light of the results obtained during the first, general stage of the assessment, the examiner makes a decision as to which areas of functioning are to be examined more closely. Functions that have so far proven intact should not necessarily be scrutinized further, while functions that have appeared possibly or positively affected are brought into focus. In practice, the examiner often will have already formulated one or more diagnostic hypotheses that he or she attempts to test during the continued assessment.

Luria stated that the objective of the first, general stage of the assessment is a preliminary identification of the primary defect (or defects). In the second, specific stage of the assessment, a further exploration and explication of the nature of the primary defect, as well as a clarification of the *systemic* consequences of the disorder, is undertaken. Thus, the neuropsychologist is now attempting to determine which functional systems are affected by the primary defect and in which way. The patient's use of intact resources and techniques of compensation also may be illustrated during this stage of the assessment procedure. If a patient cannot solve a test within a reasonable time limit, the conditions for the problem solving are modified in order to clarify the nature of the patient's difficulties and to find how to bypass these difficulties, if possible. The patient may be asked to slow down his or her speed, to split up the task

[7]A partial exception from this hierarchical approach is found within "intellectual processes," where only relatively complex activities, such as concept formation and problem solving, are examined.

TABLE 8.2. Summary of Luria's Neuropsychological Investigation

- Cerebral dominance
- Motor functions
  - Motor functions of the hands
  - Oral praxis
  - Speech regulation of the motor act
- Audiomotor organization
  - Perception and reproduction of pitch relationships
  - Perception and reproduction of rhythmic structures
- Cutaneous and kinesthetic functions
  - Cutaneous sensation
  - Muscle and joint sensation
  - Stereognosis
- Visuospatial functions
  - Visual perception of objects and pictures
  - Spatial orientation
  - Intellectual operations in space
- Impressive speech
  - Phonemic hearing
  - Word comprehension
  - Understanding of simple sentences
  - Understanding of grammatical structures
- Expressive speech
  - Articulation of speech sounds
  - Repetitive speech
  - The nominative function of speech
  - Narrative speech
- Writing and reading
  - Phonetic analysis and synthesis of words
  - Writing
  - Reading
- Arithmetical skill
  - Comprehension of number structure
  - Arithmetical operations
- Mnestic processes
  - The learning process
  - Retention and retrieval
  - Logical memorizing
- Intellectual processes
  - Understanding of thematic pictures and texts
  - Concept formation
  - Discursive intellectual activity

into smaller components, to accompany his or her behavior with verbalization, and so on. If the stability of the level of functioning is in question, it might be necessary to repeat the same tests at a later assessment.

The second stage of the neuropsychological assessment thus has a distinctly individualized character, often contains more complex tests than the first stage, and makes higher demands on the flexibility of the examiner, his or her clinical experience, and diagnostic knowledge.

Comparative Analysis of Test Results

As mentioned above, Luria considered it insufficient to conclude the neuropsychological assessment with a quantitative statement of test results compared with normative data. He recommended that all three levels of analysis should be included in the summary, if possible: identification of the primary defect, description of the effects on one or more functional systems, and nosological classification of the condition in the form of a diagnosis or syndrome. Considerations concerning the localization of any circumscribed lesions form part of the summary. The attempts to localize any lesions on the basis of the neuropsychological assessment were obviously of greater importance at the time Luria worked as a clinician than today, when advanced imaging techniques are routinely employed in neurology. Every single assessment is, in other words, viewed experimentally and *casuistically.* That is, the examiner's task is to analyze and define which functional deficits are charateristic for this specific patient, and which individual methods of compensation he or she uses. Luria's approach to assessment can be considered as aimed at the identification and description of the great variability that might characterize functional deficits caused by cerebral pathology. For the experienced examiner, it will often be possible to obtain a comprehensive and coherent understanding of the condition, even in cases where a nosological classification of the condition is uncertain.

CASES

The following cases illustrate, more specifically, the clinical application of Luria's approach.

Patient 1

The patient was a 38-year-old psychiatric nurse. She had given birth to a daughter when she was 30 and married. This marriage was dissolved 3 years later. She entered a second relationship 2 months before her illness.

Medical History

The patient's blood pressure had been elevated since she was 24, but it was controlled effectively by medication. She collapsed suddenly during physical exercise, with loss of consciousness. A computed tomography (CT) scan showed a subarachnoid hemorrhage with a small hematoma in the left Sylvian fissure. Cerebral angiography revealed the hemorrhage to be from a middle cerebral artery aneurysm and also showed another aneurysm of the bifurcation of the internal carotid artery, which had not hemorrhaged. Both aneurysms were ligated, leaving a postoperative right-sided hemiparesis/hemiparalysis most pronounced in the upper extremity.

rCBF measurement was undertaken 2 years postoperatively for the purpose of correlating the neuropsychological test findings with the brain lesion. The pattern showed a global blood flow level within the lower part of the normal range, and a lower hemispheric mean on the left side. A marked focal flow decrease was seen temporally on the left side. During activation by speech, the normal elevation in the frontal areas was absent, indicating disturbance that may be explained by a weakened connection between temporal areas and the left frontal lobe.

Primary Defect

The fundamental symptom of the patient when examined 2 years postoperatively was severe speech difficulty. Sensorimotor disturbances of the mouth, as well as ideopractic disturbances for complex oral movements, were found, whereas disturbances for the upper extremity were only slight. Spontaneous speech consisted predominantly of single words expressed in telegraphic style. Receptive speech seemed uncompromised, but investigation of the acoustic span revealed that not more than two or three acoustic signals, phonemes, or words were captured.

The patient was highly motivated and showed intelligent and compensatory behavior using mimicry, signs, and gesticulation. Visual function was not problematic, and her memory was excellent.

Systemic Consequences

The absence of oral expression affected reading and writing. She appeared to have learned, by heart, a vocabulary of words that were easy to articulate and highly frequent. When she tried to find new words, she groped for the right position of her articulatory apparatus. She seemed to have preserved an automatic ability to write, but the sequence of phonemes was often disturbed. Furthermore, the lack of expressive possibilities seemed to restrict her range of experience, preventing a nuanced and abstract categorization.

Classification

The aphasia presented corresponds in Luria's terminology to afferent-motor aphasia, in this case complicated by the restricted acoustic span. The intact parieto-occipital cortical areas and medial structures made it possible for the patient to compensate effectively in all functions in which her limited speech was not of primary influence.

Patient 2

The patient was a 25-year-old goldsmith with a premorbidly normal intelligence and good social adjustment.

Medical History

The patient suffered an anoxic cerebral injury caused by poisoning with carbon monoxide (CO). No CT scan or other neuroradiological data were available, but as a result of the poisoning, bilateral damage to the hippocampal region was expected.[8] In cases of more severe CO poisoning, diffuse damage of the cerebrum would also be expected.

At neuropsychological assessment almost 2 years postinjury, the patient complained of severe learning difficulties. He also experienced difficulties in recalling events prior to the poisoning, difficulties in recognizing previous friends and acquaintances, and problems with retrieval of previously learned facts and knowledge.

Primary Defect

The essential primary defect was a markedly poor ability to store new impressions and sensory input. There were no disorders of perception, and analysis of input and the auditory span were fully intact. It appeared that fresh inputs were registered in a normal way, but they were not held for more than a brief time interval. The length of this interval appeared to be determined mainly by when the patient received additional input. Thus, there was a pronounced sensitivity to interference, meaning that the most recent impressions almost completely wiped out previous impressions. For example, the patient experienced no difficulties when repeating an 8- to 10-word sentence, but if presented with two different sentences with no semantic interconnection, he was capable only of repeating the one most recently presented. The ability to retrieve life history events and previously learned knowledge was also affected, though to a less severe degree. The patient's active knowledge on matters of geography, politics, and culture was clearly below the premorbid level, as was his active vocabulary.

Systemic Consequences

The failing ability to store impressions resulted in severe difficulties in later retrieval of verbal and visuospatial material. The difficulties were multimodal and general, and thus also characterized immediate learning of short motor sequences. The difficulties in retrieval of general knowledge gave rise to a subtle language disorder in the form of defective retrieval of words and difficulties in naming. In complex problem-solving tests requiring simultaneous information processing and application of strategies over time, performance appeared reduced. These difficulties were presumed to be, in part, determined by the enhanced sensitivity to interference, although

[8]Simplified, the mechanism involved is as follows. The CO molecules have affinity for the red blood cells responsible for the transport of oxygen to the brain. The saturation of the red blood cells with CO therefore results in a failing supply of oxygen. Animal experiments have shown that the hippocampus is particularly vulnerable to lack of oxygen. Experimentally induced ischemia in rats causes severe damage to the CA1 region in the hippocampus and results in chronic defects of learning and memory (Squire & Zola-Morgan, 1991).

other types of cognitive disorders resulting from diffuse cerebral injury could also be suspected.

Classification

The condition can be described as an amnestic syndrome accompanied by subtle problems with retrieval of words (remains of a slight amnestic aphasia) and a reduced ability for complex problem solving. The patient was highly motivated for resuming his former work, and after approximately a year of training, he reestablished the specific technical skills required for a goldsmith. He had forgotten the common routines of work, including the use of special tools, but these skills reemerged relatively effortlessly and quickly. It appeared that motor skills and procedures were considerably better preserved than his general knowledge, probably due to a higher degree of automation. Also, motor skills could be reestablished at a faster pace than intellectual skills.[9]

PERSPECTIVES FOR REHABILITATION

It is our experience that Luria's approach to neuropsychological assessment holds valuable opportunities for planning of cognitive remediation and rehabilitation. As mentioned above, Luria's qualitative approach provides information concerning intact versus affected functions. Additionally, it provides information on the patient's working methods and identifies possibilities for compensation for deficits.

In his book *Restoration of Function after Brain Injury,* Luria outlined a theoretical model for the reorganization of complex cognitive functions (Luria, 1963). As discussed above, the organization of functional systems has, according to Luria, some degree of individuality depending on the kinds of influences the individual has received during the years of growth. Functional systems also are supposed to be characterized by a certain degree of plasticity, meaning that they might be *reorganized* in case of changes in their cerebral basis or in external social conditions. This flexibility of function can be used during rehabilitation after brain injury.

On the basis of experience from clinical practice, Luria discriminated among three different types of reorganization of mental functions:

1. Elementary intrasystemic reorganization
2. Intrasystemic conceptual reorganization
3. Intersystemic reorganization

The *elementary intrasystemic reorganization* takes place on an automatic, nonconscious level. This is seen typically after a lesion in one of the primary sensory or motor projection areas of the cortex. Hemiparesis of the dominant (right) arm might

[9]The clinical impression of this patient seems to confirm the hypothesis that procedural and declarative memory represent separate cognitive systems (Salmon & Butters, 1987).

result in a gradual reorganization of the functional system of movement of the upper extremities, so that the nondominant hand takes over more and more of the activities formerly performed by the dominant hand. Luria's examples of elementary intrasystemic reorganization are connected to basic motor and sensory functions, and it is not clear if this elementary form of reorganization is of any practical importance in relation to restoration of cognitive functions proper such as attention, concentration, and learning, among others.

A lesion in one of the secondary cortical zones (modally specific areas of analysis and synthesis) will, according to Luria, result in disturbances of more complex cognitive functions. Restoration of complex cognitive functions takes place through a process called *intrasystemic conceptual reorganization,* expressing a conscious, goal-directed reorganization of the functional system supporting the activities in question. In the normal brain, many cognitive processes instrumental to our thinking, such as learning, recalling, retrieval of words, and concept formation, appear to take place mainly on a semiautomatic or automatic, nonconscious level. Intrasystemic conceptual reorganization is characterized by raising the cognitive processes involved in a given cognitive function to a more conscious and "conceptual" level.

To illustrate the method of conceptual reorganization, Luria referred to cases of efferent aphasia, characterized by pathological inertia when trying to pronounce polysyllables (Luria, 1963). This pathological inertia might, in some cases, be overcome through increasing the conceptual "distance" between the syllables. For example, each syllable can be pronounced with a different emotional tone or can be connected associatively with different situations. Also, disruption of activities such as perception of phonemes or visual gnosis might, according to Luria, be overcome through conceptual reorganization through making the patient aware of the underlying cognitive processes and supporting them through the patient's intact ability for concept formation. As a rule, conceptual reorganization requires systematic and prolonged training.

If elements that have not previously been included in the cognitive activity are involved in the reorganization of a functional system, Luria spoke of *intersystemic reorganization.* As a rule, intersystemic reorganization takes place if one or more crucial elements in the functional system have been damaged. Luria particularly called attention to the possibilities for compensation for loss of different types of afferent feedback from the sensory systems. The afferent systems are generally so complex that loss of a specific type of afferent feedback to some extent can be compensated by other, intact afferent systems. To illustrate the method of intersystemic reorganization, Luria referred to the phenomenon that loss of proprioceptive feedback from the limbs, causing apractic difficulties, can to some extent be compensated for by increased visual feedback (Luria, 1963).

A convincing illustration of intersystemic reorganization was demonstrated in experiments by Vygotsky and Luria with patients suffering from Parkinson's disease (Luria, 1979). They were puzzled by the observation that patients who could not take two successive steps when walking on a level floor before a severe tremor sat in and made further walking impossible were able to climb stairs without difficulty. Vygotsky and Luria hypothesized that in climbing stairs, the successive automatic flow of movement that is conceived of as a subcortically organized, involuntary activity is replaced by chains of separate motor reactions set off by each step on the stairs. By placing a series of small paper cards on the floor and asking the patients to step over each one of them, they actually helped the patients to overcome the tremor and cross the room.[10]

SUMMARY

Luria's approach to neuropsychological assessment is closely connected to a general theory of development and organization of cortical functions. As an adherent of the historico-cultural tradition in psychology, Luria believed that cognitive functions are developed primarily through internalization of external cultural representational systems. Complex cognitive functions are not narrowly localized in the cerebrum, but, rather, are organized in a network of cooperating cerebral zones that Luria referred to as functional systems.

Luria's neuropsychological investigation is a qualitatively oriented, nonstandardized method rooted in the neurological examination, among other methods. The approach is hierarchical, starting with an assessment of basic sensorimotor functions and continuing with assessment of gradually more complex functions. When evaluating test performances, three levels of analysis are applied: a neurophysiological level, a systemic level, and a descriptive or classificatory level. In this context, the systemic level is the most interesting, as a dynamic analysis and description of the consequences of the brain injury for the functional systems are attempted. The analysis of the functional systems is carried out through a flexible, considerably individualized hypothesis-testing method, in which the patient's possibilities for compensation for the cognitive deficits also are explored. Regarding remediation of cognitive functions, Luria emphasized that the individuality and flexibility that are thought to characterize many functional systems can be used in connection with various kinds of reorganization of cognitive functions.

ACKNOWLEDGMENT

We wish to thank our friend and colleague Thomas W. Teasdale for his revision of the English and review of the content of this chapter.

REFERENCES

Christensen, A. L. (1984). *Luria's Neuropsychological Investigation* (2nd ed.). Copenhagen: Munksgaard.

Goldberg, E. (1990). Tribute to Alexandr Romanovich Luria (1902–1977) In E. Goldberg (Ed.), *Contemporary neuropsychology and the legacy of Luria* (pp. 1–9). Hillsdale, NJ: Lawrence Erlbaum.

Kagan, A., & Saling, M. M. (1988). *An introduction to Luria's aphasiology: Theory and application.* Johannesburg: Witwatersrand University Press.

[10]Similar experiments have been performed on akinetic patients by the American neurologist Oliver Sacks, cf. the book and motion picture *Awakenings*.

Luria, A. R. (1963). *Restoration of function after brain injury.* New York: Basic Books.

Luria, A. R. (1970). The functional organization of the brain. *Scientific American, 222,* 66–78.

Luria, A. R. (1973). *The working brain: An introduction to neuropsychology.* New York: Penguin Books.

Luria, A. R. (1979). *The making of mind: A personal account of Soviet psychology.* Boston: Harvard University Press.

Luria, A. R. (1980). *Higher cortical functions in man* (2nd ed.). New York: Basic Books.

Salmon, D. P., & Butters, N. (1987). Recent developments in learning and memory; Implications for the rehabilitation of the amnesic patient. In M. Meier, A. Benton, & L. Diller (Eds.), *Neuropsychological rehabilitation* (pp. 280–293). New York: Guilford.

Squire, L. R., & Zola-Morgan, S. (1991). The medial temporal lobe memory system. *Science, 253,* 1380–1385.

Vocate, D. R. (1987). *The theory of Luria: Functions of spoken language in the development of higher mental processes.* Hillsdale, NJ: Lawrence Erlbaum.

9

Cognitive Neuropsychology and Assessment

JANICE KAY and SUE FRANKLIN

INTRODUCTION

Cognitive neuropsychology is a relatively new discipline founded on the assumption that the study of acquired disorders of cognition can inform our understanding of cognitive processing. One of its principal objectives is to learn about what Coltheart (1985) has termed the *functional architecture* of cognitive systems—that is, the kinds of knowledge and processes involved in skills such as recognizing a neighbor in the street, putting a name to that face, speaking conversationally with a friend, writing a letter, remembering telephone numbers, and remembering what happened last week.

Many proponents of this new discipline have rightly drawn parallels between present-day cognitive neuropsychology and the approach of influential nineteenth-century localizationists such as Wernicke, Dejerine, Bastian, and Lichtheim, who sought to draw causal links between brain structures and cognitive function (e.g., Ellis, 1987; Marshall, 1984; Shallice, 1988). One important difference between the two approaches, it is claimed, is the degree of emphasis placed on elucidating links between psychological and physiological levels of function. Present-day cognitive neuropsychology has tended to stress the logical independence of these two levels (e.g., Marr, 1982; Mehler, Morton, & Jusczyk, 1984), although recent advances in neurodiagnostic techniques such as positron emission tomography (PET) and magnetic resonance imaging (MRI) have found willing converts eager to explore relationships between the brain and cognitive behavior (e.g., Howard et al., 1992; Posner, 1989).

In this chapter, we will examine the new approach that cognitive neuropsychology offers to clinical assessment. Before we begin to do that, however, we need to outline

JANICE KAY • Department of Psychology, University of Exeter, Exeter EX4 4QG, England. SUE FRANKLIN • Department of Psychology, University of York, York YO1 5DD, England.

Clinical Neuropsychological Assessment: A Cognitive Approach, edited by Robert L. Mapou and Jack Spector. Plenum Press, New York, 1995.

briefly principles and practices that underpin the whole enterprise, and this will bring us, in turn, to a brief discussion of recent theoretical advances in our understanding of cognitive systems. We will then detail a practical step-by-step guide to assessment, focusing on language processing in general and spoken word retrieval in particular. This will be followed by a brief clinical case example and a few concluding remarks.

COGNITIVE NEUROPSYCHOLOGY AND COGNITIVE PSYCHOLOGY

A primary objective of cognitive neuropsychology is to account for particular patterns observed in disorders of cognition in terms of a theory of "normal" cognitive functioning. A complementary aim is to evaluate existing cognitive models, by exploring how well they can account for and predict such patterns of impaired performance: findings from individuals with cognitive dysfunction are used as a source of evidence with which to test cognitive models, in much the same way as cognitive psychologists use evidence from experimental investigations of cognitive abilities of "normal" people.

In certain respects, the relationship between cognitive neuropsychology and cognitive psychology has been one of dependence of the former on the latter. This can be illustrated by looking at the origins of the "models" used in neuropsychologically based studies. As Coltheart (1984) notes, sometimes the model comes first. In the studies of visual agnosia reported by Humphreys and Riddoch (1987), for example, a model of normal object recognition established by Marr (1982) determined the kinds of tasks that were used to investigate patterns of impaired and preserved skills in a number of patients with recognition disorders. However, in other cases, neuropsychological data have come first and have been used to create hypotheses both of the cognitive processes involved in a particular skill and of the ways in which such processes can break down. The work of Warrington and Taylor (1978) on visual object recognition is an example of how careful studies of patients with recognition disorders have led to the development of a model intended as a description of normal visual object processing. In yet other cases, data collection and model development in each area of cognitive psychology and neuropsychology have proceeded independently and then converged. "Dual-route" models of reading developed along these lines (e.g., Coltheart, 1985), as did work into peripheral spelling processes (e.g., Ellis, 1979, 1982, 1988).

Cognitive neuropsychological studies have followed an information processing approach, which, until recently at least, has dominated the development of theory in cognitive psychology. This approach views cognitive abilities as being made up of the integrated action of a number of discrete components or *modules* (we will have more to say about this in the next section). Cognitive neuropsychological studies have generally framed their research in the context of processing models that are depicted in box-and-arrow diagrams. Such models illustrate possible ways in which simple skills such as reading single words aloud, or hearing and understanding individual words, can be decomposed into their more basic components. For example, in the highly influential model of Patterson and Shewell (1987), concerned with reading, hearing, speaking, and writing single words (see Figure 9.1), there is a "box" for analyzing visual/written input (which involves transforming marks on a page into a more abstract form, independent of writing style and letter case), a "box" for identifying written words (known as an orthographic input lexicon), and, separately, a system for locating word meanings. "Boxes" have two types of function. First, they store knowledge, and second, they process information. Thus, in order to decide that *word* is a word, one must find its entry in an orthographic input lexicon. Not only must there be a representation for it in the lexicon, but there must also be a procedure that enables the representation to be found from among scores of other word forms there. "Arrows" allow communication between the boxes. Thus, once the entry for *word* has been found in the orthographic input lexicon, some form of communication from this system

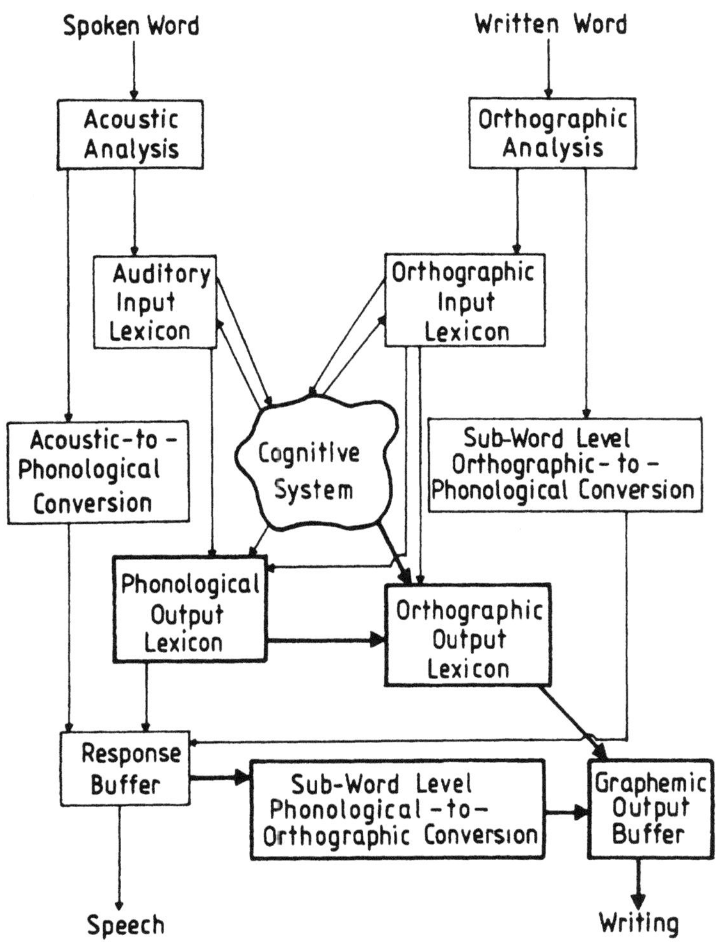

FIGURE 9.1. A simple process model for the recognition, comprehension, and production of spoken and written words and nonwords.

to the semantic system will be needed if the reader is to know what the word means.

The diagrams themselves are intended to be little more than convenient, easily communicable ways of representing how functional architectures of particular skills may be organized. They are not brain based; that is, they do not relate to notions about localizable centers and interconnections between centers in the brain. In this respect, they are unlike similar "box-and-arrow" diagrams of the nineteenth-century localizationists (Morton, 1984).

One must, however, acknowledge limitations to the usefulness of such diagrams. They cannot signal the time course of operation of particular systems within the model, for example. They cannot easily depict higher level functions such as inferential reasoning and syntactic planning, nor do they deal with specific proposals concerning how knowledge is represented and how processing is carried out. More important, however, critics have argued that such difficulties are mirrored in the models themselves. Thus, Seidenberg (1988) has written that the focus of cognitive neuropsychology on deriving a "functional architecture," with its necessary concentration on a *broad* characterization of ways in which components of particular systems interact, has often been at the expense of details about how information is represented, accessed, or transformed. Baldly stated, the criticism is that "models of the functional architecture cannot advance much beyond the description of [cognitive] functions provided by intuition unless these issues of detail are taken seriously" (pp. 407–408). Of course, Seidenberg's criticisms of the theoretical laxity observed in cognitive *neuro*-psychology may just as easily be applied to some of the work in cognitive psychology itself. Indeed, the experiments he discusses in connection with the validity of hypotheses of how lexical information (frequency, word class, imageability) is encoded within lexical representations are mainstream cognitive psychology experiments (Balota & Chumbley, 1985; McCann & Besner, 1987). Moreover, Seidenberg himself goes on to mention cognitive neuropsychological investigations that delve more deeply into the workings of cognitive systems, rather than appearing merely to glance at the blueprints of their operation. Such examples (e.g., Bub, Black, Howell, & Kertesz, 1987; Shallice, 1987) have the virtue of linking neuropsychological data, and theoretical interpretations of these data, with an independently motivated theoretical account derived from experimental studies. To counter Seidenberg's criticisms then, cognitive neuropsychological investigations cannot focus solely on trying to reveal the functional architecture of cognitive systems, but must also attempt to explain the detail of how such systems might operate. This work stresses the need to search for *converging operations* in hypothesis testing (Gardner, Hake, & Eriksen, 1956), that is, evidence that converges on the same conclusions from both experimental and neuropsychological sources.

As well as close theoretical links between cognitive psychology and neuropsychology, there are also close methodological links: practitioners in cognitive neuropsychology use a range of tasks often developed in cognitive psychology (e.g., "lexical decision" tasks given across the desk, "on-line" sentence processing tasks), together with techniques concerning experimental design and statistical analysis. Indeed, given the importance of converging operations, it is not unusual to find researchers moving between neuropsychological and experimental studies to test a particular empirical question (e.g., Ellis, Young, & Flude, 1987; Patterson & Morton, 1985).

PRINCIPLES AND PRACTICES OF COGNITIVE NEUROPSYCHOLOGY

Single-Case Methodology and Case-Series Design

The emphasis in cognitive neuropsychology is on detailed investigations of individual cases rather than on group studies. Traditional neuropsychological investigations of cognitive disorders have tended to use groups of patients who are classified according to syndrome-based diagnoses (e.g., Broca's aphasia, amnesia, visual agnostic and visuospatial disorders). Classificatory schemes have been criticized as not being specific or sophisticated enough to distinguish patients with different underlying deficits, even though gross patterns of performance may be similar (e.g., Byng, Kay, Edmundson, & Scott, 1990). Furthermore, classifications are often based on symptoms that occur for anatomical rather than functional reasons (that is, symptoms that co-occur because of damage to contiguous brain areas, rather than because they share similar processing components). In the section on assessment, below, we have tried to demonstrate how existing assessment batteries that are based on syndrome diagnoses can fail to uncover important cognitive deficits. This is critical for a number of reasons, not the least being, as Byng et al. (1990) argue, that appropriate treatment can be instituted only when the nature and degree of the deficit are understood.

In practical terms, grouping patients under a broad category label can result in important differences between individual members of the group being lost in the "averaging-out" process (just as they are in experiments with non-brain-damaged individuals, but in this case, it is to remove systematically noise in the data due to irrelevant factors). Some cognitive neuropsychologists have approached this problem by using what they believe to be more precise—cognitively driven—categories, as in the syndrome-complexes of "deep" and "surface" dyslexia, agrammatism, or dysgraphia (e.g., Coltheart, 1985). Their critics point out that the same kinds of difficulty still apply: such disorders become further fractionated (see Shallice, 1988, for discussion of input, central, and output forms of deep dyslexia, for example), without a payoff in terms of a greater theoretical understanding of the root causes of these disorders. One response to this difficulty is provided by Ellis (1987), who states that "cognitive neuropsychologists must learn (or relearn) to treat single patients like single experiments." By this, Ellis does not mean that neuropsychologists should work with only a single patient at a time, but that the findings from each patient should be used separately as a test of the theory under consideration. This is because even patients who share a similar symptom may actually show different underlying reasons for that symptom. Working with patients with similar symptomatology in a case-series design may be one way of pointing this out, but the design still operates fundamentally at the level of the individual. What this means in practical terms is that care must be taken to chart variations in performance over time and to ensure internal validity of the results (including replication of critical effects).

Theoretical Assumptions

Explicit in a cognitive neuropsychological approach are four primary assumptions: that cognitive systems are organized in a modular way (*modularity*); that brain damage can result in the *fractionation* of individual modules; that brain damage does not result in the creation of new systems, but in the operation of existing systems minus those that have been impaired (*subtractivity*); and finally, that there is *transparency* in the nature and function of individual modules. We will briefly discuss each of these assumptions in turn.

According to the principle of *modularity*, mental abilities are made up of separable cognitive subsystems or modules. Thus, the operation of spoken word retrieval may be made up of one set of modules, written word recognition another, and visual object recognition yet another. What follows from this is a second assumption, that individual modules can *fractionate*, so that acquired brain damage can selectively impair some modules while leaving others intact (Caramazza, 1984). Thus, one might expect to observe cases, for example, in which spoken word retrieval is disordered, while written word recognition remains relatively preserved. One might also expect to observe instances of selective damage within sets of modules, so that, for example, within the domain of spoken word retrieval, one might discover a case in which naming pictures is impaired, while reading picture names is considerably more successful (e.g., Hillis & Caramazza, 1992).

Underpinning careful cognitive neuropsychological studies that aim to reveal precise patterns of impairment (and abilities that appear to remain intact, or relatively so) is the assumption of *subtractivity*, the view that the performance of an individual patient reveals the usual cognitive apparatus employed in a particular task, minus those systems that have been damaged (Caramazza, 1984). The final assumption, that of *transparency*, holds that the nature and function of a particular cognitive component will be reflected in an undistorted way in the patterns of acquired disorder that are observed to occur. Now, as Caramazza (1984) has cogently noted, performance on a task after brain damage reflects a variety of factors, including disruption to processing systems other than the component one has targeted, and including strategic and compensatory mechanisms that do not normally come into play (collectively, what Seidenberg [1988] calls the sidestreets, rather than the expressways, of performance). One way of ensuring "expressway" investigation, as we have indicated, is to seek confirmatory data from experimental studies (converging operations), and another is to search for reliability and validity through replication of results.

Modularity, Fodor, and Weak Modularity

A logical justification for the assumption that cognitive systems are organized in a modular way is to be found in the vision research work of Marr (1982), who argued persuasively that complex systems (whether one is thinking about the human brain or state-of-the-art computer technology) are easier to "debug" (to detect and correct system errors) and to "upgrade" (to add to, or to improve) if they are organized in a modular way. If they are not, argues Marr, then "a small change to improve one part has to be accompanied by many simultaneous compensatory changes elsewhere" (Marr, 1976). Empirical evidence from neuropsychological studies, showing a wide array of different selective impairments observed in individual neurological cases, appears strongly to support the notion of modularity. Cognitive neuropsychological studies search for patterns of *dissociation*, in which one aspect of performance is impaired, while another is preserved. Such patterns may indicate that the two aspects involve different sets of cognitive processes. However, Shallice (1979) has stressed the importance of *double dissociations* as more reliable indicators that two tasks are handled by different modules. A well-known example is that after brain damage, one person is able to read words competently but is newly unable to construct pronunciations for novel letter strings. The dissociability of these tasks may reflect differences in underlying processing mechanisms, but it may rather simply indicate that the first task (word reading) is easier than the second (novel word reading). The first assumption becomes more plausible, however, if a second patient is observed who can read aloud novel letter strings but has an acquired difficulty in reading words. Thus, double dissociations play an important role in the methodology of cognitive neuropsychology and have also been used to support arguments that cognitive systems are organized in a modular way.

There have been supportive arguments, too, from cognitive psychology. Allport (1980), for example, claims that the results of *dual-task* experiments can reveal the operation of independent processing components. Dual-task experiments examine the degree to which performance is affected when two tasks are carried out at the same time. If two tasks do *not* involve common processing components, then substantial decrements to performance would not be expected, compared with tasks that are believed to involve shared modules. Thus, Shallice, McLeod, and Lewis (1985) addressed the issue of whether there are separate phonological input and output systems, by asking subjects to read arbitrarily chosen words at a rapid rate, while at the same time requiring them to detect particular targets from among words spoken to them at approximately the same rate. Shallice and his colleagues found that performance was only marginally affected when the tasks were combined, compared with each task carried out separately. In contrast, detecting a heard target word while shadowing, both of which involve auditory input processing, were tasks that could not be combined. The authors suggest that dual-task methodology supports the claim that separate auditory input and phonological output systems exist, and it parallels similar findings drawn from neuropsychological data (e.g., Blumstein, Cooper, Zurif, & Caramazza, 1977).

Fodor (1983, 1985) argues, largely on philosophical grounds, for the coexistence of modular and nonmodular systems within cognition. Relatively peripheral mechanisms concerned with input processes are, he suggests, organized in a modular way. They are "highly specialised computational mechanisms," and they embody the property of *informational encapsulation*, which, in simple terms, means that neither the representational knowledge they contain nor their processing operations are accessible to other modules. Examples of such modules are systems for processing different types of visual stimuli, such as objects and words. Modules also accept as their input only one type of information: they are *domain-specific*. Thus, input to a module or modules concerned with word reading consists of written alphabetical material (at least in alphabetical reading systems), rather than more general visual symbols (e.g., line drawings, pictograms). These two properties have been accepted by some as relatively uncontroversial (though, as Schwartz and Schwartz [1984, p. 41] note, "the various components of perceptual systems, including language, may exhibit the properties of modules to different degrees, and in different combinations"). Rather more hotly debated have been two further claims. The first is that information processing in modular systems is not under voluntary control—that given the necessary input, processing will proceed in an inevitable or *mandatory* way. While there is evidence that this may be the case in some systems (in processing auditory perceptual input, for example), it is less strong in other cases. Thus, as Ellis and Young (1988) observe, if we see a familiar person in the street, we can recognize him or her as familiar immediately, but we are not always automatically able to retrieve his or her name. Indeed, we do seem to have some strategic control over the amount of information about the name that we can retrieve. The second claim is that cognitive modules are *innate*—that, as a result of being neuronally and computationally hardwired, they spring into action fully formed, like a reflex, rather than assembled gradually from more basic processes. Although some abilities, like auditory perception, appear, phenomenologically at least, to arise in this way, others like reading, writing, and mental arthmetic skills do not—yet there is evidence that they are all organized in a modular way and are each capable of being selectively impaired.

Perhaps the most controversial of Fodor's claims is the view that while input systems (and possibly output systems, too) are organized in a modular way, central cognitive systems to do with higher level thought processes (reasoning and decision making, beliefs and moral judgments) are *not* modular in their operation (i.e., processing is not informationally encapsulated, not domain-specific, not mandatory, etc.) and may work on quite different principles. This makes them substantially less amenable to scientific study (indeed, there may be good reasons to believe that they never will be). As Shallice (1988) notes, in order to evaluate this claim critically, it is important to establish what the boundaries between input and central processes might be. Using the criteria of informational encapsulation, domain specificity, and mandatory processing, for example, one might conclude that given a heard sentence, the syntactic parse that is carried out is under modular control, while its interpretation requires central systems. However, Shallice (1988) provides neuropsychological data to suggest that at least some central processes (e.g., high-level memory functions, sentence processing skills) may be organized in as modular and dissociable a way as lower level input systems. Further, Schwartz and Schwartz (1984) note that some central processes, "by virtue of repeated experience, or explicit tutoring, or whatever, become . . . modular in practice."

What if the functional architecture of cognitive systems, even at the level of input and output, is not organized in such a tightly modular way? Over the last decade, parallel distributed processing (PDP) or *neural network* models of cognition have increasingly gained in popularity. Unlike information processing accounts, they are computationally based models fundamentally bound up with concepts derived from current understanding of neuronal function (although they differ from actual neural networks in important ways). Neural networks do not consist of independent, informationally encapsulated modules. Instead, they function under what some authors have termed *weak modularity* (Kosslyn & Koenig, 1992), by which they mean that although a particular network may be yoked to one particular cognitive function and receive one kind of input, some parts of the system may be involved in other networks as well (just as letters from assembled words in a Scrabble game can be used to build other words). Kosslyn and Koenig (1992) have described differences between information processing and neural network models by using florid imagery: information processing characterizes mental events without regard to the brain, an approach they call "dry mind"; neural networks assume that facts about the brain are needed to characterize mental events accurately, an approach they call "wet mind." There is little doubt that cognitive neuropsychological investigations will increasingly take a "wet mind" approach. In the next section, we will consider in a little more detail how this is beginning to happen.

Cognitive Neuropsychology: Health Tips to Avoid Premature Death

In previous sections, we have discussed how cognitive psychology and cognitive neuropsychology are disciplines that are inextricably bound together, both theoretically and methodologically. We have stated how the theoretical assumptions of modularity, fractionation, subtractivity, and transparency have underpinned the building and testing of information processing models in these cognate disciplines (and we have briefly mentioned how the assumption of strict modularity is relaxed in neural network models of cognition). We have described how cognitive neuropsychological studies have focused on thorough and precise investigations of individual cases (sometimes using a case-series design). We would now like to take stock of what we think are the major contributions of this area to our understanding of acquired disorders of cognitive function. Because space is necessarily limited, we will focus primarily on acquired disorders of reading as a specific exemplar of our general point.

The somewhat whimsical heading for this section stems from the ominous note sounded by Seidenberg (1988) in his critique of cognitive neuropsychological studies of language: "One of the ironic aspects of science is that a body of work that is successful in changing the way we think about a problem can (some say inevitably will) lead to discoveries that result in its eventual displacement." Seidenberg's "health tip" is that cognitive neuropsychology must develop more computationally explicit models. There are indications that, in the few years since Seidenberg's comments, the field (along with proponents from mother disciplines such as cognitive psychology and related disciplines such as neuropsychology) is attempting to do just that.

In 1973, Marshall and Newcombe published a paper on acquired disorders of reading that had a powerful and enduring impact. In the paper, on the basis of single-case studies of individual patients, they distinguished different kinds of reading disorder that had different characteristic signatures. *Deep dyslexia*, for example, was associated with a complete inability to read novel letter strings, while word reading was characterized primarily by the production of semantic errors (e.g., *city* read as *town*). (For a more recent summary of work on deep dyslexia, see Coltheart, Patterson, and Marshall [1987].) Later on, Beauvois and Derouesne (1979) described an apparently "purer" disorder, termed *phonological dyslexia,* in which novel letter string reading was impaired, while word reading remained relatively intact.

In contrast, *surface dyslexia* was associated with a reasonable ability (though somewhat impaired) to construct pronunciations for novel letter strings, while reading words like *castle,* with unusual spelling–sound patterns, was severely impaired. Word reading in surface dyslexia—unlike in deep dyslexia—appeared to rely on the same processes that were used to assemble nonword pronunciations. These reading patterns, then, appeared to be doubly dissociated. (Indeed, the terms—somewhat opaque now—were held to reflect disturbances to what Chomsky [1964] referred to as deep and surface structures of language.) They were interpreted within a cognitive model of reading in which there were two routes from print to pronunciation: one was a lexical (or word-specific) route via meaning, and the second was nonlexical, requiring procedures for converting letters or letter units into corresponding sounds. Neuropsychological data converged with independent evidence from experimental studies of speeded naming that revealed there are reaction-time costs to read aloud exception words (like *castle*), compared with rule-governed regular words (like *candle*), and to read aloud novel words (like *dusp*), compared with familiar words (like *dust*). Further evidence from later studies indicated that the experimental distinction between "exception" and "regular" words was too simple: regular words like *bead* with visually similar neighbors with different pronunciations (e.g., *head, bread*) took longer to pronounce than regular words like *bean* with neighbors with consistent pronunciations. Furthermore, novel words like *tead* derived from "inconsistent" words took longer to pronounce than "consistent" nonwords like *tean.* Such findings were mirrored in detailed neuropsychological investigations of surface dyslexia (e.g., Shallice, Warrington, & McCarthy, 1983). Some investigators claimed that these findings supported the view that word and novel word pronunciations alike were assembled by analogy with visually and phonologically similar words (Glushko, 1979; Marcel, 1980). Since this view required only a single reading route, it proposed a direct challenge to dual-route theorists. It was, however, both theoretically and computationally underspecified, and when dual-route theorists elaborated their models to suggest that the nonlexical procedures comprised not only letter–sound patterns, but also larger spelling–sound units such as *-ead* and *-ean,* there were few motivated grounds on which to choose between them (Norris & Brown, 1985). More recently, the scales have been somewhat tipped in favor of the single-route hypothesis with the development of the PDP connectionist model of Seidenberg and McClelland (1989). They claim that "our model, and others like it, offers an alternative that dispenses with this two-route view in favour of a single system that also seems to do a better job of accounting for the behavioral data" (p. 564). By behavioral data, Seidenberg and McClelland mean not only experimental data, but also findings from surface dyslexia and deep/phonological dyslexia as well. Neuropsychological evidence not only has contributed critical empirical data, but also has been instrumental in the model's theoretical development (Patterson, Seidenberg, & McClelland, 1990). We cannot say that this is the end of this particular argument, however, since Coltheart, Curtis, Atkins, and Haller (in press) have recently put forward a computationally implemented "dual-route cascade" model of reading aloud.

Connectionist models have also recently been used to investigate several of the effects observed in deep dyslexia, focusing on the genesis of semantic and visual errors and the effects of imageability/abstractness (e.g., Hinton & Shallice, 1991; Plaut & Shallice, 1991). They have not restricted their sphere of interest to language processing, however, but cover other areas of cognition such as face processing and its disorders (e.g., Burton & Bruce, 1992), and visual object processing and its disorders (e.g., Humphreys & Riddoch, 1987). In fact, the signs are that cognitive neuropsychology is flourishing at present. Indeed, its influence appears to be spreading to cognate disciplines such as psychiatry, with recent work on the cognitive neuropsychology of schizophrenia (e.g., Frith, 1993) and other delusional states (e.g., Ellis & Young, 1990).

The general point that we wish to make here is that cognitively based investigations of acquired disorders of cognition *have* contributed to our greater understanding of normal cognitive processing as well as of the disorders themselves, by helping in the development and testing of model-based theories, including recent connectionist and neural network models. The rigor with which such investigations have been carried out has led to the development of new assessments and treatment programs as we will see below.

COGNITIVE NEUROPSYCHOLOGICAL ASSESSMENT: A PRACTICAL GUIDE

While current standardized batteries often fail to reveal the true *cognitive* basis of acquired cognitive deficits, assessment based on cognitive neuropsychological methods is a much more accurate means of achieving this aim. In this section, we will attempt to persuade you why assessment of acquired disorders of cognition *must* be cognitively based.

Assessment in cognitive neuropsychology can be seen as a process of *hypothesis testing*. Thus, an exploration of individual patterns of performance (relatively spared versus relatively impaired abilities) should be guided by predictions that follow logically from the particular model one is using. The process itself is *iterative*: detailed testing of a particular aspect of performance under consideration will lead to further questions. Each one must be pursued, by reference to the model, until one arrives at a detailed profile of the performance characteristics. We can demonstrate what we mean by using investigation of word retrieval disorders as a specific example of the general approach. Let's start, though, by reviewing how classification of word retrieval disorders has commonly been carried out.

Anomia is a term that is used interchangeably with word-finding difficulty to describe a particular symptom of a patient's language behavior. In this sense, anomia is an almost universal feature of dysphasic production. Somewhat confusingly, anomia is also itself a syndrome label, in which a difficulty in word finding is the preeminent feature. In most current approaches to aphasia assessment (e.g., Goodglass & Kaplan, 1983), the syndrome of anomia is regarded as a *unitary* disorder. Low scores on word-finding subtests relative to the level of severity of dysphasia, combined with good comprehension and repetition abilities, are sufficient to produce a diagnosis of the syndrome, regardless of the particular pattern of word retrieval difficulty shown by an individual patient. However, we will show that neither the symptom of anomia (when isolated from other aspects of performance) nor the use of anomia as a syndrome are reliable indicators of the cognitive basis of the difficulty in word retrieval (cf. Ellis, Kay, & Franklin, 1992).

Syndrome-based schools of dysphasia classification have long held that major aphasia syndromes—Broca's, Wernicke's, conduction, and anomic aphasia—display different characteristic patterns of word-finding disorder. Such patterns are thereby tied not only to a particular syndrome diagnosis, but also to a hypothesized location of anatomical abnormality. Linguistically, the patterns are assumed to vary according to error type and also to other factors, such as response to cuing (e.g., Benson, 1979; Goodglass & Geschwind, 1976; Goodglass, Kaplan, Weintraub, & Ackerman, 1976; Pease & Goodglass, 1978). Convincing evidence linking pattern of word retrieval disorder to syndrome type has proved hard to find, however. On the contrary, semantic paraphasias, circumlocutions, and phonological paraphasias can be observed in all aphasic syndromes (e.g., Kohn & Goodglass, 1985; Mitchum, Ritgert, Sandson, & Berndt, 1990). Kohn and Goodglass (1985), for example, showed that when the level of severity of naming impairment is controlled across aphasic subgroups, there are no significant differences between the syndromes in the production of either semantic or phonological paraphasias, though these error categories were the two largest in the total corpus of naming errors (36% and 33%, respectively). Neither does the efficacy of particular types of cue relate to syndrome type in any straightforward way (e.g., Goodglass, Kaplan, Weintraub, & Ackerman, 1976).

There are, of course, several factors that could obscure any correlation between syndrome and performance profile: individual patients under the same umbrella "syndrome" may have been misclassified initially, for example, or may have partially recovered and no longer be "typical" of a particular syndrome type (e.g., Kohn & Goodglass, 1985). However, Laine, Kujala, Niemi, and Uusipaikka (1992) recently studied the naming ability of 10 patients who were purported to be typical representatives of classical aphasia syndromes: Broca's, Wernicke's, conduction, and anomic aphasia. Their investigation revealed individual variations in performance that bore no discernible relationship to syndrome classification. Such variations can best be captured, we would argue, by framing assessment within the context of a cognitive model of word retrieval. And what applies to word retrieval in particular also applies to other cognitive skills in general.

Information processing models of speech production (e.g., Ellis, 1985; Ellis, Kay, & Franklin, 1992) claim that a number of separable modules are involved in comprehension and word retrieval (see also Dell [1986] and Plaut and Shallice [1991], for a different perspective on this problem). Such accounts are similar in essence to that put forward by Benson (1979, 1988), and we will focus on his proposal as an example of a cognitively based model. Benson views the act of word retrieval (following a particular stimulus input, such as a picture, for example) as a necessary progression through a series of steps: sensory registration and perception, sensory association (involving word meanings), word selection, motor speech planning, and production. He distinguishes four types of word-finding disorders that reflect different deficits at different stages of the model: word production anomia, word selection anomia, semantic anomia, and disconnection anomia.

According to Benson, *word production anomia* is characterized by problems with motoric production. He suggests that these can be of two kinds. One, associated with both Broca's and transcortical motor aphasia, is tied to the problems in finding substantive words that are observed in agrammatic speech. He suggests that the patient often appears to know the word but cannot initiate articulation without prompting. With prompting (in the form of a phonemic cue or even the merest hint of an appropriate lip movement), the word can often be produced immediately, indicating that the difficulty is one of initiation rather than prior selection. A second kind of production disturbance results in paraphasias that are phonologically related to the intended word, but can also be so distorted that any phonological relationship is unclear. In this type of disturbance, associated with conduction aphasia, errors may have the same number of syllables as the intended word and be appropriately inflected. Prompting may be of little help, though the patient may produce successively closer attempts to the target.

In *word selection anomia*, Benson claims that neither motor production nor word comprehension is significantly impaired (spoken repetition can be well preserved, for example). Rather, the difficulty appears to be one of selecting a specific target; when a selection fails, performance is characterized by pauses, compensatory circumlocutions, and outright failures to name. Benson also states that the word-finding difficulty of word selection anomia is not ameliorated by prompts, such as contextual or phonemic cues. This pattern of disorder is associated with the syndrome of anomic aphasia.

In contrast with difficulties in word selection and word production, patients with *semantic anomia* have difficulties with meaning that lead not only to problems in production, but also to deficits in comprehension. Benson (1988) claims that "in the most characteristic cases, the patient repeats the name correctly but fails to interpret the meaning of the word. . . . The word no longer represents the object, a true semantic deficit" (p. 23). He does not go into the type of errors that one might expect to find with "a true semantic deficit," though it is not unreasonable to assume that it may be associated with the production of semantically related paraphasias. Benson suggests that the disorder is observed in transcortical sensory aphasia, but is also associated with nonfocal pathology found in progressive dementing disorders such as Alzheimer's disease and Pick's disease.

Benson's final category, *disconnection anomia*, is associated with difficulties in producing words that belong to a specific category, or when the input is presented in a particular modality. As examples of category-specific anomias, he points to specific difficulty in retrieving body part names, and to color agnosia (or color naming disturbance), in which there is an inordinate difficulty in naming colors to confrontation or pointing to colors when the name is presented (e.g., Benson, 1989; Damasio, 1985; Geschwind & Fusillo, 1966; Oxbury, Oxbury, & Humphrey, 1969). Modality-specific anomias are characterized by an inability to name objects when presented in just one sensory modality. Benson groups category-specific and modality-specific deficits together because they appear to depend on the disconnection of "a primary sensory or sensory association area from the major language areas."

Benson's framework is useful because it provides a way of thinking about different *functional* patterns that can occur when word retrieval is disrupted. Assessment should be directed at discovering whether a particular pattern can be accounted for by difficulties at any one or more of these levels. Finding out whether a patient has difficulties in semantic comprehension of words, for example, or in word selection, has a number of important consequences for *diagnosis* of the word-finding problem, because it will have implications for what else might be impaired and the path that assessment should take. In these terms, *"diagnosis" refers to a conceptual understanding of the cognitive deficit.* This, in turn, has important implications for *therapy,* because it will provide guidelines for the design of remediation programs (e.g., Howard, Patterson, Franklin, Orchard-Lisle, & Morton, 1985a, 1985b; Jones, 1990; Nettleton & Lesser, 1991, for specific examples of treatment programs for word retrieval difficulties).

Pertinent to the development of cognitive models in general have been the ways in which cognitive variables such as visual complexity, imageability/picturability, concept familiarity, and age of acquisition can be used to reveal underlying cognitive impairments. Whether variables such as these play any part in governing naming performance, for example, has often been investigated in previous research studies: word frequency (Howes, 1964; Rochford & Williams, 1965), age of acquisition (Rochford & Williams, 1962), picturability (Goodglass, Hyde, & Blumstein, 1969), sensory modality (Goodglass, Barton, & Kaplan, 1968), semantic field (Goodglass & Baker, 1976), and operativity (Gardner, 1973). However, unlike more recent cognitive neuropsychological investigations, these studies do *not* make explicit connections between particular variables and their hypothesized role in producing particular patterns of performance. Detailed investigation of individual patients shows that such links can often be established—and, moreover, that particular error patterns can be tied to the influence of particular variables (e.g., Nickels, in press).

In the following sections we will describe how cognitive neuropsychological assessments are carried out, again using word retrieval as our example. Assessments such as these are complemented by rigorous design features borrowed from cognitive psychology, such as the use of appropriate control materials and balancing of noncritical variables across conditions.

EXAMPLES OF COGNITIVE NEUROPSYCHOLOGICAL ASSESSMENT: WORD RETRIEVAL ABILITIES

We will illustrate a general cognitive neuropsychological approach to assessment by focusing on a range of examples from language assessment, including some from two recent batteries that we have been involved in designing: PALPA (Psycholinguistic Assessments of Language Processing in Aphasia) (Kay, Lesser, & Coltheart, 1992) and the ADA Comprehension Battery (Franklin, Turner, & Ellis, 1992) (see also Caplan, Chapter 4, this volume). It is important to emphasize that the principles involved in designing assessment tasks (careful investigation of the factors and variables that affect correct and error performance) *apply generally to all investigations of cognitive disorder,* even though the specific examples relate to assessment of word-finding difficulties. We will frame our discussion by referring to the four patterns of anomia described by Benson (1988), but we will also set it in the context of what has been learned from current cognitive neuropsychological case studies in terms of model-based interpretation.

Prior to beginning, we would like to emphasize several elements of good methodology and practice, which should be stressed in carrying out assessment tasks. Again, these apply not only to the example to be presented, but to cognitive neuropsychological assessment in general. First, *to avoid carryover and practice effects, different versions of the same task should not be given in the same session.* Second, in assessment, *patients should not be made aware of items on which they have made errors, nor should they be provided with the correct response.* This will allow for retesting in a different modality or for a posttherapy assessment of the same items. Third, *for the purposes of adequate statistical analysis, a large number of items should be used in each assessment test.* This is particularly important for tests with carefully balanced sets (e.g., high- and low-frequency words). Fourth, *time should be spent ensuring that the patient fully understands the task requirements*; this may require lots of practice and modeling or shaping the procedure. Finally, *tests using similar procedures, but with different assessment purposes, should not be given one after another in a clinical session.* An ABBA, or Latin square, design is commonly used in assessment. For example, in attempting to discover whether a certain cue helps naming more than simply allowing extra time, the examiner may give the half of the items in the no-cue condition (Condition A), followed by half of the items given with cues (Condition B), followed by the remaining materials from each condition, reversing the order of presentation.

The conventional way of examining word retrieval difficulties is to use a standard visual confrontation naming task, such as the Boston Naming Test (Kaplan, Goodglass, & Weintraub, 1983) or the Graded Naming Test (McKenna & Warrington, 1983). Both of these tests consist of black-and-white line drawings of pictures that are graded according to hypothesized orderings of difficulty. They allow the examiner to observe the kinds of errors that are made and to measure responsiveness to prompts such as semantic and phonemic cues, but they do not test or control for psycholinguistic variables such as semantic category, word frequency, and syllable length. Confrontation naming tasks that are designed from a cognitive neuropsychological standpoint build in such variables, and these help to *maximize* the amount of information that can be gathered about factors that govern word retrieval ability. If one variable is manipulated, others are kept constant across conditions. Thus, if one is interested in finding whether there is an effect of word frequency on naming ability, one might select pictures whose names fall into high-, medium-, and low-frequency bands, ensuring that across these bands words are matched for syllable length and morphological complexity (e.g., *table, lemon, camel*). Sometimes variables are varied orthogonally (e.g., high- and low-frequency words of either one, two, or three syllables in length). The PALPA assessments have two confrontation naming tasks: one examines an effect of word frequency on picture naming; the other allows a comparison of spoken picture naming with repetition and reading of the picture name set, written picture naming, and writing the names to dictation. The latter is particularly useful when assessing difficulties in word retrieval that stem from word selection and word production impairments.

The effects of cue type on naming performance can also be investigated experimentally (see p. 257). Thus, the influence of the correct initial phoneme cue in producing a naming response can be compared with a "miscue" (the first sound in the name of a semantic coordinate) and an unrelated sound cue. (It should be stressed that it is sometimes helpful to know whether a "miscue" will precipitate semantic errors in naming; this condition would be included only as part of a specific assessment program with a particular patient, rather than in the usual run of clinical work.) As well as initial phoneme cues, the effect of semantic cues can also be investigated. People who benefit from extra semantic information when attempting to name a picture may not be able to obtain enough information about the item from the picture alone. This may be due to problems in processing the picture itself, in accessing semantic information from the picture or to a deficit within a semantic store.

The types of errors that are produced in naming can also be investigated experimentally. A cognitive neuropsychological approach aims to tie error types to particular cognitive deficits. For example, semantic errors may arise because of a semantic-level deficit. Thus, Coltheart (1980) suggests that "shared feature" errors, in which the error belongs to the same category as the target, either as a superordinate (e.g., robin → "bird"), for example, or as a coordinate (e.g., cow → "donkey"), occur because a distinguishing feature or features (between category members at different levels of a semantic hierarchy, or within category members at the same level) are lost or inaccessible, at least temporarily. Circumlocutions, in which a description of the target is provided that may be accurate, or lacking in specificity, may arise from the same level. Phonological errors, on the other hand, in which a phonological resemblance can be readily identified between the sought-after target and the actual response, appear to arise later in the sequence of word retrieval: the correct target has been appropriately located, but not realized appropriately. Neuropsychological evidence has shown, however, that there is no necessary *exclusive* relationship between error type and locus of impairment. The same error type may arise from a number of different underlying causes. Semantic errors in picture naming, for example, may stem from difficulties either within a semantic system itself, or in access to correct word phonology from semantic representations, or from difficulties within a system of word selection (a speech output lexicon) (e.g., Caramazza & Hillis, 1990). Circumlocutions may similarly arise from semantic-level damage or from access to word phonology from relatively intact semantic representations. Even phonological errors may result from a semantic-level deficit, in which information "cascades" from semantic to phonological retrieval processes (e.g., Schwartz, 1987). Using error typing as the sole means of deducing the nature of the language impairment is therefore fraught with difficulty, unless accompanied by converging evidence from the *profile* of performance on word retrieval and comprehension tasks. Individual patients may produce a variety of error types, and even classification itself is not always straightforward: for example, semantic errors in which a single related word is produced in lieu of the target may on occasion be more appropriately characterized as a single-word circumlocution, or description, of the target word, rather than as a miscomprehension of it.

As well as arriving at a particular profile of a patient's naming ability using confrontation naming and error analysis, it is also necessary to test other skills that may require access to word selection processes. Thus, picture naming performance can be compared with repetition and oral reading of the same items (as in one of the PALPA tasks described above). Although successful repetition (and oral reading) may be carried out by understanding what is heard (or read) and then translating it into a form compatible with speech output, it is also clear that we can repeat and read aloud by using cognitive procedures that do not involve semantic and word-based knowledge. We can repeat or read aloud something that we have never heard or never seen written down before by using a system that constructs, *de novo,* speech forms from auditory or written input (sublexical acoustic–phonology conversion, and sublexical orthography–phonology conversion). Because of the availability of a number of different routines for repeating and reading aloud both words and unfamiliar words, and for producing spoken words in picture naming, word production must be assessed in a variety of tasks (e.g., spoken picture naming, repetition of spoken picture names) and using a variety of materials (e.g., words and unfamiliar words). Comparison of performance across these tasks can provide information about where the deficit lies: for example, impaired picture naming in the absence of significant repetition problems suggests that the locus of the disorder does not lie in actual word production, but may arise from difficulties in word selection (see below).

Word Selection Anomias

Some dysphasic patients appear to have little difficulty on comprehension tasks involving picturable material and single words, so that a semantic-level impairment is not a convincing account of their particular problems in word retrieval; rather, their difficulty seems to be one of *word selection*. Benson (1988) suggests that when word selection breaks down, performance is characterized by compensatory circumlocutions and outright failures to name. However, the characteristics of the word selection problem depend on exactly *how* word selection procedures are impaired, and this may differ from patient to patient. It is clear that "word selection" involves a number of separable procedures, such as access to a phonological word store (or speech output lexicon) and selection of the appropriate target word. It is likely that each of these procedures can be damaged in a number of different ways, with different consequences for the outward manifestation of a naming deficit. Thus, while it is reasonable to expect circumlocutory descriptions of the target word when a patient has a precise target in mind, one might also expect that the accuracy of the description will be mediated by both the nature and the severity of the deficit. "Outright failures to name" may result from an inability to access, or activate, any lexical target, though it is unclear that this is an inevitable consequence of a word selection difficulty, nor that this is the only precipitant of naming failures.

Kay and Ellis (1987) suggested that selection difficulties arising from problems in phonological access are characterized by frequency effects and by phonological errors in picture naming. However, since we know that word frequency can exert its effects at a variety of different levels (more frequent items may be associated with "richer" semantic structures, for example, or with "stronger" phonological activation), it appears to have limited localizing power. Moreover, recent cases have been described of patients who appear to show word selection problems. They have good comprehension abilities, for example, and they show strong frequency effects in naming, but they do not tend also to make phonological errors (Hirsh, Ellis, & McCloskey, 1990; Miceli, Giustolisi, & Caramazza, 1991; Zingeser & Berndt, 1988). It therefore appears that frequency effects and phonological errors may not be linked causally in word retrieval disorders.

Word Production Anomias

While phonological errors may result from disturbances that affect lexical representations in a speech output lexicon, they may also arise from postlexical retrieval stages, at which phonemes are ordered and translated into articulatory commands (e.g., Ellis, Kay, & Franklin, 1992). As we mentioned above, one way of distinguishing between these alternatives is to consider performance on a variety of output tasks (e.g., word repetition and reading aloud), using both word and nonword materials. Impairment of postlexical production routines would be expected to affect output tasks to the same extent, regardless of the materials used. One would also expect to find similar patterns of phonological errors across all tasks (e.g., Caplan, Vanier, & Baker, 1986). Since word production disorders involve disruption to the procedures of construction, assembly, and maintenance of phonologically coded strings, effects of phonological variables such as syllable length should be assessed.

Assessing Word and Picture Semantics

Word-finding difficulties revealed by a confrontation naming task may reflect problems in semantic comprehension. An effective way of revealing comprehension deficits in word and picture semantics is by using a carefully designed word-to-picture matching task. To test whether a person is able to make relatively fine-grained semantic judgments, distractor pictures should be included that are related closely in meaning to the target (such as members of the same coordinate category). Thus, in the 40-item word-to-picture matching task from the PALPA battery, the patient is asked to point to the picture of an *ax*, for example, with a picture of a coordinate word, such as *hammer*, as distractor. The degree of difficulty of the task can be manipulated in a number of ways. For example, the level of specificity of semantic knowledge available to a patient can be examined by manipulating the degree of semantic relatedness. While some dysphasic patients tend to make errors that apparently reflect lapses of quite precise semantic knowledge (e.g., Patient J.C.U. reported by Howard and Orchard-Lisle [1984], tended to make coordinate errors in comprehension), others show semantic deficits that result in the deterioration of all but broad semantic categories, or "spheres" of meaning (e.g., Caramazza & Berndt, 1978; Goodglass, 1980; Zurif, Caramazza, Myerson, & Galvin, 1974). For this reason, the PALPA test includes not only coordinate pictures, but also ones that are more distantly related to the target; thus, using our current example, the patient hears the word *ax* and is required to choose among pictures of an *ax,* a *hammer,* and a *pair of scissors.* The task enables the examiner to find whether a patient tends to choose either the correct picture or its coordinate, or whether choices are distributed more broadly over the related picture set.

Dysphasic patients may have more difficulty in distiguishing the target and the coordinate picture if the two are not only semantically related, but also structurally related (Bishop & Byng, 1984); thus, *ax* and *hammer* not only are close semantic coordinates, but also have similar visual features. In the PALPA test, an effect of visual and semantic similarity, over and above one of semantic similarity, is tested for by using 20 pairs that have similar meanings and also look similar (e.g., *ax, hammer*), and 20 pairs that have similar meanings but are visually quite distinct (e.g., *carrot, cabbage*).

The range of impairments that such a task can pick up can be widened further by adding yet more distractor types. (This has an additional advantage of not completely constraining the kinds of errors that patients can make; thus, if a test only makes use of semantic distractors, then *any* errors will be attributed to a semantic cause.) Pictures that are visually similar to the target, but not related in meaning, can be used to screen for visually based perception and identification difficulties. Thus, in the PALPA test, the patient hears the word *ax* and is required to choose among pictures of an *ax,* a *hammer,* a *pair of scissors,* a *flag* (which visually resembles the ax), and a *kite* (which is unrelated in any way to an ax) (see Figure 9.2). Pictures whose names are phonologically similar to the target word can be used to identify auditorily based disorders of perception, identification, and comprehension. In a word-to-picture matching test from the ADA battery, for example, distractors can be phonologically related to the target (e.g., *socks–fox*), phonologically and semantically related (e.g., *snake–snail*), or purely semantically related to the target (e.g., *beard–hair*).

It is important to administer a word-to-picture matching task in a written word version and in a spoken word version, so that performance can be compared across modalities. The Pyramids and Palm Trees test (PPT), devised by Howard and Patterson (1992), allows one to test comprehension ability using not only *cross-modal* (i.e., word–picture) matching, but also matching *within the same modality* (i.e., picture–picture and word–word). In all versions of the PPT, the patient is asked to decide, by pointing, which of a pair of items, such as a *palm tree* or a *pine tree,* goes better with a third (a *pyramid*). The stimulus can be a written or spoken word or a picture; the target and distractor can be pictures or written words. The basis of the match is a semantic association; in this case, the palm tree "goes with" the pyramid, on the grounds that both are found in hot climates, or that both are found in Egypt. Although there may be some room for subjectivity in deciding on the "correct" association, Howard and Patterson report that non-brain-damaged control subjects make three er-

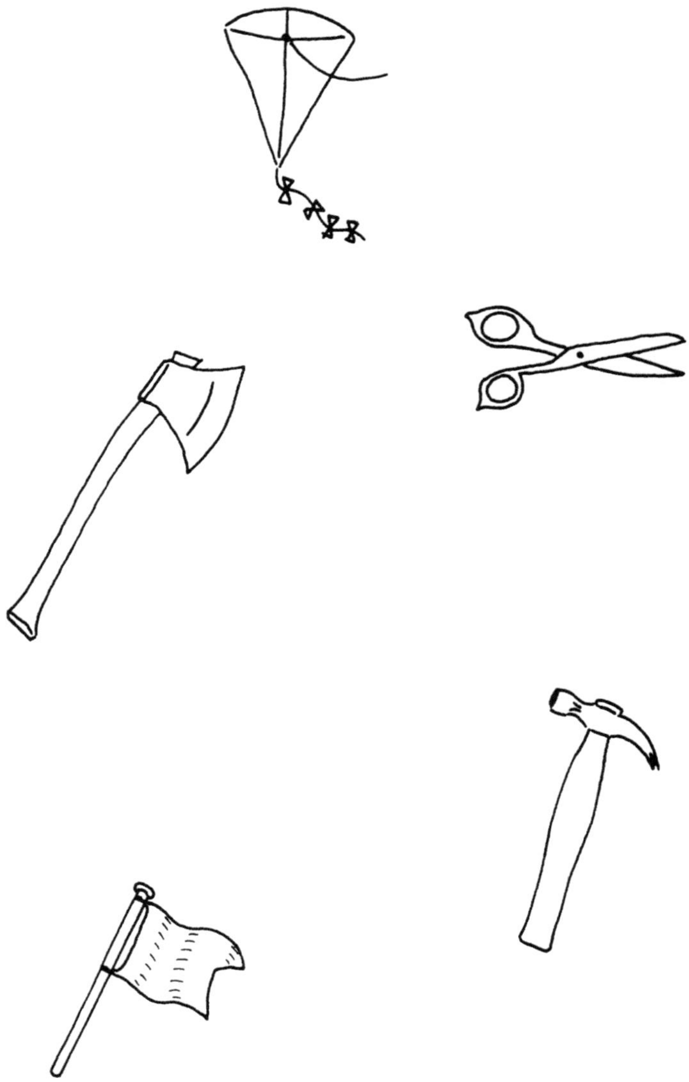

FIGURE 9.2. Example of materials from the Word–Picture Matching task in the PALPA (Kay, Lesser, & Coltheart, 1992).

rors or fewer on the 52-item task. Target and distractor are semantic coordinates, so a correct decision requires semantic knowledge sufficient to make an association between stimulus and target and sufficient to distinguish target from coordinate.

Some authors have proposed that information about the meanings of objects and words is represented in separate semantic stores. Picturable material accesses an object semantic system, while verbal material (spoken and written words) accesses a lexical semantic system (e.g., Beauvois, 1982; Shallice, 1987; Warrington, 1975). To other researchers, the existence of multiple semantic stores is controversial. They postulate a central semantic store that takes input from pictures and words, regardless of modality of input and the nature of the stimuli (e.g., Gainotti, 1982; Riddoch, Humphreys, Coltheart, & Funnell, 1988). We do not need to engage this debate here. What is important for present purposes is to note that the PPT task allows for independent assessment of "object semantic" knowledge (three-picture version), "lexical semantic" knowledge (three-word version), and transfer of information between the two semantic systems (word/picture versions).

As well as using tasks to compare across input modalities for word and picture comprehension, it is informative to use the same materials for both comprehension and naming. A similar profile of performance in comprehension and naming, for example, suggests that anomic difficulties may stem from an underlying comprehension impairment (e.g., Caramazza, Hillis, Rapp, & Romani, 1990; Howard & Orchard-Lisle, 1984), while differential profiles (e.g., impaired naming in the absence of significant comprehension of picture names) indicate that naming problems do not result from problems in picture comprehension (e.g., Caramazza & Hillis, 1990; Kay & Ellis, 1987; Zingeser & Berndt, 1988). Moreover, the same target pictures used in matching and association tasks can be presented for naming to confrontation to give information about consistency of response. A simple task that allows easy comparison across comprehension and production is *picture name judgment* (e.g., Howard & Franklin, 1988; Howard & Orchard-Lisle, 1984). In this test, a single picture is shown along with a single spoken, or written, word. The word can be either the correct name, a semantically related word, or an unrelated word. For example, the patient may be presented with a picture of a *lion* and asked on different occasions, "Is it a lion?" "Is it a tiger?" or, "Is it a pencil?" In a production task, the patient is asked merely to generate the name or, in cases in which there is difficulty in producing a spoken output, is given a cue. The cue can be the correct initial sound of the target (e.g., "luh," for *lion*, in the example), or a wrong sound cue (e.g., "tuh" for *tiger*), or the first sound of an unrelated word (e.g., "puh" for *pencil*). This is to see not only whether a patient will make semantic errors in comprehension (or unrelated errors), but also whether the patient can be induced to make semantic errors in naming. The degree of semantic relatedness, or the nature of the semantic relationship (e.g., paradigmatic versus syntagmatic), can be readily manipulated in the choice of semantically related word. It is an easy and flexible task to construct, not least because any pictures can be used and it can be readily customized. Thus, Howard and Franklin (1988) used not only semantically related foils, but also phonologically related word foils (e.g., Is it an *iron*?) and phonologically related nonword foils (e.g., Is it a *pion*?) to test a patient with suspected auditory comprehension difficulties. Picture name judgment tasks may be more demanding than word-to-picture matching tasks because the person cannot try to work out the correct answer by elimination (Best, personal communication). On the other hand, it may underestimate comprehension abilities if the person fails to grasp the task requirements and believes that semantically related names should be accepted as correct.

If a person performs well on tasks like word-to-picture matching and picture name judgment, then one should test ability on more demanding comprehension tasks. Many dysphasic patients have particular difficulty in dealing with words that are low in imageability. One test that uses only single-word materials and manipulates the degree of imageability of items is a *synonym judgment* test. In this test, the patient listens to (or reads) two words and has to decide whether they are closely related in meaning. The two words are either synonyms (e.g., *marriage–wedding*) or unrelated pairs (e.g., *marriage–ship*). Half of the items are high in imageability (e.g., *marriage–wedding*), and half are low in imageability (e.g., *safety–security*). Both sets should be matched on word frequency (or orthogonally varied by frequency) and other pertinent variables. Versions of this task can be found in both the PALPA and ADA assessments.

It is, of course, important to be able to say whether a particular score on a particular task is impaired, and how far it is impaired. In tasks in which there is a forced choice between items or a yes/no decision (e.g., PPT, picture name judgment, and synonym judgment), a score of 50% is expected by chance. Whether a score is better than chance can be calculated by using a binomial test. On tasks such as word-to-picture matching, working out "chance" estimates is slightly less straightforward. For example, on the 40-item word-to-picture matching task from PALPA, with five pictures to choose from, a patient making choices in a random manner will have a 1 in 5 chance of picking the correct picture. However, if the patient has some (though not necessarily complete) semantic knowledge, the chance of picking the correct picture may be 1 in 3, or even 1 in 2, when the patient is simply undecided between the target and the close semantic distractor. Some tasks supply normative data from control groups of non-brain-damaged adults. However, one should bear in mind that non-brain-damaged adults may be performing at ceiling on these tasks, and it is unwise to conclude that a patient who behaves within "normal" limits is showing unimpaired performance.

Central Semantic Deficits and Semantic Anomia

Varieties of comprehension impairments will be associated with different characteristic signatures. For example, a patient may make errors on matching and association tasks regardless of whether items are presented as pictures, as written words, or cross-modally, as words and pictures or spoken words and written words. This suggests that the difficulty may be a *central semantic deficit,* rather than one of *access* to meaning. Like Benson (1988), if one assumes that a central system of meaning governs word production as well as comprehension, then impairment to this system would result in semantic errors in production as well as in comprehension. Hillis, Rapp, Romani, and Caramazza (1990) claim that their dysphasic patient, K.E., has a central semantic deficit. K.E. made semantic errors in spoken and written word-to-picture matching and semantic paraphasias in spoken picture naming, oral reading, written picture naming, and writing to dictation. Note, however, that if a patient makes semantic errors in comprehension across all modes of presentation, it is not beyond the realms of possibility that the problem is in fact one of access to meaning—a number of impairments that affect access across all modalities tested. Semantic errors occurring also in production would, by the same argument, be explained as a disconnection, or partial disconnection, between meaning and output systems. Although one might choose on the grounds of parsimony to posit a single locus of impairment, rather than multiple loci, researchers have appealed to theoretically based criteria to distinguish access versus central store deficits. According to Shallice (1987), for example, impairment to a central store may result in "degraded" semantic representations. A degraded store deficit should result in *consistent responses* across test sessions. No matter how or when semantic information about a particular concept is tested, if it has become degraded in some way, it will be consistently impaired. There should also be relatively invariant order in which information is lost. *Degradation will affect more specific levels of information before it affects more general information* (distinctions between *hat* and *cap*, for example, will be lost before more general knowledge about *headware* and *clothing*). Shallice suggests that *more frequent concepts are more robust* because they will have richer semantic structures than less common concepts. Warrington and McCarthy (1987) claim that, in the long term, central store impairments show *little expectation of recovery*. These criteria (testing for consistency across tasks and across sessions; testing for item frequency or familiarity) can be built into any language assessment program. As one might expect, the patient in the study by Hillis et al. (1990) showed a high degree of consistency in her responses. However, one should also bear in mind that these criteria are not hard and fast. Humphreys and Riddoch (1988), for example, have pointed out that although consistency may be associated with central store deficits, one might also find similar effects with other types of impairment (such as noise in access routes).

Modality-Specific Deficits and Disconnection Anomia

Some patients will present with comprehension difficulties that affect a particular modality or modalities of input. This kind of impairment falls into Benson's category of disconnection anomia and, more particularly, modality-specific anomia. Benson (1988) suggests that "the modality-specific syndromes produce a notable word-finding defect that is correctly intepreted as an agnosia but truly represents a word finding problem." In fact, difficulty in naming that is restricted to just one modality can be produced by impairments at any one of a number of different levels, in perceptual processing, for example, or because of problems at more abstract levels of recognition and identification. Take the case of a person who is considerably more impaired in carrying out the PPT task when it is given as three pictures, compared with picture-to-word and word-to-word versions. Her difficulty may indeed reflect relatively peripheral problems in processing pictorial material, such as a visual agnosic deficit. On the other hand, it may reveal a *modality-specific access impairment*. That is, the difficulty might stem from a problem in accessing information about the meaning of picturable material, even though semantic comprehension abilities appear to be well preserved (to judge from performance on written words), and it can be demonstrated through other tasks that the patient is not impaired in picture processing. Some researchers who argue for multiple semantic systems (e.g., Shallice, 1987) have claimed that modality-specific access impairments can be explained by postulating central semantic difficulties, but in just one semantic system (e.g., in object semantics or in lexical semantics) or in translation between them. Examples of patients who demonstrate modality-specific difficulties that do *not* appear to be agnosic in character have been reported by Beauvois (1982); Beauvois, Saillant, Meininger, and Lhermitte (1978); Denes and Semenza (1975); and Riddoch and Humphreys (1987).

Category-Specific Deficits and Disconnection Anomia

Zingeser and Berndt (1988) observed that their patient with word selection anomia had particular difficulty in producing nouns compared with frequency-matched verbs. Caramazza and Hillis (1990) report a similar finding for their patient. Benson (1988) suggests that such "category-specific anomias" should be described as *disconnection anomias,* in which the difficulty is one of finding the name for items belonging to a specific category or categories. He groups category-specific and modality-specific deficits together because both types appear to depend on a disconnection between particular sensory systems and more abstract linguistic knowledge systems. In fact, more precisely, category-specific deficits appear to say something about the nature of the organization both of semantic memory and of word selection routines. Silveri and Gainotti (1988) report the case of a patient who had particular problems in comprehending and producing animal, fruit, flower, and food names, but not names of body parts. Similarly, Hart, Berndt, and Caramazza (1985) describe a patient who had especial difficulty in dealing with fruit and vegetable names, but while he was certainly unable to produce the names of exemplars from these categories, he was apparently well able to understand what they were and the fine-grained differences between them. Whereas the performance of Silveri and Gainotti's patient is consistent with a central store deficit, that of the patient in the study by Hart et al. would appear to arise at a later word selection stage.

SUMMARY

We have discussed how to carry out assessment within the framework of a cognitive neuropsychological approach, by using acquired disorders of word retrieval as our example. From the standpoint of rehabilitation of cognitive disorders, this approach emphasizes that in order to treat any cognitive impairment, one must first understand what has gone wrong. And what is meant by "understanding," here, is being able to characterize the nature of the disorder in *processing* terms. Given the complexity of any cognitive system, there will be a large number of different ways in which it can break down, and this will correspond with many different patterns of impairments. The purpose of assessment is both to describe and to explain the nature of these impairments as completely as possible. Relating assessment to a hypothesized theoretical account of the system under consideration provides a *logical basis* with which to proceed. Of course, each different pattern of impairment will require a different pattern of treatment, and this is one reason why rehabilitation programs and, indeed, assessments themselves, are customized to the individual with whom one is working (for more on cognitive neuropsychological rehabilitation studies, see Riddoch and Humphreys [1993b]). Emphasis on a single-case approach (or case-series design) raises questions about appropriate statistical methods and experimental designs; for detail on these matters, the interested reader is directed to Howard (1986) and Pring (1986).

CASE EXAMPLE: L.E.—A CASE OF LEXICAL SELECTION ANOMIA

This section illustrates how one might set about a brief assessment using the techniques we have described, again with word retrieval difficulties as our example.

L.E. had a cerebrovascular accident (CVA) in February 1988, when she was 41 years old. Prior to her illness, she worked as a domestic assistant at a local hospital. No neurological details are available. Initially, L.E. presented as totally aphasic, with a dense right hemiplegia. The hemiplegia resolved sufficiently for her to walk, but she regained little functional use of her right hand. When the assessment described here took place, approximately 18 months after the CVA, L.E. presented with moderately nonfluent and anomic speech. She had good functional auditory comprehension but limited reading comprehension. A severe agraphia meant she was able to write only two or three very common words. Her oral reading was also affected, and conformed to the pattern of "phonological dyslexia"; that is, her word reading was significantly better than her nonword reading.

L.E. was given the 100 Picture Naming Test (Howard & Franklin, 1988) for spoken naming. She was able to name 78 of the pictures correctly and self-corrected a further 5 words. One error was phonologically related (*rake* → *rail*). All other errors were circumlocutions or semantic errors (Table 9.1 illustrates her incorrect naming responses). A mixed phonological and semantic cue was often successful in eliciting those words L.E. was unable to produce. What was the nature of the impairment that gave rise to this anomia?

Semantic Processing

Some of the circumlocutory errors suggested that L.E. had accessed the meaning of the picture. For example,

> *mayor* → "it's a man, and it's . . . quite high up"
> *crook* → "outside, and it's sheep farmer, and it's . . ."

However, we were uncertain whether she had accessed the actual meaning or just a related one. So, we gave her an auditory comprehension test, the Synonym Judgments task from the ADA Comprehension Battery, in order to establish whether she had a semantic processing deficit. She made 148/160 correct judgments on this test, which is within the normal range (albeit at the lower end); there was no effect of imageability or frequency (see Table 9.2). L.E.'s good performance on this test supports the notion that there was no central semantic impairment underlying her anomia.

TABLE 9.1. L.E.'s Errors from 100 Picture Naming Test

Self-corrected
egg → "hen"
mermaid → "woman's body"
pig → "cow"
stool → "I got one in there"
tent → "outside"

Incorrect
arch → "ancient, and it's very old, and it's . . ."
cotton → "spool"
crook → "outside, and it's sheep farmer, and it's . . ."
globe → "world"
hoof → "foot, horse's foot"
hose → "thing on the tap . . . I got one in my shed"
lamp → "lampshade"
mayor → "it's a man, and it's . . . quite high up"
pepper → "vegetable, it's green"
pyramid → "in the desert, and it [name of husband] knows it"
rabbit → "it's outside, and it's [name of son] has it"
rake → "rail"
sword → "knife'
toe → "foot"
water → "tap"
wool → "ball of st . . . knitting"
worm → "garden, it's a snail"

Phonological Processing

The types of errors L.E. made in naming and her performance on auditory comprehension testing suggest that she had an output anomia. This could be the result of either a lexical selection deficit or a word production anomia. Given the rarity of phonological errors in L.E.'s naming, it seemed unlikely that it was a word production anomia. To confirm this, L.E.'s naming was compared with her oral reading of the same items. If her anomia was at the level of word production, then error rates on both tasks should have been identical, irrespective of input mode.

L.E. was given the Hirsh Naming Screener (1992), which consists of 16 words each of high, medium, and low frequency (a similar test to one in the PALPA) for both

TABLE 9.2. Synonym Judgments: Auditory Presentation

Total correct: 148/160	(Non-brain-damaged controls: 148–158)
By word type (proportion correct)	
High imageability	.95
Low imageability	.93
High frequency	.90
Low frequency	.93

picture naming and reading. Although L.E. is dyslexic, her oral reading on this test was significantly better than her naming (45/48 versus 38/48; McNemar Test, p = .02). This confirmed that her naming errors are not due to an impairment of phonological word production. This is further supported by the observation that she had almost no impairment in word repetition.

Diagnosis and Outcome

Since there is no obvious impairment of either semantics or phonology, it is plausible that L.E. has a word selection anomia. This is supported by the fact that her success in naming is affected by word frequency (Hirsh Naming Screener, high frequency 15/16, medium frequency 13/16, low frequency 10/16). L.E. was often able to cue herself semantically to produce the correct word and responded to cuing from others. This, with the existence of the word frequency effect, suggested that there was a good prognosis for her word finding, as long as she continued to practice naming and using her cuing strategies. Her performance on the 100 Picture Naming Test approximately 1 year later bears this out: the only "errors" she made were actually synonyms (e.g., dress → "frock").

CONCLUSIONS

In this chapter, we have discussed how cognitive neuropsychology has proved useful to our understanding of acquired disorders of cognition, and using varieties of naming impairment as an example, we have shown how it provides a rigorous approach to assessment. Our claim is that to understand the nature of functional impairments in acquired disorders of cognition, assessments must be cognitively based. We have described some of the assessments that have been constructed and are currently available for language testing in dysphasia and other neurological disorders. There are others that are designed for other cognitive impairments (e.g., Birmingham Object Recognition Battery [BORB]; Riddoch & Humphreys, 1983a). We must point out, however, that one must also be prepared to develop additional tests in order to evaluate specific hypotheses concerning particular impairments. One of the themes of this paper has been to reflect on how cognitive neuropsychology developed from cognitive psychology, and we have stressed the elements of this approach that derive from the rigorous methodologies employed in cognitive psychology.

In describing the development of cognitive neuropsychology, we described two of its main objectives. We have neglected a third, which is concerned with using models of cognitive function and dysfunction to plan rehabilitation programs. Howard and Hatfield (1987), writing about aphasia therapy, emphasize that "if therapy is organised in this way it can be made both rational and specific . . .; then we can develop theory that relates to therapy and therapy that relates to theory. If we motivate, specify and test our therapy it will get better; it needs to" (p. 135). We echo their claim; we also have tried to suggest how we believe assessment should be organized.

ACKNOWLEDGMENTS

This work has been supported by a Wellcome Trust University Award to Janice Kay and by an MRC Project Grant to Sue Franklin.

REFERENCES

Allport, D. A. (1980). Attention and performance. In G. Claxton (Ed.), *New directions in cognitive psychology.* London: Routledge and Kegan Paul.

Balota, D. A., & Chumbley, J. I. (1985). The locus of the word frequency effect in the pronunciation task: Lexical access and/or production. *Journal of Memory and Language, 24,* 89–106.

Beauvois, M.-F. (1982). Optic aphasia: A process of interaction between vision and language. *Proceedings of the Royal Society (London), B298,* 35–47.

Beauvois, M.-F., & Derouesne, J. (1979). Phonological dyslexia: Three dissociations. *Journal of Neurology, Neurosurgery, and Psychiatry, 42,* 1115–1124.

Beauvois, M.-F., Saillant, B., Meininger, V., & Lhermitte, F. (1978). Bilateral tactile aphasia: A tacto-verbal dysfunction. *Brain, 101,* 381–401.

Benson, D. F. (1979). Neurologic correlates of anomia. In H. Whitaker & H. A. Whitaker (Eds.), *Studies in neurolinguistics (Vol. 4).* New York: Academic Press.

Benson, D. F. (1988). Anomia in aphasia. *Aphasiology, 2,* 229–236.

Benson, D. F. (1989). Luria on naming defects. *Journal of Neurolinguistics, 4,* 19–35.

Bishop, D. V. M., & Byng, S. (1984). Assessing semantic comprehension: Methodological considerations and a new clinical test. *Cognitive Neuropsychology, 1,* 233–244.

Blumstein, S. E., Cooper, W. E., Zurif, E. B., & Caramazza, A. (1977). The perception and production of voice-onset time in aphasia. *Neuropsychologia, 15,* 371–383.

Bub, D., Black, S., Howell, J., & Kertesz, A. (1987). Speech output processes and reading. In M. Coltheart, G. Sartori, & R. Job (Eds.), *The cognitive neuropsychology of language* (pp. 79–110). London: Lawrence Erlbaum.

Burton, A. M., & Bruce, V. (1992). I recognise your face, but I can't remember your name: A simple explanation. *British Journal of Psychology, 81*(1), 45–61.

Byng, S., Kay, J., Edmundson, A., & Scott, C. (1990). Aphasia tests reconsidered. *Aphasiology, 4,* 67–91.

Caplan, D., Vanier, M., & Baker, D. (1986). A case study of reproduction conduction aphasia. *Cognitive Neuropsychology, 3,* 99–128.

Caramazza, A. (1984). The logic of neuropsychological research and the problem of patient classification in aphasia. *Brain and Language, 21,* 9–20.

Caramazza, A., & Berndt, R. S. (1978). Semantic and syntactic processes in aphasia: A review of the literature. *Psychological Bulletin, 85,* 898–918.

Caramazza, A., & Hillis, A. E. (1990). Where do semantic errors come from? *Cortex, 26,* 95–122.

Caramazza, A., Hillis, A. E., Rapp, B. C., & Romani, C. (1990). Multiple semantic or multiple confusions? *Cognitive Neuropsychology, 7,* 161–168.

Chomsky, N. (1964). *Current issues in linguistic theory.* The Hague: Mouton.

Coltheart, M. (1980). The semantic error: Types and theories. In M. Coltheart, K. E. Patterson, & J. C. Marshall (Eds.), *Deep dyslexia.* London: Routledge and Kegan Paul.

Coltheart, M. (1984). Editorial. *Cognitive Neuropsychology, 1,* 1–8.

Coltheart, M. (1985). Cognitive neuropsychology and the study of reading. In M. Posner & O. S. M. Marin (Eds.), *Attention and performance XI* (pp. 3–37). Hillsdale, N.J.: Lawrence Erlbaum.

Coltheart, M., Curtis, B., Atkins, P., & Haller, M. (in press). Models of reading aloud: Dual-route and parallel-distributed-processing approaches. *Psychological Review.*

Coltheart, M., Patterson, K. E., & Marshall, J. C. (1987). *Deep dyslexia* (2nd ed.). London: Routledge and Kegan Paul.

Damasio, A. R. (1985). Disorders of complex visual processing: Agnosias, achromatopsia, Balint's syndrome and related difficulties of orientation and construction. In M-M. Mesulam (Ed.), *Principles of behavioral neurology*. Philadelphia: F. A. Davis.

Dell, G. (1986). A spreading activation theory of retrieval in sentence production. *Psychological Review, 93*, 283–321.

Denes, G., & Semenza, C. (1975). Auditory modality-specific anomia: Evidence from a case study of pure word deafness. *Cortex, 11*, 401–411.

Ellis, A. W. (1979). Slips of the pen. *Visible Language, 13*, 265–282.

Ellis, A. W., (1982). Spelling and writing (and reading and speaking). In A. W. Ellis (Ed.), *Normality and pathology in cognitive function*. London: Academic Press.

Ellis, A. W. (1985). The production of spoken words: A cognitive neuropsychological perspective. In A. W. Ellis (Ed.), *Progress in the psychology of language, 2*. London: Lawrence Erlbaum.

Ellis, A. W. (1987). Intimations of modularity, or, the modularity of mind. In M. Coltheart, G. Sartori, & R. Job (Eds.), *The cognitive neuropsychology of language* (pp. 397–408). London: Lawrence Erlbaum.

Ellis, A. W. (1988). Normal writing processes and peripheral acquired dysgraphias. *Language and Cognitive Processes, 3*, 99–127.

Ellis, A. W., Kay, J., & Franklin, S. (1992). Anomia: Differentiating between semantic and phonological deficits. In D. I. Margolin (Ed.), *Cognitive neuropsychology in clinical practice*. Cary: Oxford University Press.

Ellis, A. W., & Young, A. W. (1988). *Human cognitive neuropsychology*. London: Lawrence Erlbaum.

Ellis, A. W., Young, A. W., & Flude, B. (1987). "Afferent dysgraphia" and the role of feedback in the motor control of handwriting. *Cognitive Neuropsychology, 4*, 465–486.

Ellis, H., & Young, A. W. (1990). Accounting for delusional misidentifications. *British Journal of Psychiatry, 157*, 239–248.

Fodor, J. A. (1983). *The modularity of mind*. Cambridge, MA: MIT Press.

Fodor, J. A. (1985). Precis of *The modularity of mind* (with commentaries). *Behavioral and Brain Sciences, 8*, 1–42.

Franklin, S., Turner, J., & Ellis, A. W. (1992). The ADA Comprehension Battery. London: Action for Dysphasic Adults.

Frith, C. D. (1993). *The cognitive neuropsychology of schizophrenia*. Hove: Lawrence Erlbaum.

Gainotti, G. (1982). Some aspects of semantic-lexical impairment in aphasia. *Applied Psycholinguistics, 3*, 279–294.

Gardner, H. (1973). The contribution of operativity to naming capacity in aphasic patients. *Neuropsychologia, 2*, 213–220.

Gardner, W. R., Hake, H. W., & Eriksen, C. W. (1956). Operationalism and the concept of perception. *Psychological Review, 63*, 149–159.

Geschwind, N., & Fusillo, M. (1966). Color naming defects in association with alexia. *Archives of Neurology, 15*, 137–146.

Glushko, R. J. (1979). The organization and activation of orthographic knowledge in reading aloud. *Journal of Experimental Psychology: Human Perception and Performance, 5*, 674–691.

Goodglass, H. (1980). Disorders of naming following brain injury. *American Scientist, 68*, 647–655.

Goodglass, H., & Baker, E. (1976). Semantic field naming and auditory comprehension in aphasia. *Brain and Language, 3*, 359–374.

Goodglass, H., Barton, M. I., & Kaplan, E. (1968). Sensory modality and object naming. *Journal of Speech and Hearing Research, 11*, 488–496.

Goodglass, H., & Geschwind, N. (1976). Language disturbance (aphasia). In E. C. Carterette & M. Friedman (Eds.), *Handbook of perception* (Vol. 7). New York: Academic Press.

Goodglass, H., Hyde, M. R., & Blumstein, S. (1969). Frequency, pictureability, and availability of nouns in aphasia. *Cortex, 5*, 104–119.

Goodglass, H., & Kaplan, E. (1983). *The assessment of aphasia and related disorders.* Philadelphia: Lea & Febiger.

Goodglass, H., Kaplan, E., Weintraub, S., & Ackerman, N. (1976). The "tip-of-the-tongue" phenomenon in aphasia. *Cortex, 12,* 145–153.

Hart, J., Berndt, R. S., & Caramazza, A. (1985). Category-specific naming deficit following cerebral infarction. *Nature, 316,* 439–440.

Hillis, A. E., & Caramazza, A. (1992). The reading process and its disorders. In D. I. Margolin (Ed.), *Cognitive neuropsychology in clinical practice.* Cary, NY: Oxford University Press.

Hillis, A. E., Rapp, B., Romani, C., & Caramazza, A. (1990). Selective impairment of semantics in lexical processing. *Cognitive Neuropsychology, 7,* 191–244.

Hinton, G. E., & Shallice, T. (1991). Lesioning an attractor network: Investigations of acquired dyslexia. *Psychological Review, 98*(1), 74–95.

Hirsh, K. W. (1992). Hirsh Naming Screener. Unpublished manuscript, York University, York, England.

Hirsh, K. W., Ellis, A. W., & McCloskey, M. (1990, July). *Naming and word frequency: Predicting success but not error type.* Paper presented to the Experimental Psychology Society, Oxford, England.

Howard, D. (1986). Beyond randomised controlled trials: The case for effective case studies of the effects of treatment in aphasia. *British Journal of Disorders of Communication, 21,* 89–102.

Howard, D., & Franklin, S. (1988). *Missing the meaning.* Cambridge, MA: MIT Press.

Howard, D., & Hatfield, F. M. (1987). *Aphasia therapy.* London: Lawrence Erlbaum.

Howard, D., & Orchard-Lisle, V. (1984). On the origin of semantic errors in naming: Evidence from the case of a global aphasic. *Cognitive Neuropsychology, 1,* 163–190.

Howard, D., & Patterson, K. E. (1992). *The Pyramids and Palm Trees Test.* Bury St. Edmunds, England: Thames Valley Test Company.

Howard, D., Patterson, K. E., Franklin, S., Orchard-Lisle, V., & Morton, J. (1985a). The facilitation of picture naming in aphasia. *Cognitive Neuropsychology, 2,* 49–80.

Howard, D., Patterson, K. E., Franklin, S., Orchard-Lisle, V., & Morton, J. (1985b). The treatment of word retrieval deficits in aphasia: A comparison of two therapy methods. *Brain, 108,* 817–829.

Howard, D., Patterson, K. E., Wise, R., Brown, W. D., Friston, K., Weiller, C., & Frackowiak, R. (1992). The coritical localization of the lexicons: Positron emission tomography evidence. *Brain, 115,* 1769–1782.

Howes, D. (1964). Application of the word frequency concept to aphasia. In A. V. S. De Reuck & M. O'Connor (Eds.), *Disorders of Language* (Ciba Foundation Symposium). London: Churchill Livingstone.

Humphreys, G. W., & Riddoch, M. J. (1987). *Visual object processing.* London: Lawrence Erlbaum.

Humphreys, G. W., & Riddoch, M. J. (1988). On the case for multiple semantic systems: A reply to Shallice. *Cognitive Neuropyschology, 5,* 143–150.

Jones, E. V. (1990). A year in the life of EVJ and PC. In *Advances in aphasia therapy in the clinical setting: Proceedings of the 1989 summer conference of the British Aphasiology Society,* Cambridge, England.

Kaplan, E., Goodglass, H., & Weintraub, S. (1983). *Boston Naming Test.* Philadelphia: Lea & Febiger.

Kay, J., & Ellis, A. W. (1987). A cognitive neuropsychological case study of anomia: Implications for psychological models of word retrieval. *Brain, 110,* 613–629.

Kay, J., Lesser, R., & Coltheart, M. (1992). *PALPA: Psycholinguistic Assessments of Language Processing in Aphasia.* Hove, England: Lawrence Erlbaum.

Kohn, S. E., & Goodglass, H. (1985). Picture naming in aphasia. *Brain and Language, 24,* 266–283.

Kosslyn, S. M., & Koenig, O. (1992). *Wet mind: The new cognitive neuroscience.* New York: Free Press.

Laine, M., Kujala, P., Niemi, J., & Uusipaikka, E. (1992). On the nature of naming difficulities in aphasia. *Cortex, 28,* 537–554.

Marcel, A. J. (1980). Surface dyslexia and beginning reading: A revised hypothesis of the pronunciation of print and its impairments. In M. Coltheart, K. E. Patterson, & J. C. Marshall (Eds.), *Deep dyslexia*. London: Routledge and Kegan Paul.

Marr, D. (1976). Early processing of visual information. *Philosophical Transactions of the Royal Society (London), B290*, 199–218.

Marr, D. (1982). *Vision*. San Francisco: W. H. Freeman.

Marshall, J. C. (1984). Multiple perspectives on modularity. *Cognition, 17*, 209–176.

Marshall, J. C., & Newcombe, F. (1973). Patterns of paralexia. *Journal of Psycholinguistic Research, 2*, 175–195.

McCann, R. S., & Besner, D. (1987). Reading pseudohomophones: Implications for models of pronunciation assembly and the locus of word-frequency effects in naming. *Journal of Experimental Psychology: Human Perception and Performance, 13*(1), 14–24.

McKenna, P., & Warrington, E. K. (1983). *The Graded Naming Test*. Windsor, England: NFER.

Mehler, J., Morton, J., & Jusczyk, P. W. (1984). On reducing language to biology. *Cognitive Neuropsychology, 1*, 83–116.

Miceli, G., Giustolisi, L., & Caramazza, A. (1991). The interaction of lexical and nonlexical processing mechanisms: Evidence from aphasia. *Cortex, 27*, 57–80.

Mitchum, C. C., Ritgert, B. A., Sandson, J., & Berndt, R. S. (1990). The use of response analysis in confrontation naming. *Aphasiology, 4*, 261–280.

Morton, J. (1984). Brain-based and non-brain-based models of language. In D. Caplan, A. R. Lecours, & A. Smith (Eds.), *Biological perspectives on language*. Cambridge, MA: MIT Press.

Nettleton, J., & Lesser, R. (1991). Therapy for naming difficulties in aphasia: Applications of a cognitive neuropsychological model. *Journal of Neurolinguistics, 6*, 139–157.

Nickels, L. (in press). Getting it right? Using aphasic naming errors to evaluate theoretical models of spoken word production. *Language and Cognitive Processes*.

Norris, D., & Brown, G. D. A. (1985). Race models and analogy theories: A dead heat. A reply to Seidenberg. *Cognition, 20*, 155–168.

Oxbury, J. M., Oxbury, S. M., & Humphrey, N. K. (1969). Varieties of color anomia. *Brain, 9*, 847–860.

Pease, D. M., & Goodglass, H. (1978). The effects of cuing on picture naming in aphasia. *Cortex, 14*, 178–189.

Patterson, K. E., & Morton, J. (1985). From orthography to phonology: An attempt at an old interpretation. In K. E. Patterson, J. C. Marshall, & M. Coltheart (Eds.), *Surface dyslexia*. London: Lawrence Erlbaum.

Patterson, K. E., Seidenberg, M., & McClelland, J. L. (1990). Connections and disconnections: Acquired dyslexia in a computational model of reading processes. In R. G. M. Morris (Ed.), *Parallel distributed processing: Implications for psychology and neuroscience*. London: Oxford University Press.

Patterson, K. E., & Shewell, C. (1987). Speak and spell: Dissociations and word-class effects. In M. Coltheart, G. Sartori, & R. Job (Eds.), *The cognitive neuropsychology of language* (pp. 273–294). London: Lawrence Erlbaum.

Plaut, D. C., & Shallice, T. (1991). *Deep dyslexia: A case study of connectionist neuropsychology* (Tech. Rep. No. CRG-TR-91-3). Department of Computer Science, University of Toronto, Canada.

Posner, M. I. (1989). *Foundations of cognitive science*. Cambridge, MA: MIT Press.

Pring, T. R. (1986). Evaluating the effects of speech therapy for aphasics and volunteers: Developing the single case methodology. *British Journal of Disorders of Communication, 21*, 103–115.

Riddoch, M. J., & Humphreys, G. W. (1987). Visual object processing in optic aphasia: A case of semantic access agnosia. *Cognitive Neuropsychology, 4*, 131–185.

Riddoch, M. J., & Humphreys, G. (1993a). *BORB: Birmingham Object Recognition Battery*. Hove, England: Lawrence Erlbaum.

Riddoch, M. J., & Humphreys, G. (1993b). *Cognitive neuropsychology and cognitive rehabilitation*. Hove, England: Lawrence Erlbaum.

Riddoch, M. J., Humphreys, G. W., Coltheart, M., & Funnell, E. (1988). Semantic system or systems? Neuropsychological evidence reexamined. *Cognitive Neuropsychology, 5,* 3–25.

Rochford, G., & Williams, M. (1962). Studies in the development and breakdown of the use of names: I: Relationship between nominal dysphasia and the acquisition of vocabulary in childhood. *Journal of Neurology, Neurosurgery, and Psychiatry, 25,* 222–227.

Rochford, G., & Williams, M. (1965). Studies in the development and breakdown of the use of names, IV: The effects of word frequency. *Journal of Neurology, Neurosurgery and Psychiatry, 28,* 407–413.

Schwartz, M. (1987). Patterns of speech production deficit within and across aphasia syndromes: Application of a psycholinguistic model. In M. Coltheart, G. Sartori, & R. Job (Eds.), *The cognitive neuropsychology of language* (pp. 163–199). London: Lawrence Erlbaum.

Schwartz, M. F., & Schwartz, B. (1984). In defence of organology. *Cognitive Neuropsychology, 1,* 25–42.

Seidenberg, M. (1988). Cognitive neuropsychology and language: The state of the art. *Cognitive Neuropsychology, 5,* 403–426.

Seidenberg, M., & McClelland, J. L. (1989). A distributed, developmental model of word recognition and naming. *Psychological Review, 96,* 523–568.

Shallice T. (1979). Case study approach in neuropsychological research. *Journal of Clinical Neuropsychology, 1,* 183–211.

Shallice, T. (1987). Impairments of semantic processing: Multiple dissociations. In M. Coltheart, G. Sartori, & R. Job (Eds.), *The cognitive neuropsychology of language* (pp. 111–127). London: Lawrence Erlbarum.

Shallice, T. (1988). *From neuropsychology to mental structure.* Cambridge, England: Cambridge University Press.

Shallice, T., McLeod, P., & Lewis, K. (1985). Isolating cognitive modules with the dual-task paradigm: Are speech perception and production processes separate? *Quarterly Journal of Experimental Psychology, 37A,* 507–532.

Shallice, T., Warrington, E. K., & McCarthy, R. (1983). Reading without semantics. *Quarterly Journal of Experimental Psychology, 35A,* 111–138.

Silveri, M. C., & Gainotti, G. (1988). Interaction between vision and language in category-specific impairment. *Cognitive Neuropsychology, 5,* 677–709.

Warrington, E. K. (1975). The selective impairment of semantic memory. *Quarterly Journal of Experimental Psychology, 27,* 635–657.

Warrington, E. K., & McCarthy, R. (1987). Categories of knowledge: Further fractionation and an attempted integration. *Brain, 110,* 1273–1296.

Warrington, E. K., & Taylor, A. M. (1978). Two categorical stages of object recognition. *Perception, 7,* 695–705.

Zingeser, L. B., & Berndt, R. S. (1988). Grammatical class and context effects in a case of pure anomia: Implications for models of language production. *Cognitive Neuropsychology, 5,* 473–516.

Zurif, E. B., Caramazza, A., Myerson, R., & Galvin, J. (1974). Semantic feature representations for normal and aphasic language. *Brain and Language, 1,* 167–187.

10

A Hypothesis-Testing Approach to Assessment

KEVIN W. WALSH

Neuropsychological evaluation is no longer limited to earlier considerations of "brain damage" or of regional diagnosis. Present-day emphasis, instead, is on an understanding of the ways in which psychological functions are compromised or spared by neurological disorders. One goal of such an evaluation is to provide a basis for developing strategies of compensation or retraining, which will allow the individual with acquired deficits to function more effectively. Thus, there is a need for flexibility to cover all types of cases likely to be presented. Hypothesis-testing methodology is seen as an efficient way to pursue this aim. Centered on the examination of single cases, it regards clinical neuropsychology as an applied science. As such, it calls on *all* relevant knowledge from neuropsychology and related disciplines, such as neurology and neuropathology, as well as cognate areas of psychology.

The purpose of this chapter is to introduce the reader to hypothesis-testing methodology in clinical neuropsychology. Because the concepts of hypothesis-testing methodology may be applied to many neuropsychological instruments, less time will be spent discussing particular instruments, while more time will be devoted to discussion of theoretical and practical implications of the approach, as illustrated through case examples. First, general methodological considerations will be presented. It will be shown how a hypothesis-testing approach may help the clinician circumvent some of the limitations of "fixed battery" or strictly quantitative approaches to assessment. Second, some of the pitfalls of interpretation based on scores alone will be presented, using case illustrations. Assumptions regarding the meaning of test failure, as exemplified in scores, will be challenged, and the use of qualitative information to understand sources of failure will be illustrated. Third, there will be a brief discussion of the assessment and written report. Finally, the chapter will conclude with three case

---

KEVIN W. WALSH • Austin Hospital, Heidelberg 3084, Melbourne, Australia.

Clinical Neuropsychological Assessment: A Cognitive Approach, edited by Robert L. Mapou and Jack Spector. Plenum Press, New York, 1995.

illustrations of hypothesis-testing methodology. These cases are presented in considerable detail, to offer the reader a sense of the hypothesis-testing process.

METHODOLOGICAL CONSIDERATIONS

The basis of the method requires the clinician to develop a frame of reference made up of two major elements: (1) familiarity with the current body of knowledge of neuropsychological findings and their relationship to neurological disorders, and (2) a personal experience of as wide a range of these disorders as possible, examined at various stages of their evolution and resolution. The method allows the ready incorporation of newly emerging descriptions of syndromes or disorders and constantly clarifies the ways in which these are, or are likely to be, reflected in tests, particularly those of cognition (see case S.A., below).

Admittedly, the most difficult feature in the application of clinical methods that combine different classes of data is the relative weighting to be given to the various pieces of information. Much of this is dependent on supervised case analysis. As advocated elsewhere for training in clinical psychology (Dana, 1966), supervision in report writing can form a central part of training for assessment, especially in getting rid of faulty interpretation based on reading into the data one's own ideas, rather than using a reasoned argument closely tied to the data. As Dana (1966) suggested, reports from skilled clinicians can and should be used as models. Unfortunately, the dearth of skilled supervision sets serious limits on the potential of individual practitioners in many centers to acquire the second part of this broad base for operations.

The assessment of the individual case is essentially the inductive–deductive approach used in medicine. Here, assessment is seen "as a logical, sequential decision making process rather than as simply the administration of a fixed battery of tests" (Benton, 1985). Such an approach was commended to clinical psychology by Shapiro (1967):

> A score from even one of the best validated tests can usually be regarded as the basis of a plausible hypothesis about the subject; the result cannot lead to firm unqualified conclusions. Such hypotheses must, if time and facilities permit, be tested by various methods, such as clinical observations of the patient's behavior and skills, further investigations and experiments. (p. 1039)

While the method has proven difficult to apply in clinical psychology, the nature of disorders in neuropsychology makes it much more germane. A reciprocal relationship between knowledge emerging from both clinical and experimental research in the understanding of individuals is exemplified in the work of Warrington and her colleagues (McCarthy & Warrington, 1990; see also Chapters 4, 5, and 9, in this volume); this "flexible and eclectic" method shares much of the philosophy described here. Likewise, there are similarities with Benton's (1985) suggestion of the use of a core battery followed by the "exploration of specific possibilities . . . depending on both the specific referral question and the patient's pattern of performance on the core battery." However, this latter method still means that in some instances the core battery may miss the point through lack of relevance. Even the primary examination should be directed by the history. The discovery that certain tests prove useful time and time again should not lead to their unthinking use in all cases. As the practitioner becomes more expert, a very wide range of test procedures from which to select will need to be known and available. While expertise in the method requires application and training, many hypotheses tend to recur in clinical practice, so that appropriate measures and observations can be quickly used, leading to greater effectiveness and economy of the clinician's time. Fixed examination systems tend to be wasteful, since in some situations tests will be used that are not appropriate and hence unproductive. On the other hand, even extensive batteries may err in the opposite direction, since even hours of examination may fail to address the central issue. This model of practice retains the strengths of statistical data while avoiding some of the weaknesses of purely quantitatively based methods.

One of the disadvantages of some neuropsychological methods that are based strictly on quantitative data is that they will miss the case where the signs or deficits are minimal, that is, not significantly deviant statistically. This is crucial in progressive disorders, where early detection may be of paramount importance, and also in conditions where the deficit is subtle but incapacitating. This is not to deny the value of quantitative data, but merely to point out that negative instances should be viewed with caution. Also the low frequency of occurrence of some conditions may mean that there will never be sufficient cases documented to use statistically based systems.

One approach to this early detection is to exemplify to trainees what the neuropsychiatrist Emil Kraepelin termed the "method of extreme cases." The method involves training the clinician first to recognize a disorder in its obvious form, so that he or she will develop the ability to recognize the same disorder when the indicators are less than optimal. Likewise, a principal limitation of some purely psychometric approaches to cognitive evaluation is that they are unable to deal meaningfully with the concept of a multifactorial syndrome or disorder, although there are obvious difficulties with the concept. Nevertheless, the concept has proved useful when dealing with complex clinical phenomena. The salient feature is that the syndrome has significance only as a gestalt, and to look at the component features in isolation is to destroy this significance.

THE ASSESSMENT

The principal aspects of the evaluation are the history and the application of cognitive measures.

History

The history should determine the form and the content of the examination. The flexibility that is one of the advantages of the method begins here. It has been suggested that "extra time spent on the history is likely to be more profitable than extra time spent on the examination" (Hampton, Harrison, Mitchell, Pritchard, & Seymour,

1975, p. 489). The overemphasis on assessment as a nomothetic process has meant the neglect in some cases of careful appraisal of the history.

It is important to obtain confirmation of major historical features, especially in situations where the true facts may be difficult to ascertain. In interpreting the medical history, the significance of certain events or facts may be missed or their significance given insufficient weight unless the neuropsychologist has a grasp of cognate discipline; hence, the importance of case discussions.

Since the medical history will not always be adequate for neuropsychological purposes, extra information often will have to be obtained from the patient and other observers. The neuropsychologist should check for congruence between findings from different sources and for consistency with the usual course of known or suspected disorders. In particular, the emergence of new complaints after a "latent" period should be examined carefully.

Cognitive Measures

In a very real sense, there are no such things as neuropsychological tests, only tests of cognition that are used to test questions. The fundamental point is that the selection of measures will depend on the hypotheses being considered. The specific measures will be a product of test knowledge and availability, and the practitioner should seek to constantly expand command of an enlarging armamentarium. Examination not only should seek confirmatory evidence for a particular point of view but should also elicit information to confirm or disconfirm competing hypotheses or diagnoses. It is assumed that the reader will have familiarity with a wide range of neuropsychological measures. Reference may be made to Lezak (1983), to Spreen and Strauss (1991), or to the recent literature in journals such as *The Clinical Neuropsychologist,* in order to obtain the latest information on extant neuropsychological measures.

PITFALLS OF INTERPRETATION

It should be stressed that hypothesis-testing methodology should not be seen as denying the importance of standardized tests of cognition, only in warning against uncritical interpretation based on the sole use of quantitative measures. An expanded treatment of this topic can be found in Walsh (1991).

The Danger of Aggregate or Summarizing Measures

In speaking of the most widely used summarizing measure, namely the intelligence quotient derived from the Wechsler scales, Lezak (1988) wrote, "Its [the IQs] use—and that of any scores representing sums or averages of disparate data obtained from tests of brain functions and mental abilities—can obscure specific facets of a subject's neuropsychological status or misrepresent it generally." Combining data, whether within or between tests, often results in loss of information of crucial significance. For example, only one subtest of a scale may show a lower than expected score. Simply summing the items within one subtest may overlook the significance of certain failures. Particular failures are of signal importance in pseudoneurological cases (Walsh, 1991). It is not uncommon in such cases to observe failures on simple items of tests graded in order of difficulty, whereas more difficult items are handled with ease. If one invokes the commonsense principle that the difficult subsumes the easy, then a score that combines this differing information means that the key to understanding of the individual case may be lost.

A typical example was provided by a young accident victim claiming compensation for brain impairment, even though there appeared to have been no significant head injury. Almost from the start of the examination, he evinced a strange pattern of failure that was repeated on several tests. For example, on the Porteus Maze Test, he failed quite simple items at the 6-, 10-, and 11-year-old levels. Although this met criteria for test discontinuation, the neuropsychologist continued the test, and the man completed the Adult level on the first attempt in the most facile manner. Failure on the simpler problems was most unlikely to be due to neural incapacity, and the hypothesis that he was probably enacting was strongly supported by his behavior on subsequent tests including symptom validity testing (see Binder & Pankratz, 1987; Walsh, 1991).

Another common mistake is to take summary scores to mean the same thing in the brain injured as would be valid in those with intact nervous systems. Wechsler (1944) defined intelligence as "the aggregate or global capacity of the individual to act purposefully, to think rationally, and to deal effectively with the environment." While there is little doubt that a reasonable correlation does exist between the Wechsler measures and intelligent behavior in people with intact brains, the same cannot be said of those who have brain pathology. If we try to apply Wechsler's definition to those with closed head injuries, we frequently observe that they fail *to act purposefully,* do not always *think rationally,* and are totally unable to *deal effectively with the environment* despite obtaining high scores on the intelligence scales. This means that in this situation, the intelligence scales must be low on measures of these essential attributes. Such a situation holds for Case B.A., described below.

A second example of the loss of sensitivity of summary measures comes from the allied Wechsler Memory Scale (WMS). A 57-year-old woman suffered a stroke affecting the deep portions of the left temporal and occipital lobes, which resulted in loss of the right half of each visual field and severe memory difficulty. There were no other neurological signs or symptoms. After several weeks of confusion her sensorium cleared, and she seemed relatively well oriented, but was described at home as very forgetful. Tested 3 months after her stroke, she had a memory quotient (MQ) of 122. Despite the clear history, she was described in a psychological report as having a relatively good memory performance, presumably on the basis of the MQ.

Her WMS Form 1 performance was as follows:

Information	6	Digits Total	12
Orientation	4	Visual Reproduction	12
Mental Control	9	Associate Learning	10
Logical Memory	11		

The raw data showed that the score of 10 on Associate Learning over the three trials was due to her ability to repeat all six easy pairs immediately ("old" material), while being virtually unable to learn the hard pairs ("new" material). This was confirmed on extended testing. Moreover, what little she learned was lost with the slightest interference or delay. Thus, the single Associate Learning score, as well as the MQ, both grossly misrepresented the situation.

Face Validity and the Law of Parsimony

There is still a tendency to take tests at their face value and to be seduced into inferring that failure on a test necessarily means that the subject has a deficit in the function that the test is purported to measure. This would be true if there were only one reason for failing the test. In fact, some psychologists have long been skeptical of a simple relationship between tests scores and functions. For example, Shapiro (1967) wrote, "Most tests have only an indirect relationship with the variables they are supposed to measure."

This state of affairs comes about because most tests are multifactorial in their composition and thus may be failed for any one of a number of reasons. Some of these reasons may be determined by observing the qualitative features of the subject's performance. On other occasions, hypotheses must be generated about the possible reasons for failure on the particular test. If failure is due to a certain functional deficit, this can be ascertained by giving one or more tasks, in which the stated function is the central or major component.

The obverse of this argument is that there should also be caution in taking the similarity of scores from different tests to indicate an identity of causation, as "different individuals may obtain the same score on a particular test for very different reasons" (Ryan & Butters, 1980). Some of these issues will now be addressed in more detail.

Logical Constraints

In a brief but important note, Miller (1983) pointed to what can be termed "paralogical thinking" when drawing conclusions from test findings. In support, he cited a number of studies, such as one that argued that since normal elderly subjects did less well on tests that have been shown to be sensitive to right-hemisphere pathology, the right hemisphere ages more rapidly than the left.

Miller pointed out that while damage to a structure may produce a change on a test, this does not mean that the converse follows. He stated:

> In fact the logical status of this argument is the same as arguing that because a horse meets the test of being a large animal with four legs that any newly encountered large animal with four legs must be a horse. The newly encountered specimen could of course be a cow or hippopotamus and still meet the same test. (Miller, 1983, p. 131)

The implication is obvious: discovering that a particular group (e.g., the elderly) manifests impairment on measures that are found in other groups (e.g., stroke patients) to be sensitive to particular types of dysfunction does not permit one to conclude that the former group has the same type of brain dysfunction as the latter.

Qualitative Information

As noted, the use of quantitative data alone leaves out important information. A test response is not a score; scores, where applicable, are abstractions designed to facilitate intraindividual and interindividual comparisons, and as such they are extremely useful in clinical testing. However to reason, or to do research, only in terms of scores or score patterns is to do violence to the nature of the raw material. The scores do not communicate the responses in full (Schafer, as quoted in Shapiro, 1951).

More recently, Goldberg and Costa (1986) restated this truism, writing, "The behavior that generates scorable responses is, however, far richer and more varied than any scoring system will allow." While it is desirable to use quantification where possible, some clinically relevant information does not lend itself readily to such quantification, particularly in the early stages of development of a clinical discipline, as is the case at present with neuropsychology.

One way of coping with the shortcoming of using scores alone is to attempt to capture the behavior more fully by noting the quality and patterning of responses during evaluation. Ryan and Butters (1980) advised that "information about the neuropsychological processes which underlie a subject's performance can only be provided by a detailed qualitative analysis." This position is shared by Kaplan and her colleagues (Kaplan, 1983, 1988), whose development of the Boston Process Approach is described elsewhere.

The study of qualitative features may be observations of performance on standardized tests or may be extended to include less formal tests and general behavioral observation. Such observations may suggest a nonorganic cause for failure or point to a specific form of neuropsychological disorder, for example, a visuospatial or executive difficulty. Two simple examples of the former will illustrate the basic concept.

Case 1. A young woman was referred by a clinical psychologist as having a very short memory span. This followed a minor motor vehicle accident, in which she sustained no apparent head injury but was seeking compensation. The referring psychologist postulated an attention disorder, as reflected in a digit span of only three. This poor performance was confirmed when the neuropsychologist repeated the test. However, when the series was extended in length it soon became apparent that although still *failing* all of the items, the patient could often get all but the last two digits of a sequence correct, even the first eight of a series of ten! The failures consisted of either reversing the last two digits or adding a new one. It was quite clear that whatever her problem was, it was not one of being unable to hold any more than three items. The answer lay in areas other than neural incapacity.

Case 2. A 30-year-old man, who was being counseled for marital difficulties, was referred by his therapist with a complaint of failing memory over the preceding 6 months. On the Associate Learning subtest of the WMS, his score of 13 consisted of the following: 3,3; 4,3; 3,4 (the two figures for each trial represent easy and hard pairs). Several qualitative features stood out. Although he still failed to learn easy pairs such as *metal–iron* after three trails, he mastered three of the four hard pairs on the first trial and retained them. His three responses to metal were "don't know," "tin," and "zinc," while those to fruit were "pear," "peach," and "don't know." Numerous other nonneurological types of response were produced on other tests. The psychologist was advised that there was no organic disorder likely to hinder therapy.

Test Failures versus Functional Deficits

Following failure on a number of tests, patients are often described as having multiple deficits. It is wise to remember that the law of parsimony has never been repealed. Usually patients have only a small number of deficits, and they fail on a variety of tasks because apparently different tasks have one or more of the deficient factors in common. The key question to ask is what could cause failure on these seemingly disparate tasks. Again, this leads to setting up one or more hypotheses for inspecting the information already available from tests completed, or for guiding selection of additional measures. The hypothesis may also receive support or otherwise from known facts of the history.

Fluctuation of Function

Differences of opinion sometimes arise between clinicians when patients return different levels of performance on like-named tests at different times. This may suggest to one of them that the person's ability is fluctuating. The difference may arise from the fact that while the two tests share a good deal in common, one test may tap a factor that provides difficulty for the patient while the other test does not require this factor for its successful solution. Thus, awareness of the component cognitive functions required for completion of each task may help to resolve the apparent discrepancy.

COMMUNICATING THE RESULTS OF EVALUATION

Many professionals, particularly neurologists, will find the method of presenting specific hypotheses to be directly in line with their normal mode of operating. The types of questions for which the neuropsychologist will be able to provide help will become clearer as the two professionals interact over a number of cases. Two main methods assist the process: (1) the written report, and (2) the professional conference.

The Written Report

Where the method is unfamiliar, it is essential for neuropsychologists to indicate via clearly written reports the type of information they are able to provide and the logical arguments used in support of their conclusions (see Chapter 7, Walsh, 1991). Where the data themselves may be understood by the reader, these may be provided in an addendum. This process is at first time consuming for busy practitioners, but proves beneficial in forcing the examiner to exteriorize thinking processes. This, in turn, can lead to further development of clinical competence.

The report should comment not only on the qualitative and quantitative aspects of the formal assessment but also on such matters as the congruence between similar measures of the same function and congruence among test performance, other behavior at the interview, and reports of everyday behavior. Reports must not contain comments outside the area of the clinician's personal experience unless citing well-established facts in the literature.

The Professional Conference

When possible, it often proves mutually helpful to clarify reports verbally. The case conference with other professionals is the ideal vehicle for this purpose, although brief talks with the referring clinician often suffice. The sequential nature of the problem-solving process often means that these brief exchanges of shared information may well modify the next step in the investigation procedures of both parties, leading to economy of time and effort.

In sum, hypothesis-testing methodology offers a number of advantages over "fixed-battery" approaches to assessment. These are only a few of the ideas that contribute to hypothesis-testing methodology. The reader is referred to Walsh (1991) for a more comprehensive discussion of these issues.

CASE EXAMPLES

The following case examples serve to illustrate hypothesis-testing methodology in more depth.

Checking a Presented Hypothesis

Case S.G.

This analysis is condensed from the full case report in Walsh (1991). This 45-year-old man was referred in 1983 by a neurologist to check the validity of his complaints of weakness of memory. Several weeks earlier, he had been involved in a rear-end collision, in which his neck was severely flexed after his stationary car was struck from behind. He was seeking monetary compensation through litigation. In fact, his legal counsel rang the neuropsychologist and expressed a not uncommon skepticism of the reality of complaints following whiplash injuries.

History. The patient impressed the examiner as being a well-educated person who expressed his difficulties in a moderate fashion. He was a little unclear about the details of the first few hours after the accident, but his wife, who was also in the car, gave a lucid account that agreed with records of the accident. The patient also produced photographs, one showing severe damage to the rear of his car, and another one showing the driver's headrest bent at right angles to the seat back, which itself had been broken and was parallel to the floor. As the man was wearing a seat belt, it could be assumed that his neck had been very strongly flexed.

The wife stated that neither of them had lost consciousness for any measurable time. She reported, however, that shortly after getting out of the car and for 6 hours or so thereafter, her husband repeated a series of questions that were no sooner put than they were asked again, as though S.G. were totally unaware of having asked them before. This feature cleared rapidly later in the day, while he was in the hospital under observation. The only physical aftermath was a sore neck, which was also tender to touch, and S.G. was a trifle dizzy on sudden movement. After some hours of observation, he was allowed to leave the hospital and was examined by a neurologist a week later.

Previous medical history gave nothing of relevance. The patient described himself as a fitness fanatic. After completing high school, he went on to obtain a diploma of engineering.

S.G. reported to the neurologist that his memory was faulty, but said that it had improved. Physically, apart from neck stiffness, he complained that his tongue was heavy, with some numbness on the left side, but that this was improving. His wife had commented that for several days he had tended to mumble, but that this, too, was improving.

Neurological Examination. This was reported as normal with only the following exceptions: "When he protruded his tongue it did protrude slightly to the left; there was a suggestion of mild impairment of rapid repetitive movements and fasciculation of the tongue bilaterally; slight tenderness on palpation of cervical muscles." A brief mental status examination revealed minor memory weakness, but no detailed examination was made.

The neurologist's letter provided a very clear hypothesis. Moreover, the neurologist had gone as far as to provide further supporting evidence. First, he recognized the similarity of the wife's description to cases of transient global amnesia and pointed to a then recent case of whiplash described by Fisher (1982), which seemed very similar to the present case. Second, subsequent radiological investigation of the neck revealed narrowing of one of the cervical disc spaces with some bony encroachment on the intervertebral foramina (through which the vertebral arteries travel on their way to join to form the basilar artery, which supplies the posterior parts of the brain including the hippocampal complex).

The neurologist thus hypothesized that flexion of the neck may have temporarily compromised the posterior circulation to the brain and brainstem, resulting in memory difficulty and minor neurological signs. Record of brainstem evoked potentials was, indeed, mildly abnormal at the time.

Hypotheses. The principal neuropsychological hypothesis for confirmation was a form of organic amnesic syndrome. A competing hypothesis was that the memory complaint was a form of nonorganic difficulty seen not infrequently after motor vehicle accidents (see Walsh, 1991). Standard tests of memory function were thought to be adequate to test between these.

Added History. On his return to work, S.G. was conscious of his memory being below par, especially as his job involved keeping track of rapidly changing information concerning machine models and parts and required him to travel frequently to keep up with developments. For the first time, he became dependent on frequent note taking to support his memory in day-to-day affairs.

Neuropsychological Examination. Selected results were as follows:

WMS Form 1 (at 3 weeks)

Information	5	Digits Total	12 (8,4)
Orientation	5	Visual Reproduction	14
Mental Control	9	Associate Learning	10 (4,1; 5,1; 5,1)
Logical Memory	8		
MQ 112			

Several findings are of note. First, although the summary measure (the MQ) would seem to suggest no great difficulty, subsequent testing with the Wechsler Adult Intelligence Scale-Revised (WAIS-R) gave him an IQ of around 125. It is our experience that such superior individuals commonly reach the ceiling of the memory scale at 147, and thus his MQ of 112 suggested a significant fall-off in memory performance. Second, the following features were consistent with an impoverished memory performance and inconsistent with other possible bases for his complaints such as neurosis or enactment: (1) near-perfect scores on the first three subtests measuring orientation and routine mental operations, together with a maximum score for visual memory of a simple nature involving immediate recall, and an excellent score on digits forward contrasting with, (2) comparatively poor performance on recall of prose material (Logical Memory) and great difficulty with acquisition of the novel (difficult) pairs of the Associate Learning task with relatively little difficulty in acquiring the easy pairs, which are based on well-learned associations. This is a pattern constantly seen with most forms of organic amnesic syndromes.

On the more lengthy Rey Auditory Verbal Learning Test (RAVLT), S.G. also encountered difficulty in learning the entire list, a task he believed would have been easy for him before his injury. Results were as follows:

			List A			List B	List A	
Trials	1	2	3	4	5	Recall	Recall	Recognition
Correct	6	9	10	11	11	6	4	15

Again, this had the characteristics of a moderate amnesic disorder. The learning curve peaked well below expectation based on his background, and was followed by a considerable fall-off in recall after the presentation of the interfering list B, but a perfect recognition memory score for the re-presentation of the first list. This pattern is exactly what has been experienced in amnesic populations with confirmed pathology and is certainly not the configuration seen in neurotic or enacting individuals.

In this case, the examination would have been improved by the introduction of further measures of forgetting, since some individuals with this degree of acquisition difficulty also show a very rapid rate of forgetting for the material that they have rather laboriously acquired. This rapid forgetting seems to correlate more with the patient's complaints than the acquisition capability, which, without verification, might lead the inexperienced examiner to think that the problem was not serious.

Other tests confirmed the presence of a mild to moderate amnesic difficulty that persisted from this time. S.G. found it difficult to cope at his previous level of work, as this was highly dependent on good memory performance. At a later stage, he actually took recreation leave to which he was due, but returned to his office to cope with some of the backlog of work in his own time. Reexamination at 15 weeks revealed no change. He subsequently took a lower level position in another firm, where the demands on his memory were not so great.

Evaluating the Hypotheses. In arguing the medico-legal case, we supported the neurologist's original hypothesis, namely, that this man had been left with a "fragility of memory." The neurological and neuropsychological examinations seemed to be congruent with the events as described by the patient and his wife, and at no time did a neuropsychological examination of other areas of cognitive function produce evidence of other functional deficit. In the ensuing period before settlement of his claim, other very similar cases appeared in the literature (Hofstad & Gjerde, 1985; Matias-Guiu, Buenaventura, & Codina, 1985).

Checking Competing Hypotheses

The essence in some situations is to test the congruence of the findings with divergent points of view. This is typical of medico-legal cases, where the opposing opinions (hypotheses) are thrown into strong contrast.

Case B.A.

This 48-year-old senior executive in an engineering firm was a survivor in a head-on collision in which both drivers and front seat passengers were killed. B.A. and another rear-seat passenger survived, although both sustained severe injuries. The acute management of the patient was carried out at an adjacent country hospital before he was transferred some 6 hours later to a metropolitan facility. The first admission records were incomplete, merely noting that he was unconscious at the scene about 45 minutes after the accident but was "conscious though confused" when transferred to the city hospital. B.A. sustained facial injuries, fractured ribs with a pneumothorax, a fractured femur, and bruising to his legs and chest. These conditions required operation and sedation over ensuing days.

History. The history was taken in separate interviews with the patient, his wife, and several senior members of his company. There were no major discrepancies.

B.A. had graduated in mechanical engineering. After 10 years in the design department of a large multinational corporation, he had become a director on the board of management. His work took him overseas to professional and business meetings. His colleagues described his personality before the accident as that of a pleasant, quietly confident person who was somewhat reserved in social contacts.

His wife described him as a formerly mature, quiet, friendly individual who remained "unruffled" by difficulties. He had been an attentive, considerate father. His only pastime was golf, which he played regularly, and he and his wife were both members of the social activities committee. B.A. estimated his daily alcohol consumption as some six standard drinks, usually beer taken with colleagues before returning home to dinner. His wife said that he was intoxicated "a little" two or three times a year, usually at large parties, but she did not consider alcohol to be a problem.

On his return from the hospital, B.A.'s wife described her husband as completely changed. He was verbally aggressive to her for the first time and had "lost all his finesse," so that friends kept away from the house. He was intolerant of waiting for anything and could not delay sexual gratification, which she found embarrassing. His impulse buying had also threatened the family budget. They separated after 2 years, during which there had been little essential alteration in what she described as "his new personality."

B.A.'s colleagues confirmed this marked change, citing his insensitive handling of employees and his interruptions and rude comments at meetings. These comments were not always pertinent to the matters at hand. He was verbose and repetitive in discussions, a marked difference from his incisive approach beforehand. They were also surprised by mistakes that he had made since his return, some of these being on quite elementary tasks. They felt that they could no longer rely on him in a senior management position. The patient himself was puzzled by these lapses but continued to make them.

At the interview, B.A. admitted to the neuropsychologist that he was aware that he had changed, but he showed incomplete insight into the effect these changes had on others. He also said that his grasp of the technical side of his job was not as good as before, but he could not explain the difficulty and tended to play this down.

Hypotheses. The principal hypothesis suggested by the history was that the changes seemed characteristic of traumatic damage of closed head injury, affecting the anterior portions of the brain. Since the personality changes appeared almost pathognomonic, the examination was designed to confirm the hypothesis by evaluating aspects of adaptive behavior with appropriate and sensitive measures described in the literature (see Chapter 5, Walsh, 1991). This was imperative, since an alternate cause, namely alcohol-related brain damage, had been suggested by a physician and given some support by a clinical psychologist.

Neuropsychological Examination. Two examinations were conducted, 2 and 3 years after the injury. As there were no essential differences between them, the main features are combined. The WAIS results shown are taken from an examination by another psychologist, completed at the request of opposing counsel in the litigation process over compensation (also 3 years after the event). It was believed that nothing was to be gained from repeating these standard measures.

Information	12	Picture Completion	12
Comprehension	13	Object Assembly	11
Arithmetic	12	Block Design	12
Digit Span	13	Digit Symbol	14
Similarities	15	Picture Arrangement	12
Verbal IQ 120		Performance IQ 126	
Full Scale IQ 124			

One of the most sensitive cognitive measures was used first, namely, the Milner pathway on the Austin Maze Test (Walsh, 1991). The second testing at 3 years showed no essential improvement from a year before.

Over the first 10 trials, B.A. steadily eradicated his errors and appeared to be on the verge of "learning" the pathway.

Trial	1	2	3	4	5	6	7	8	9	10
Errors	16	8	10	6	5	4	3	4	2	1

Nevertheless, despite obvious eagerness to demonstrate his mastery, he continued to make errors, even reverting to errors after he had achieved one error-free trial. He became very frustrated with himself, cursing mildly at his failures when he had it "nearly right" and was loath to quit when the examiner discontinued the exercise.

Trial	11	12	13	14	15	16	17	18	19	20
Errors	2	1	7	3	1	1	1	1	1	0

Trial	21	22	23	24	25	26	27	28	29
Errors	1	2	1	2	2	1	1	1	1

This is a classical pattern, whereby patients with anterior damage from whatever reason find it difficult, if not impossible, to eradicate all errors from their programs of behavior. Moreover, he was not just perseverating on one particular error. B.A. made different errors on different occasions, some of which he had not made previously for many trials. All of this occurred, despite the fact that he said that he recognized that he was making errors.

On the Rey Figure, the copy was complete (Copy score 34), but executed in an unsystematic way. After a 3-minute delay, there was considerable impoverishment of his reproduction from memory (Recall score 12), and he added several features that had not been present in the model.

On a measure of verbal fluency, he managed to average only 10 words for each of the three presented letters, which placed him just below the 25th percentile, considerably below expectation based on his history. He also broke the rules several times, although he was able to repeat these rules for the examiner.

The first four problems of the Tower of London (Shallice, 1982, 1988) were solved easily. He solved problems five and seven, although slowly, and failed on item six and the final four items. Although some of his difficulty may have arisen from a planning deficit, some failures seemed clearly due to his inability to inhibit response tendencies, since after the test he was able to verbalize what he should have done on at least one of the intermediate items. Again, it appeared to be not a basic incapacity but an inability to regulate his programs of action.

Part A of the Trail Making Test was performed accurately and rapidly (24 seconds), but he was considerably slower on Part B (124 seconds), although he made no errors. On the Colour-Form Sorting Test, he sorted immediately according to shape and began to do so again before making the shift to color.

The WMS Form 1 yielded the following scores:

Information	6	Digits Total	12 (8,4)
Orientation	5	Visual Reproduction	14
Mental Control	9	Associate Learning	17 (6,1; 6,3; 6,4)
Logical Memory	11		
MQ 120			

On this test his performance seemed close to expectation. After a 30-minute delay, he recalled 9 of the 10 pairs in the Associate Learning subtest, and a relatively intact memory was shown on the RAVLT below.

			List A			List B	List A	
Trials	1	2	3	4	5	Recall	Recall	Recognition
Correct	8	11	13	12	13	7	9	15

Discussion. One common area of difference of opinion in such cases concerns the degree of brain injury sustained or likely to have been sustained in the type of accident described. Since there was no skull fracture, any injury would come under the classification of a closed head injury, and based on numerous large-group studies, it is generally agreed that the severity of such an injury can be gauged by the length of the period of unconsciousness or, better still, by the period of posttraumatic amnesia (PTA) which may be defined as the time from the injury to the time when the person begins to establish stable memories. The longer the period of PTA, the more likely it is that the person will have lasting sequelae. However, while this is a clinically useful generalization, it is far from a perfect correlation. Cases are recorded where there has been only a relatively short period of unconsciousness, for instance, a matter of hours, and only a few days of confusion or PTA. Yet, in such cases, there has been clear radiological evidence of brain contusion maximal in the anterior regions of the brain, and concomitant finding of neuropsychological deficits, particularly in the form of personality changes, deficits of complex cognitive functions, and difficulties in adaptive behavior (Levin, Eisenberg, & Benton, 1989).

In the present case, the medical records were far from ideal, since documentation was not precise. For example, no standard PTA scale was employed. This man appears to have been unconscious at first and confused for several days. B.A. said that he remembered little or nothing of his first 2 weeks in the hospital. His wife estimated that there were 2 weeks of rapid forgetting before his memory returned to normal. As often happens with trauma cases, no accurate estimate is possible, since in the first few days after the event he had an operation to set his fractures and was under sedation because of the pain resulting from his multiple injuries.

Evaluating the Hypotheses. Several features of the results argue in favor of the head-injury hypothesis. Psychometric preservation, that is, the absence of seriously depressed scaled scores, particularly on the Wechsler tests, is seen commonly in subjects of previously high intelligence and advanced education or training. By adulthood, such individuals have developed a repertoire of programs or strategies that allow them to deal with a variety of situations, provided that these do not call for modifying the programs to deal with changing situations. On the other hand, B.A. showed consistent and characteristic executive difficulties accompanying his personality changes, particularly disinhibition. Both sets of changes appeared for the first time immediately after the injury. There was no evidence of attempts to exaggerate or enact other deficits.

In contrast, several feature militate against the alcohol impairment hypothesis. First, none of the observed changes of personality or cognition were reported by any observers to be present before the injury, even in retrospect. Changes with alcohol-related brain damage are slow and insidious, never of sudden onset. Second, the type of change in personality is uncharacteristic of alcohol-related brain impairment but highly characteristic of traumatic damage. There is often reduced sex drive with alcohol, and intolerance of gratification delay seen in B.A. is also not typical. Third, although changes in adaptive behavior and problem solving largely dependent on cognitive loss are a feature of alcohol damage, they occur against a background of more widespread cognitive deterioration. In all cases in our experience, these changes lead to a lowering of some subtests of the Performance Scale of the WAIS or WAIS-R, in particular Object Assembly, Block Design, and Picture Arrangement. Fourth, while it is often difficult to gain a true estimate of the degree of an individual's drinking, there was no evidence of the usual sort put forward even by those supporting this hypothesis. Fifth, mild atrophy, which had been seen on the CT scan, might be consistent with alcohol damage, but there was also a localized area in the front of the brain more consistent with trauma, although, of course, head injuries are very common in alcoholics.

The court ruled in favor of head injury as the cause of the man's changes.

Updating the Frame of Reference

One of the advantages of the hypothesis-testing method is that newly emerging facts and concepts from the literature can be incorporated, with a result of improved understanding of subsequent cases. The method necessarily places demands on practitioners of the method to keep abreast of developments if they are to achieve maximum effectiveness.

One area that illustrates this clearly is that of presenile dementia. Neary (1990) has stressed that it is time to reject "the notion that dementia represents a non-specific breakdown in intellect and memory" but, instead, reflects a set of "distinct neuropsychological syndromes characterising particular cerebral disorders," each of which appears to possess distinguishable pathological and pathophysiological features.

One such emerging entity has been termed *dementia of the frontal-lobe type* (DFT). This disorder appears at an earlier age than other types of dementia and has a strong association with a history of dementia in one parent. Like many conditions based largely in anterior cerebral pathology the deficits, particularly in the early stages, tend to be subtle. For this reason, it is now apparent that many cases may have been overlooked in the past. Neary (1990) has estimated that the ratio of incidence of DFT to the more common Alzheimer's disease may be as high as 1 to 4. Brun (1987) described predominant frontal or frontotemporal atrophy in 26 of a prospective series of 158 cases, and only 4 of these could be classified as Pick's disease on pathological grounds.

The clinical picture emerging from different centers is very similar (Gustafson, 1987; Johanson & Hagberg, 1989; Knopman et al., 1989; Neary, Snowden, Northen, & Goulding, 1988). The onset is insidious, the first signs being a set of personality changes that may have a characteristic frontal flavor. There is frequently a loss of interest in usual activities coupled with a bland indifference, which is followed by loss of interest in personal care. This self-neglect may be marked long before any cognitive changes are apparent to observers (Orrell, Sahakian, & Bergman, 1989). In other cases, there may be an insensitivity for others, disinhibition, and uncharacteristic rudeness, which indicate serious changes in functioning to friends and relatives.

A clear difference from Alzheimer's disease is the relative preservation of memory. Patients show an ability to retain some new material on formal testing after the personality changes have been obvious for some time. At the same time, all of those tests that have proven useful in the detection of frontal disorders are usually performed badly, with the characteristic qualitative features of such anterior lesions. Also common are changes in speech and language without frank aphasia. More characteristic is reduction of speech with stereotypy and verbal adynamia. As with all conditions affecting the left frontal region, tests of associative verbal fluency are sensitive early.

The electroencephalogram (EEG) is almost invariably abnormal in Alzheimer's disease but normal in DFT. While using the term *DFT,* one should realize that several subgroups (including Pick's disease) with differing clinical pictures are probably included at present.

Case S.A.

This 40-year-old science graduate had successfully worked on research projects for some years before taking up administrative posts in which he was described as capable and efficient. However, he was without a job when his position was made redundant in an economic recession, and he was still without work when seen about a year later. His wife and father described changes in his personality around this time. He had become withdrawn and largely uncommunicative, a marked difference from his prior outgoing, gregarious character.

Two separate examinations could find no typical psychiatric disorder. A trial of antidepressant medication made no difference in his state. He was then referred to a neurologist whose examination revealed no abnormal clinical signs. The neurologist noted that he was unable to elicit any "complaint of cerebral disarray" from the patient, whom he described as "most unforthcoming." The neurologist thought that a tumor or a degenerative process should be investigated. The latter possibility was strengthened when the neurologist talked to S.A.'s father, who described "an obvious deterioration in mental sharpness and in the élan of his conversation and social address to family, friends, and acquaintances" over a year or more. S.A. was referred to a neuropsychologist for diagnostic help.

Hypotheses. The primary hypothesis was that S.A. was suffering from a form of DFT. Alternate hypotheses included other neurologically based sources of personality change, such as a different type of degenerative dementia or a tumor.

Neuropsychological Examination. At the interview, S.A. was once again very reticent and appeared to have no insight into the changes described. He merely said that his wife got upset at times because, "I eat too much and am a bit lazy." Tests used comprised four subtests of the WAIS-R, the WMS Form 1, Verbal Fluency, the Trail Making Test, the Rey Figure, and the Austin Maze (Milner pathway).

The neuropsychologist commented that he was unable to find reproducible evidence of intellectual or memory decline; the patient performed normally "on tasks noted for their sensitivity," including the maze test. He believed that "the questions raised by the man's general presentation were not supported by the neuropsychological findings." However, certain disparities were noted. For example, despite his background, S.A. stated that water boiled "at 110 degrees F or about 40 degrees C." His arithmetical responses were cavalier and impulsive. Although his prose recall was excellent, on Associate Learning he "exhibited a rapid learning of the material, and then a sudden forgetting of it." He was said to have no difficulty with the verbal fluency task.

Repeat testing was advised, and a second neuropsychologist saw him 4 weeks later. Details of the first examination were not yet on hand, although the essence of the above report was known. It was decided to repeat the interview and to use the maze test to observe the man's behavior before discussing the earlier results. Because of their descriptive detail, portions of this evaluation are quoted in full. The second neuropsychologist wrote, "This man presents a subtle problem. To my surprise, as soon as I met him I felt there was something neurological in the wind. I was quite astounded, knowing his past history, to find him both fatuous and vacuous. His conversation was almost devoid of content, and the further we went in the interview the more apparent it was that he had absolutely no insight into what must be quite considerable changes in him over the last year or more. His responses to my few pleasantries seemed excessive. As at former interviews, he stated blandly that there was nothing amiss with him and passively accepted any suggestion I put to him without the slightest show of affect. At the same time, I was tolerably well convinced that he was in no way depressed and, in one sense, I would not even describe him as apathetic.

"It seemed to me that he was like patients I have seen with frontal lobe degeneration of an extensive kind and the old truism came to mind that 'frontal' patients may appear essentially normal until you sit down and test them, test them, that is, with appropriate tests. Of course, I was then confronted with the verbal information I had been given about some of his test performances, which might seem to render the frontal hypothesis unlikely.

"Nevertheless, I thought it would be helpful to repeat at least the Austin Maze examination and to push it a bit further. To my increasing surprise, he gave a quite classical 'frontal' performance [as shown below]:

Trials	1	2	3	4	5	6	7	8	9	10	11
Errors	8	7	5	8	3	2	1	2	1	2	2

Trials	12	13	14	15	16	17	18	19	20	21
Errors	1	2	0	1	1	1	1	1	0	0

"He demonstrated that he was familiar with the rules by answering my queries correctly and, concentrating well, he reduced his errors to only one after seven trials but took another seven to reach his first error-free performance. However, unlike the previous occasion for Dr. H. only a month before, he then immediately reverted to making an error. Even when I stopped him and asked him to indicate where he was going wrong, he was able to indicate the place without difficulty but then repeated the identical error five times before reaching another error-free trial. There was now no doubt in my mind that he was showing the classical 'dissociation between knowing and doing,' together with the problem of error utilization pathognomonic of frontal lesions."

The examination was then deferred until discussion of earlier testing could take place. These former results included:

WAIS-R			
Information	14	Picture Completion	11
Arithmetic	9	Block Design	12
WMS Form 1			
Information	6	Digits Total	10
Orientation	5	Visual Reproduction	13
Mental Control	6	Associate Learning	14 (6,2; 6,3; 6,0)
Logical Memory	16		
MQ 124			

Verbal Fluency: F-11, A-7, S-9, total 27 with three errors.
Trail Making Test: Part A, 34 seconds; Part B, 67 seconds.
Austin Maze (Milner pathway): Errors on 10 trials were 15, 9, 8, 7, 6, 3, 3, 3, 0, 0.

This review brought out the following features, which were not inconsistent with the second neuropsychologist's hypothesis of DFT. First, the Verbal Fluency result was thought to be very poor for S.A.'s background, based on his history and the richness of his responses on the Information subtest. This score ranks between the 11th and the 22nd percentiles (Lezak, 1983). He also made three rule-breaking errors. Second, the low score on Arithmetic was the result of failing the last three items through impulsive errors. Third, having acquired three of the four difficult pairs on the Associate Learning subtest, he lost them on the next trial despite the fact that he appeared to be attending and cooperating with the examination.

Arrangements were being made for further neuropsychological evaluation when the patient left the area. However, at this time a CT scan revealed atrophic changes in the frontal regions with mild enlargement of the anterior horns of the lateral ventricles. An EEG and a second neurological examination were normal.

Six months later, although his previous symptoms had gradually worsened, S.A. cooperated well enough for a third examiner at another hospital to complete both the Wechsler intelligence and memory scales. Results were as follows:

WAIS-R			
Information	16	Picture Completion	13
Digit Span	7	Picture Arrangement	13
Vocabulary	11	Block Design	11
Arithmetic	10	Object Assembly	18
Comprehension	8	Digit Symbol	10
VIQ 97		PIQ 117	

The WMS MQ was 114. He was described as having good general information but "a weaker ability to reason in an abstract and conceptual manner." On the RAVLT, the patient reached a plateau of nine on the fifth trial with the same score on recognition.

This same neuropsychologist reexamined S.A. a year later. S.A. was restless and sometimes stood up to do the tests and wandered in and out of the room. Nevertheless, he completed some of the Wechsler subtests again as well as the Trail Making Test. Some of the neuropsychologist's detailed comments are quoted verbatim, as they provide an excellent view of his progress.

On this occasion, the patient's MQ had fallen to 89, although this may have been due, in part, to his attentional difficulties. Prose recall and digit span were much poorer than on examination 6 months before. As on previous occasions, his Visual Reproduction was very good. The PIQ estimated from three subtests was 94. Six and 12 months earlier, PIQ had been 105 and 117, respectively. Qualitative features were noted: "On the Picture Completion subtest he was able to name quite complex items that were missing from the pictures, and this was unusual in someone who performed so badly in other ways. On the Block Design subtest, he gave up after the sixth item, but prior to that he had done some quite quickly and managed others with a little encouragement. He had to be constantly pushed to do the tests. He did the Object

Assembly items very quickly. He was quite unreflective; he just rushed in and put things together, but basically he managed to get them correct and obtained his best score at a near-average level."

This neuropsychologist believed that there had been "a very significant deterioration" from her earlier examinations, but that S.A. did not have any disorder of visual perceptual or constructional skills. She went on by noting, "What seems to be lacking is the ability to regulate, to monitor, and to check what he is doing in a normal manner. Throughout, he seemed to have the ability to continue with a task once he had started going on it, but then when he gave up or stopped, he could not self-direct back to it."

About this time, repeat CT scan showed an increase in the frontal atrophy noted earlier with ventricular enlargement, prominence of the Sylvian fissures, and other features seen in Pick's disease.

Progress. The major signs of blunted affect, poverty of speech, lack of insight, restless wandering, and disinhibition (such as undressing in public) gradually worsened, and he was hospitalized in a closed psychiatric center. There had been no response to antipsychotic medication. Despite this progression, S.A. remained oriented, and 2 years after his original presentation (i.e., some 3 years after onset), he registered and repeated three words after 3 minutes. Once or twice he voiced odd ideas such as the fact that he heard his wife's voice and was controlled by her. Neurological examination was still essentially normal, but over time primitive reflexes had emerged.

Examining the Hypotheses. Observations of personality change, findings on neuropsychological evaluation, CT scan results, and progressive deterioration over time all supported the initial hypothesis of DFT. The relative preservation of language and memory argued against Alzheimer's disease, and CT findings ruled out the presence of a tumor.

Although this case presents a difficult problem, if one considers it to be essentially one of Pick's disease or DFT, one is struck with the similarity to certain schizophrenic conditions. An almost identical case presenting the differential diagnosis of Pick's disease versus schizophrenia was described recently by Buisson (1989). Certainly there appears to be early preservation of at least many functions necessary to produce good psychometric scores on a range of tasks. The picture is in keeping with the observation that in "classical psychological terms, one could say that if in AD (Alzheimer's disease) the intellectual faculties are disturbed, in PD (Pick's disease) their utilization is faulty" (Tissot, Constantinidis, & Richard, 1985, p. 233). Such cases warn us that we should not dismiss the possibility of a dementing process on the basis of scores alone, especially without periodic review. Every attempt should be made to employ tests that are sensitive to disruption of the use of effective intelligence such as the Tower of London test (Shallice, 1982) and the Wisconsin Card Sorting Test. As we approach the time when therapy for such degenerative conditions may arrest or even partially reverse them, it is important for neuropsychologists to learn more about the early detection of these emerging categories of deficit. This may depend on deriving new tasks based on research findings.

REFERENCES

Benton, A. L. (1985). Some problems associated with neuropsychological assessment. *Bulletin of Clinical Neurosciences, 50,* 11–15.

Binder, L., & Pankratz, L. (1987). Neuropsychological evidence of a fictitious memory complaint. *Journal of Clinical and Experimental Neuropsychology, 9,* 167–171.

Brun, A. (1987). Frontal lobe degeneration of non-Alzheimer type, I: Neuropathology. *Archives of Gerontology and Geriatrics, 6,* 193–208.

Buisson, G. (1989). A props d'un cas d'état démentiel précoce: Maladie de Pick ou schizophrenie? *Annales Medico-Psychologiques, 147,* 121–124.

Dana, R. H. (1966). Eisegesis and assessment. *Journal of Projective Techniques, 30,* 215–222.

Fisher, C. M. (1982). Whiplash amnesia. *Neurology, 32,* 667–668.

Goldberg, E., & Costa, L. D. (1986). Qualitative indices in neuropsychological assessment. An extension of Luria's approach to executive deficit following prefrontal lesions. In I. Grant & K. M. Adams (Eds.), *Neuropsychological assessment of neuropsychiatric disorders* (pp. 48–64). New York: Oxford University Press.

Gustafson, L. (1987). Frontal lobe degeneration of non-Alzheimer type, II: Clinical picture and differential diagnosis. *Archives of Gerontology and Geriatrics, 6,* 209–223.

Hampton, J. R., Harrison, M. J. G., Mitchell, J. R. A., Pritchard, J. S., & Seymour, C. (1975). Relative contributions of history taking, physical examination, and laboratory investigation to diagnosis and management of medical out-patients. *British Medical Journal, ii,* 486–489.

Hofstad, H., & Gjerde, I. O. (1985). Transient global amnesia after whiplash injury. *Journal of Neurology, Neurosurgery, and Psychiatry, 48,* 956–957.

Johanson, A., & Hagberg, B. (1989). Psychometric characteristics in patients with frontal lobe degeneration of non-Alzheimer type. *Archives of Gerontology and Geriatrics, 8,* 129–137.

Kaplan, E. (1983). Process and achievement revisted. In S. Wapner & B. Kaplan (Eds.), *Toward a holistic developmental psychology* (pp. 143–156). Hillsdale, NJ: Lawrence Erlbaum.

Kaplan, E. (1988). A process approach to neuropsychological assessment. In T. Boll & B. K. Bryant (Eds.), *Clinical neuropsychology and brain function: Research, measurement, and practice* (pp. 125–167). Washington, DC: American Psychological Association.

Knopman, D. S., Christensen, K. J., Schut, L. J., Harbaugh, R. E., Reeder, T., Ngo, T., & Frey, W. (1989). The spectrum of imaging and neuropsychological findings in Pick's disease. *Neurology, 39,* 362–368.

Levin, H. S., Eisenberg, H. M., & Benton, A. L. (Eds.). (1989). *Mild head injury.* New York: Oxford University Press.

Lezak, M. D. (1983). *Neuropsychological assessment* (2nd ed.). New York: Oxford University Press.

Lezak, M. D. (1988). IQ: R. I. P. *Journal of Clinical and Experimental Neuropsychology, 10,* 351–361.

Matias-Guiu, J., Buenaventura, I., & Codina, A. (1985). Whiplash amnesia. *Neurology, 35,* 1259.

McCarthy, R. A., & Warrington, E. A. (1990). *Cognitive neuropsychology: A clinical introduction.* New York: Academic Press.

Miller, E. (1983). A note on the interpretation of data derived from neuropsychological tests. *Cortex, 19,* 131–132.

Neary, D. (1990). Non-Alzheimer's disease forms of cerebral atrophy. *Journal of Neurology, Neurosurgery, and Psychiatry, 53,* 929–931.

Neary, D., Snowden, J. S., Northen, B., & Goulding, P. (1988). Dementia of frontal type. *Journal of Neurology, Neurosurgery, and Psychiatry, 51,* 353–361.

Orrell, M. W., Sahakian, B. J., & Bergman, K. (1989). Self-neglect and frontal lobe dysfunction. *British Journal of Psychiatry, 155,* 101–105.

Ryan, C., & Butters, N. (1980). Learning and memory impairment in young and old alcoholics: Evidence for the premature aging hypothesis. *Alcoholism: Clinical and Experimental Research, 4,* 288–293.

Shallice, T. (1982). Specific impairments of planning. *Philosophical Transactions of the Royal Society of London, 298,* 199–209.

Shallice, T. (1988). *From neuropsychology to mental structure.* New York: Cambridge University Press.

Shapiro, M. B. (1951). Experimental studies of a perceptual anomaly, I: Initial experiments. *Journal of Mental Science, 97,* 90–100.

Shapiro, M. B. (1967). Intensive assessment of the single case: An inductive–deductive approach. In P. Mittler (Ed.), *The psychological assessment of mental and physical handicaps* (pp. 645–666). London: Tavistock.

Spreen, O., & Strauss, E. (1991). *A compendium of neuropsychological tests.* New York: Oxford University Press.

Tissot, R., Constantinidis, J., & Richard, J. (1985). Pick's disease. In J. A. M. Frederiks (Ed.), *Handbook of clinical neurology* (Vol. 46, pp. 233–246). Amsterdam: Elsevier.

Walsh, K. W. (1991). *Understanding brain damage: A primer of neuropsychological evaluation* (2nd ed.). Edinburgh: Churchill Livingstone.

Wechsler, D. (1944). *The measurement of human intelligence.* Baltimore: Williams & Wilkins.

III

Integration

11

A Cognitive Framework for Neuropsychological Assessment

ROBERT L. MAPOU

INTRODUCTION

Over the past decade, the emphasis of clinical neuropsychological assessment has shifted from lesion detection and localization to delineation of a patient's cognitive strengths and deficits (Hartman, 1991; Leonberger, 1989; Mapou, 1988b), in order to understand a patient's neurobehavioral competencies. Because of this increased focus on the patterns of cognitive dysfunction associated with brain disorder, it has become increasingly important to base neuropsychological assessment on empirical knowledge of human cognition. Yet, research on cognition is not always applied to clinical assessment. The frequently nonconverging paths of cognitive and clinical neuropsychology, as related to the current state of the field, have recently been described by Butters (1993):

> [The] rapid growth of interest in neuropsychological issues . . . has also led to the emergence of two factions or subdivisions of the discipline, that is, clinical and cognitive neuropsychology. Those who compose the cognitive camp often have their origins in experimental psychology or behavioral neuroscience and utilize brain-damaged patients for uncovering the anatomical and cognitive processes underlying normal language, attentional, visuoperceptual, executive, and memory functions. In contrast, those who view themselves as clinical psychologists emanate primarily from Boulder-model clincal psychology programs and tend to focus their neuropsychological research on various assessment issues. Unfortunately, cognitive neuropsychologists frequently ignore the

Disclaimer. The views and opinions expressed herein are the private views of the author and are not to be construed as official or as reflecting the views of the Henry M. Jackson Foundation for the Advancement of Military Medicine.

ROBERT L. MAPOU • Henry M. Jackson Foundation for the Advancement of Military Medicine, Walter Reed Army Medical Center, Washington, DC 20307-5001.

Clinical Neuropsychological Assessment: A Cognitive Approach, edited by Robert L. Mapou and Jack Spector. Plenum Press, New York, 1995.

> importance of their work for the identification and rehabilitation of neurologic disorders; likewise, clinical neuropsychologists dedicated to their fixed or flexible test batteries have generally eschewed the implications of their work for our understanding of normal cognition. (Butters, 1993, p. 3)

Review of recent neuropsychology textbooks confirms this impression. Although some cognitive neuropsychology texts have begun to provide a clinical perspective (e.g., McCarthy & Warrington, 1990), many instruments used by cognitive neuropsychologists still are unavailable to clinical neuropsychologists and are not easily applied to clinical practice. Such measures tend to be unpublished and lack the normative data associated with currently used standardized instruments, although this is beginning to change (e.g., Speed and Capacity of Language-Processing Test; Baddeley, Emslie, & Nimmo-Smith, 1992; Recognition Memory Test; Warrington, 1984; Visual Object and Space Perception Battery; Warrington & James, 1991). Conversely, with few exceptions, such as the California Verbal Learning Test (CVLT; Delis, Kramer, Kaplan, & Ober, 1987), most standardized clinical assessment instruments have not been developed on the basis of cognitive neuropsychological or psychological research.

Previously, these limitations have been addressed by describing an integration of clinical (Boston Process Approach) and cognitive neuropsychological assessment methods (Mapou, 1988a). This chapter is a revision and extension of this assessment approach. It is also an attempt to integrate material presented by authors in this book. The major premise of this chapter is that clinical assessment should always be guided by a *framework of cognitive and motor functioning,* based on knowledge of how these functions are disrupted by brain disorder. Review of evaluation results should proceed systematically, similar to the way in which a physician reviews results of a physical examination. The proposed framework will be presented, along with suggested instruments used to assess the various aspects of cognitive and motor functioning. The chapter will conclude with a case illustration of how the approach is applied.

OVERVIEW OF THE NEUROPSYCHOLOGICAL EVALUATION

Parallels with Medical Examination

When completing a physical examination, a physician begins by reviewing current complaints, then takes a medical history, and finally examines the patient, with particular attention to each of the different bodily systems. Although, depending on the referral question, particular attention may be given to one system, the physician generally assesses each system to some degree. Results of examination are summarized, conclusions are drawn regarding diagnosis, and recommendations are made for treatment.

Neuropsychological evaluation can be guided by and can benefit from a similar, systematic approach. Hence, the neuropsychologist would first review current complaints, then take a medical and psychosocial history, complete the evaluation using standardized instruments, and finally test limits by modifying standard procedures or using novel instruments. Results would then be reviewed systematically using a framework of cognitive and motor functioning, conclusions would be made regarding diagnosis, and recommendations would be made for treatment. Each of these evaluation components will now be described briefly.

History and Initial Interview

In addition to providing background information, taking the history provides the clinician with an opportunity to observe the patient's behavior and to develop hypotheses about the source of the patient's difficulties. Essential components of the history and initial interview are outlined in Table 11.1. The integration of historical information with results from neuropsychological testing will be illustrated in the case example, later in this chapter.

A Framework for Assessment

Following the history, the neuropsychological assessment is completed. The selection of measures and subsequent review of findings are guided by the framework illustrated in Figure 11.1. Similar to other models in this volume, this is a hierarchical framework, in which it is proposed that skills at the "higher levels" of the framework are dependent on skills at the "lower levels" for full expression.

There are several caveats to consider when using the framework. First, the framework is a heuristic device, designed to facilitate understanding and interpretation of clinical neuropsychological findings. Although derived from empirical knowledge of brain–behavior relationships and cognition, it is not to be viewed as a processing model in the strict, cognitive neuropsychological sense. Second, the framework is not *a battery of tests,* but, instead is a way of thinking about the neuropsychological functions to consider and to review in any evaluation. The amount of attention devoted to each component of functioning and the extent of standardized assessment within each component are determined by the referral question and presenting difficulties. In many instances, informal evaluation will suffice, although it is important for the examiner to consider the patient's functioning within each component. Third, the framework should not be used to guide the *order* of testing, since measures must be intermixed to (1) minimize frustration at the beginning of the evaluation; (2) minimize fatigue toward the end of evaluation; (3) minimize potential interference effects among measures, especially those of learning and memory; and (4) allow for needed delays on memory measures. Rather, the framework guides test selection and review of neuropsychological data from each component of function. Finally, the framework is not a "how to" guide to testing. It is assumed that the reader is familiar with the brain–behavior foundations of the framework and many of the instruments presented. The following is a brief overview of the framework, after which the framework will be presented in depth.

The first step necessary for understanding and interpreting evaluation results is to gauge an estimate of the patient's *global functioning.* To accomplish this, results from

TABLE 11.1. Essential Components of the Neuropsychological History

I. Current difficulty
   A. Reason for referral
   B. Patient perspective
   C. Family/significant other perspective
II. Medical history
   A. Current problem
      1. Relevant general medical information
         a. Physical examination
         b. Laboratory findings
      2. Neurological findings
         a. Neurological examination
         b. Laboratory findings (e.g., from lumbar puncture)
         c. Neuroimaging (CT, MRI, SPECT, PET)
         d. Electrophysiology (EEG, ERP, EP)
   B. Past history
      1. Neurological
      2. Psychiatric
      3. Systemic, with neurological aspects (e.g., systemic lupus erythematosus, hypertension, cardiac disease, liver disease)
III. Educational history
   A. Primary language
   B. Number of years in school
   C. Degrees received
   D. Grades
   E. Early learning difficulties
      1. Learning disability
         a. Reading
         b. Spelling and writing
         c. Arithmetic
      2. Attention-deficit/hyperactivity disorder
      3. Repeated grades and reasons
      4. Special education, tutoring, or other assistance
   F. Results of educational testing
      1. Psychoeducational testing
      2. Entrance examinations (e.g., SAT, GRE, LSAT, MCAT)
IV. Occupational history
   A. Current job
      1. Length on it
      2. Responsibilities
      3. Salary
   B. Past job history
      1. Jobs held
         a. Length
         b. Responsibilities
         c. Salary
         d. Difficulties
      2. Periods of unemployment
         a. Length
         b. Reasons

TABLE 11.1 (Continued)

V. Social history
  A. Marital or relationship status
    1. Length
    2. Children
    3. Dating (if applicable)
  B. Social support (outside of primary relationship)
  C. Recreational activities
VI. Family history
  A. Parents
    1. Living or deceased
    2. Dates of and cause of death, if applicable
    3. Education
    4. Occupation
  B. Brothers and sisters
    1. Ages
    2. Education
    3. Occupation
  C. All family members, including grandparents and parental siblings
    1. Neurological history (e.g., dementia, stroke)
    2. Psychiatric history (e.g., major psychiatric illness, hospitalization)
    3. Substance abuse history
    4. Relevant systemic illness (e.g., cardiac disease, systemic lupus erythematosus, hypertension)
VII. Substance use
  A. Alcohol
  B. Illicit drugs
  C. Cigarettes
VIII. Current medications
  A. Dosages
  B. Reasons

general intellectual and *academic achievement* measures are reviewed and are compared to expectations based on historical data. This is followed by a systematic review of data from measures at each framework level in Figure 11.1.

Foundation skills, which include *arousal and attention, sensory and motor functions,* and *executive, problem-solving, and reasoning abilities,* are reviewed first. Within Luria's (1980) conceptualization, these skills correspond to Unit One (arousal and attention), the primary and secondary zones of Units Two (sensory) and Three (motor), and the tertiary zone of Unit Three (executive, problem solving, and reasoning). Although Luria (1980) conceptualized arousal and attention as more fundamental than the executive functions, within the current framework both are characterized as "lower level," not on the basis of cognitive complexity or ontogenetic level, but rather because these skills are seen as *fundamental* to effective expression of remaining skills in the framework.

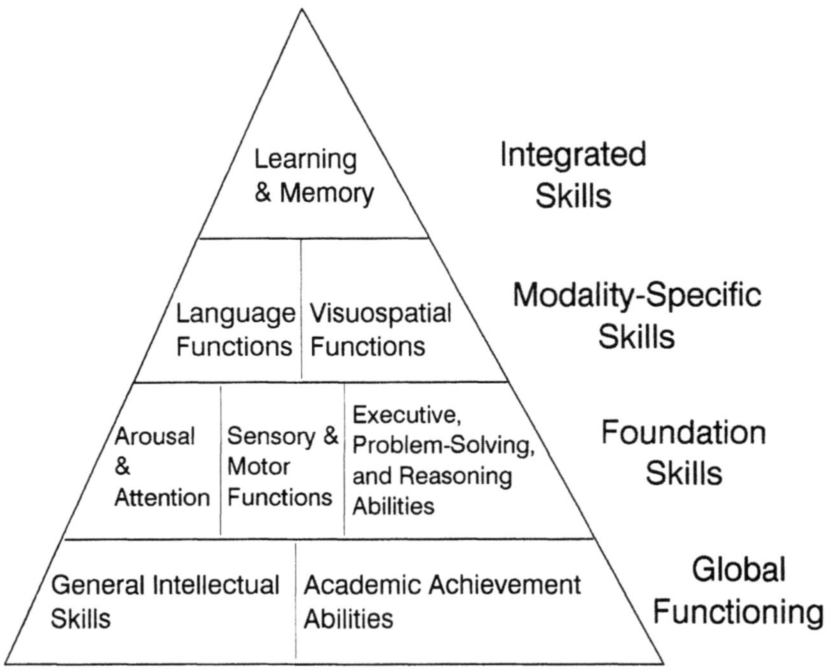

FIGURE 11.1. Schematic diagram of the framework for assessment.

Modality-specific skills, which include *language and visuospatial functions,* are at the next level of the framework. Traditionally, these abilities have been associated with functioning of the left (language) and right (visuospatial) cerebral hemispheres, although recent research has shown that visuospatial skills require the integrated functioning of both hemispheres (see Capruso, Hamsher, & Benton, this volume). Assessment of modality-specific skills provides information on the modality within which a patient functions best, provides information useful for diagnosis, and contributes to understanding breakdown in functioning at the next level of the framework.

Integrated skills, at the highest level of the framework, require interaction, integration, and coordinated functioning of skills at the lower levels of the framework. This parallels Luria's (1980) concept of functional systems (see Jørgensen and Christensen, this volume). Within the current framework, integrated skills refer specifically to learning and memory, although one could also include aspects of general intellectual abilities, academic abilities, and reasoning abilities. The reasons why these skills are included elsewhere are discussed later.

Finally, evaluation of *personality style and emotional functioning* must be included in any complete assessment. Although not part of the framework, per se, aspects of personality and emotional functioning can mediate performance on neuropsychological measures. If possible, standardized assessment instruments should be used. Sometimes, however, patients with significant cognitive or motor difficulties will be unable to complete such measures, and the clinician must rely on information obtained through observation and interviews with the patient and significant others.

Each component of the framework will now be described in detail, with examples of instruments that can be used for assessment of each component. The reader can consult the references listed, as well as Heaton, Grant, and Matthews (1991), Lezak (1983), and Spreen and Strauss (1991), for information on administration and for normative data, since most instruments will not be described in detail. Techniques to test limits and for recording qualitative information are described briefly. Several novel instruments for testing limits also are included in the lists of measures and are described briefly. The reader can consult Kaplan (1988, 1990), Kaplan, Fein, Morris, and Delis (1991), and Lezak (1983) for additional information on testing limits.

COMPONENTS OF THE FRAMEWORK

Global Functioning

Measures to evaluate *global functioning* are shown in Table 11.2. Summary scores from *general intellectual* measures can provide a global indicator of current functioning and often are required by the referral source (e.g., in cases of litigation or for establishing the presence of a learning disability). Although Lezak (1988) has noted that summary measures examined *alone* can obscure the pattaern of a patient's cognitive and motor functioning, IQ scores from the Wechsler Adult Intelligence Scale-Revised (WAIS-R; Wechsler, 1981), for example, can provide a context for gauging strengths and deficits on more specific neuropsychological measures (Leckliter & Matarazzo, 1989; Matarazzo, 1990). Standard scores from *academic achievement* measures can be used similarly.

A primary purpose of global functioning measures is to relate current global functioning to the patient's estimated premorbid skill level. The best approach is to review objective information collected prior to illness or trauma, such as school grades, standardized academic tests scores, and, when available, scores from previously administered intellectual and academic achievement tests. Comparing such information to current global functioning can then provide an indication of overall decline. Often this information is unavailable, however, and, as an alternative, data from specific global

TABLE 11.2. Global Functioning

I. General intellectual skills
   A. Wechsler Adult Intelligence Scale-Revised (WAIS-R; Wechsler, 1981)
   B. Stanford-Binet Intelligence Scale (Thorndike, Hagen, & Sattler, 1986)
   C. National Adult Reading Test (Grober & Sliwinski, 1991; Nelson & O'Connell, 1978)
II. Academic achievement abilities
   A. Woodcock-Johnson Psychoeducational Battery-Revised (WJ-R; Woodcock & Johnson, 1989)
   B. Wide Range Achievement Test 3 (WRAT 3; Wilkinson, 1993)

functioning measures can contribute to estimating the premorbid level of functioning (Lezak, 1983). For example, it has been suggested that the WAIS-R Vocabulary subtest is least vulnerable to decline and provides the single best estimate of premorbid functioning from the WAIS-R. Measures of single-word reading recognition skills, such as the National Adult Reading Test (Nelson & O'Connell, 1978; Spreen & Strauss, 1991) or the Reading subtest of the Wide Range Achievement Test 3 (Wilkinson, 1993), are also relatively invulnerable to decline following illness or trauma. Such technqiues, however, may not always be accurate (Lezak, 1983), particularly when patients have subtle language dysfunction (Stebbins, Gilley, Wilson, Bernard, & Fox, 1990; Stebbins, Wilson, Gilley, Bernard, & Fox, 1990). Thus, as a rule, results from selected general intellectual and academic achievement measures should never be used in isolation to estimate premorbid level of functioning. Instead, this information should be combined with historical information, including educational and vocational history and socioeconomic status, to arrive at an estimate of premorbid functioning. A quantitative estimate of premorbid functioning also can be established using demographic information and regression equations, although these methods are limited for the extreme ranges of skills (Barona, Reynolds, & Chastain, 1984; Eppinger, Craig, Adams, & Parsons, 1987).

Foundation Skills

Arousal and Attention

The patient's level of arousal and attention determine his or her ability to process incoming information. Hence, when deetermining the source of a patient's difficulties, test performances in this component should be considered first. As Mirsky, Fantie, and Tatman (this volume), Shum, McFarland, and Bain (1990), Sohlberg and Mateer (1989), Stuss, Stethem, and Poirier (1987), Whyte (1992a), and others have shown, attention is not a unitary function, but, rather, can be broken into different components, each of which can be impaired selectively. Thus, attention is often divided into focused or selective attention, sustained attention, complex divided attention, and encoding or attentional capacity. Construct validity of different attentional frameworks has been supported by factor-analytic studies, and similar factor structures have emerged even when tests used are slightly different (Mirsky, Fantie, & Tatman, this volume; Shum, McFarland, & Bain, 1990).

Measures to evaluate arousal and attention are shown in Table 11.3. As conceptualized here, attention is divided into two major areas. The first area, *deployment,* refers to how well a patient can channel and focus attentional resources and includes *arousal, focused attention,* and *sustained attention.* Unless a patient can deploy attention adequately, he or she may never be able to process information at a level necessary for application of other cognitive skills in the framework, such as learning and memory. The second area, *capacity/encoding,* refers to how well a patient can hold information in mind and then process it, even if distracted or required to divide attention

TABLE 11.3. Arousal and Attention

I. Deployment
   A. Arousal and level of alertness (observe)
   B. Focused attention
      1. Digit Symbol (WAIS-R; Wechsler, 1981)
      2. Trail Making Test (from the Halstead-Reitan Neuropsychological Test Battery, HRNTB; Reitan & Wolfson, 1985)
      3. Stroop Interference Test (Golden, 1978; Spreen & Strauss, 1991)
      4. Talland Letter Cancellation Task (Mirsky, Fantie, & Tatman, this volume; Lezak, 1983)
      5. Digit Vigilance (Heaton, Grant, & Matthews, 1991)
   C. Sustained attention
      1. Continuous performance tasks
         a. X and AX Tasks (Sunrise Systems; Mirsky, Fantie, & Tatman, this volume)
         b. Gordon Diagnostic System (Gordon, 1989)
         c. Test of Variables of Attention (TOVA; McCarney & Greenberg, 1990)
      2. Seashore Rhythm Test (HRNTB; Reitan & Wolfson, 1985)
      3. Digit Vigilance (Heaton et al., 1991)

II. Capacity/Encoding
   A. Span of attention
      1. Verbal
         a. Digit Span-Forwards (Wechsler Memory Scale-Revised, WMS-R; Wechsler, 1987, or WAIS-R; Wechsler, 1981)
         b. Trial 1 of verbal list learning (e.g., CVLT; Delis et al., 1987, or Rey Auditory Verbal Learning Test, RAVLT; Lezak, 1983; Spreen & Strauss, 1991)
         c. Sentence Repetition (Spreen & Benton, 1977)
         d. Logical Memory I (WMS-R; Wechsler, 1987)
      2. Nonverbal
         a. Visual Memory Span-Forwards (WMS-R; Wechsler, 1987)
         b. Seashore Rhythm Test (HRNTB; Reitan & Wolfson, 1985)
   B. Resistance to interference
      1. Consonant Trigrams (Stuss, Stethem, & Poirier, 1987)
      2. List B recall on CVLT (Delis et al., 1987) or RAVLT (Lezak, 1983; Spreen & Strauss, 1991)
   C. Mental manipulation/Divided attention
      1. Digit Span-Backwards (WMS-R; Wechsler, 1987, or WAIS-R; Wechsler, 1981)
      2. Visual Memory Span-Backwards (WMS-R; Wechsler, 1987)
      3. Arithmetic (WAIS-R; Wechsler, 1981)
      4. Mental Control (WMS-R; Wechsler, 1987)
      5. Paced Auditory Serial Addition Test (PASAT; Gronwall, 1977; Stuss et al., 1987)

among tasks. *Capacity/encoding* includes *span of attention, resistance to interference,* and *mental manipulation/divided attention.*

Although there is much overlap with the elements of attention presented by Mirsky, Fantie, and Tatman (this volume), the model presented here has some specific differences: (1) level of arousal is always observed and rated; (2) the overall model is hierarchical; (3) the encoding component is organized hierarchically, is conceptualized as multidimensional, and can be impaired at different levels; and (4) *shifting attention,* viewed as requiring control of both information input and output, is included under executive functions. By using the outline in Table 11.3, the patient's ability to deploy attention can be summarized by asking, in turn, each of a series of specific questions:

- Is the patient *awake and alert* (*arousal*)? It is particularly important to note decreases in arousal associated with disease state, sleep deprivation, medication regimens, or use of alcohol or illicit drugs.
- If the patient is awake and alert, is he or she able *to focus* attention on specific stimuli, as required by presented tasks (*focused attention*)?
- If the patient can focus attention on presented stimuli, can he or she *sustain* attention over time without fatigue or error (*sustained attention*)?

There are no standardized measures of *arousal*. Arousal is best observed and rated by the examiner, although this method may be sensitive only at the extremes (e.g., patient falling asleep; Whyte, 1992b). Instruments used to examine *focused and sustained attention* (Table 11.3) are described by Heaton, Grant, and Matthews (1991), and by Mirsky, Fantie, and Tatman (this volume). The best measure of sustained attention is the continuous performance test (Rosvold, Mirsky, Sarason, Bransome, & Beck, 1956), of which there are now many different versions. Some, however, are too brief to provide indications of a vigilance decrement, unless excessive demands are placed on processing (Parasuraman, 1984). A relatively new computer-based measure, the Test of Variables of Attention (McCarney & Greenberg, 1990), runs for approximately 25 minutes, allowing enough time to observe lapses in sustained attention, even when deficits are subtle.

In addition to formal assessment, it is important to note whether the patient is visibly distracted by external stimuli and whether he or she is able to focus attention well within the structured, one-on-one testing setting. The examiner should also note whether the patient can sustain his or her attention during lengthy testing sessions, without fatigue or increased errors, and whether the patient requires frequent breaks to "regain energy."

Having determined the degree to which the patient can deploy attentional resources adequately, it is important to determine if he or she can encode information as required for further processing. *Capacity/encoding* is organized hierarchically, and the clinician, again, can ask a series of specific questions of the patient's skills:

- Is the patient able simply *to hold information in mind* for brief periods of time (*span of attention*)?

When evaluating *span of attention*, it is important to note what happens as the patient is presented with increasing amounts of information. For example, a progressive decline in performance as the amount of information presented increases from individual digits or words, to sentences, and then to short paragraphs can indicate "overloading," that is, an inability to process information, as the amount presented exceeds the patient's span. In contrast, poor performance on immediate retention of individual items (digits, words), relative to preserved retention of paragraphs, suggests that the patient can benefit from the increased organization of material and can compensate for deficits in span by use of organizational strategies. Each pattern of findings has different implications for diagnosis and treatment.

- If the patient can hold information in mind, can he or she be distracted from it briefly, *without disruption or loss of information* (*resistance to inteference*)?

Even when span of attention is unimpaired, as may be the case in early Alzheimer's disease, mild traumatic brain injury, or Korsakoff's disease, it can be difficult for a patient to encode information when he or she is distracted briefly from it. The Brown-Peterson, or Consonant Trigrams task (Brown, 1958; Peterson & Peterson, 1959), has been used frequently in research, particularly to examine memory decay in different types of amnesias (Butters & Cermak, 1980; Squire & Butters, 1992; Warrington, 1982). Stuss, Stethem, Hugenholtz, and Richard (1989), however, have demonstrated the usefulness of Consonant Trigrams for assessing subtle attentional deficit following traumatic brain injury. They have also collected age-based normative data and have recommended the clinical use of the procedure (Stuss et al., 1987). Evidence of intact span of attention, but impaired resistance to interference, suggests that although a patient can hold information briefly in mind, he or she cannot cope with any sort of external distraction and can be vulnerable to the effects of proactive interference. This, in turn, will have a substantial impact on the patient's ability to learn and remember new information.

- If the patient can be distracted briefly from information, can he or she *hold information in mind, perform mental operations on it, and output a result* (*mental manipulation/divided attention*)?

Impairment of *mental manipulation/divided attention* can affect the patient's ability to complete complex tasks mentally or to function in an environment in which multiple, simultaneous demands are placed on attention. The Paced Auditory Serial Addition Test (Gronwall, 1977) is particularly sensitive to subtle deficits in divided attention, as it places multiple demands on span of attention, resistance to interference, mental manipulation, and speed of processing. Other less complex measures of mental manipulation/divided attention are listed in Table 11.3.

In summary, by reviewing each of these attentional components, the neuropsychologist can parse out attentional impairment from impairment in other functions. Because higher levels of cognitive processing are dependent on adequate attentional processing, the current framework is heavily weighted toward attentional assessment.

Sensory and Motor Functions

Measures to evaluate sensory and motor skills are shown in Table 11.4. *Sensory functions* are divided into *visual, auditory,* and *somatosensory* realms. Changes in olfaction and gustatory sensation are also important to note, but assessment of these sensory realms is not included in the current framework. Because there are few standardized measures of primary sensory functions, the neuropsychologist may have to

TABLE 11.4. Sensory and Motor Functions

I. Sensory functions (input)
  A. Visual: Sensory Perceptual Examination—Visual Fields (HRNTB; Reitan & Wolfson, 1985)
  B. Auditory: Sensory Perceptual Examination—Auditory Extinction (HRNTB; Reitan & Wolfson, 1985)
  C. Somatosensory
    1. Gross discrimination: Astereognosis (HRNTB; Reitan & Wolfson, 1985)
    2. Neglect: Double Simultaneous Stimulation, Sensory Perceptual Examination (HRNTB; Reitan & Wolfson, 1985)
    3. Fine discrimination
      a. Finger Agnosia, Sensory Perceptual Examination (HRNTB; Reitan & Wolfson, 1985)
      b. Fingertip Number Writing, Sensory Perceptual Examination (HRNTB; Reitan & Wolfson, 1985)

II. Motor functions (output)
  A. Lateral dominance
    1. Lateral Dominance Examination (HRNTB; Dodrill & Thoreson, 1993; Reitan & Wolfson, 1985)
    2. Edinburgh Handedness Inventory (Oldfield, 1971)
    3. Pantomime
  B. Strength—Hand Dynamometer (HRNTB; Reitan & Wolfson, 1985)
  C. Fine motor skills
    1. Speed—Finger Tapping Test (HRNTB; Reitan & Wolfson, 1985)
    2. Dexterity
      a. Grooved Pegboard Test (Matthews & Kløve, 1964)
      b. Purdue Pegboard Test (Purdue Research Foundation, 1948)
  D. Sensorimotor integration: Tactual Performance Test (HRNTB; Reitan & Wolfson, 1985)
  E. Praxis—Praxis section of BDAE (Goodglass & Kaplan, 1983)

supplement the evaluation with information from other sources (e.g., neurological examination, occupational and physical therapy evaluations).

Primary visual skills include acuity, intactness of visual fields, and the ability to perceive color, each of which should be reviewed. Although the neuropsychologist can screen for defects in primary visual skills, optometric or ophthalmologic evaluation may sometimes be required. Even when the neuropsychologist does not test these skills directly, there are several important points to consider. The clinician should always maximize the patient's acuity, for example, by inquiring whether the patient needs glasses for reading or for other visual work, and ensuring that the patient uses glasses as necessary during the evaluation. One must also determine whether the patient has visual neglect, although this is viewed more correctly as an attentional rather than a visual impairment, especially since it can be multimodal (Capruso, Hamsher, & Benton, this volume; Heilman, Watson, & Valenstein, 1985). If neglect is noted, then placement of visual stimuli should be modified accordingly, so that they are in the patient's nonneglected visual field. Capruso, Hamsher, and Benton (this volume) and McCarthy and Warrington (1990) have noted that primary visual disturbances other than visual neglect usually affect visuospatial perceptual and constructional skills only under specific conditions.

Basic auditory skills also should be reviewed. Problems with repetition, difficulties comprehending, or production of phonemic errors on word recall can reflect impaired hearing rather than cognitive processing deficits. Again, although the neuropsychologist can screen for basic auditory difficulties, an audiological evaluation to assess primary auditory functioning may be required to obtain detailed information.

Finally, although less essential for understsanding higher level deficits in cognition, *somatosensory skills* should be reviewed. These data can be useful for diagnosis of lateralized dysfunction or to understand problems a patient is encountering in everyday sensory tasks. When needed, information about tactile thresholds, including pain, temperature, and vibratory sensation, can be obtained from the neurological evaluation. There also are measures the neuropsychologist can use to assess gross somatosensory discrimination and higher levels of processing, including somatosensory neglect, fine somatosensory discrimination, and sensory localization. Questions regarding interhemispheric transfer of somatosensory information can be answered by having a patient feel an object in one hand and then select a matching object from a group using the other hand.

As shown in Table 11.4, *motor functions* are divided into *lateral dominance, strength, fine motor skills, sensorimotor integration,* and *praxis*. It is important to evaluate *lateral dominance,* and handedness in particular, because of the relation between handedness and certain developmental disorders (Geschwind & Behan, 1984; Geschwind & Galaburda, 1987). Formal procedures (Dodrill & Thoreson, 1993; Reitan & Davison, 1974) and structured questionnaires (Briggs & Nebes, 1975; Oldfield, 1971; Spreen & Strauss, 1991) can be used to assess handedness (Table 11.4). Dodrill and Thoreson (1993), however, have discussed limitations of questionnaire methods, with respect to reliability. A patient's lateral dominance can be established at a gross level by asking which hand the patient uses to write, eat, and throw a ball. Asking a patient to gesture an action can provide additional information. If one is pressed for time, Dodrill and Thoreson (1993) have suggested that asking a patient to write his or her name can provide a brief and reliable measure of handedness. In addition to patient handedness, it is important to inquire about familial handedness, as this information can be useful diagnostically (Geschwind & Behan, 1984; Geschwind & Galaburda, 1987).

Findings on measures of *motor strength, speed, and dexterity* can contribute to understanding a patient's particular motor strengths and weaknesses and their relation to cognitive difficulties, but one must be cautious when using results to infer lesion lateralization. A large proportion of the normal population shows preferred versus nonpreferred hand differences greater than the 10% "rule of thumb" difference, and many normal individuals can show better nonpreferred than preferred hand performance (Bornstein, 1986b). Yet, normal individuals rarely show consistent, "clinically significant" differences on two or more motor tests, while brain-lesioned patients do (Bornstein, 1986a). Thus, Bornstein (1986a) has emphasized the importance of examining the pattern of performance on two or more motor tests, rather than a single "abnormal" performance, in order to determine whether there is a lateralized difference. Hence, motor assessment should include, minimally, two different measures.

In addition to measures of strength, speed, and dexterity, *sensorimotor integration* skills can be examined when needed. Finally, although not strictly a motor skill, assessment of *praxis* can provide information that is potentially germane to the patient's functional skills and to understanding language-based deficits. Formal or informal assessment can include assessment of manual, axial, and bucco-facial praxis.

Executive, Problem-Solving, and Reasoning Abilities

The outline for assessment of executive, problem-solving, and reasoning abilities is shown in Table 11.5 and is similar to that presented by Goldstein and Green (this volume). As those authors have discussed, it is almost impossible to separate executive functions from problem-solving and reasoning abilities. One could potentially distinguish between reasoning skills, such as those assessed by subtests of the WAIS-R (Wechsler, 1981), Raven's Progressive Matrices (Raven, 1960) or subtests of the Woodcock-Johnson Tests of Cognitive Ability (Woodcock & Johnson, 1989), and executive skills, such as planning and flexibility of thinking, which are not assessed adequately by intellectual measures (Eslinger & Damasio, 1985; Lezak, 1982; Shallice & Burgess, 1991), by suggesting that the former are more influenced by education and cultural background than are the latter (Mapou, 1988a). As illustrated by Mirsky, Fantie, and Tatman (this volume), however, it is clear that culture also can have a substantial influence on executive functions. Thus, *all* of these skills are included as *foundation skills*, because the adequate expression of other skills in the framework, especially learning and memory, requires intact skills within this component. There is also overlap between the executive functions and complex attentional skills (Barkley, 1988), and it is sometimes difficult to separate the two. For this reason, the ability to shift attention is included under executive functions, as one aspect of flexibility of thinking.

As Goldstein and Green (this volume) and Lezak (1982) have discussed, assessment of executive functions is often difficult. The structure of the testing session can facilitate successful completion of many tasks, despite documented pathology and evidence of behavioral deficits in everyday functioning (Eslinger & Damasio, 1985; Shallice & Burgess, 1991). Thus, in addition to standardized assessment, the examiner must carefully observe the patient's performance throughout the evaluation and must ask family and significant others about the patient's functioning and behavior.

Executive, problem-solving, and reasoning abilities are divided into several areas: *planning; flexibility of thinking, hypothesis testing, and use of feedback; sequencing and organizational skills;* and *reasoning abilities*. There is overlap, however, among these areas. For example, planning requires flexibility of thinking and the ability to learn from one's errors, sequencing requires the ability to plan ahead, and reasoning includes components of planning, flexibility, and sequencing. Nevertheless, it is possible for a patient to be relatively more impaired in one area, and understanding differential impairment can be useful for directing treatment.

Planning abilities are required for completion of almost all tasks in the neuropsychological evaluation, and it is important to consider verbal and nonverbal planning skills independently. For example, performance on verbal planning tasks can indicate

TABLE 11.5. Executive, Problem-Solving, and Reasoning Abilities

- I. Executive functions and problem-solving abilities
  - A. Planning
    - 1. Verbal: Rule Governed Drawing (Mack, unpublished test)
    - 2. Nonverbal
      - a. Porteus Mazes (Porteus, 1965)
      - b. Tinkertoy Test (Lezak, 1983)
      - c. Tower Tests (Tower of London, Tower of Hanoi; see Goldstein & Green, this volume)
  - B. Flexibility of thinking, hypothesis testing, use of feedback
    - 1. Wisconsin Card Sorting Test (Heaton, Chelune, Talley, Kay, & Curtiss, 1993)
    - 2. Halstead Category Test (HRNTB; Reitan & Wolfson, 1985)
    - 3. Visual-Verbal Test (Feldman & Drasgow, 1981)
    - 4. Observation
  - C. Sequencing and organizational skills
    - 1. Trail Making Test (HRNTB; Reitan & Wolfson, 1985)
    - 2. Picture Arrangement (WAIS-R; Wechsler, 1981; WAIS-R as a Neuropsychological Instrument, WAIS-RNI; Kaplan et al., 1991)
    - 3. Sentence Arrangement (WAIS-RNI; Kaplan et al., 1991)
    - 4. Use of categories on California Verbal Learning Test (Delis et al., 1987)
    - 5. Comparison of letters and categories on Controlled Oral Word Association (Lezak, 1983; Spreen & Strauss, 1991)
    - 6. Approach to visuospatial constructional tasks
    - 7. Observation
- II. Reasoning abilities
  - A. Verbal
    - 1. Similarities (WAIS-R; Wechsler, 1981)
    - 2. Comprehension (WAIS-R; Wechsler, 1981)
    - 3. Verbal Analogies (WJ-R; Woodcock & Johnson, 1989)
    - 4. Proverb Interpretation (WAIS-R Comprehension; Wechsler, 1981; Proverbs Test; Gorham, 1956)
    - 5. Cognitive Estimation (Shallice & Evans, 1978)
  - B. Nonverbal: Raven's Progressive Matrices (Raven, 1960, 1965)
  - C. Verbal and visual
    - 1. Picture Completion (WAIS-R; Wechsler, 1981)
    - 2. Picture Arrangement (WAIS-R; Wechsler, 1981)
    - 3. Visual-Verbal Test (Feldman & Drasgow, 1981)
    - 4. Halstead Category Test (Reitan & Wolfson, 1985)
    - 5. Concept Formation (WJ-R; Wooccock & Johnson, 1989)

whether the patient is able to use verbal knowledge to guide planning and problem solving, and performance on nonverbal planning tasks can provide information on the patient's ability to plan ahead and to inhibit impulsivity. Goldstein and Green (this volume) have described a number of planning measures, many of which are listed in Table 11.5. There are few readily available measures of verbal planning, although Mack (unpublished test)[1] has described a measure that requires a patient to act on verbal constraints held briefly in mind. Several excellent "real-life" planning tasks, requiring verbal mediation, have been described by Shallice and Burgess (1991), and

[1]Information on Rule Governed Drawing and other cognitive neuropsychological measures can be obtained by writing to James L. Mack, Ph.D., Department of Neurology, University Hospitals, 2074 Abington Road, Cleveland, Ohio 44106.

standardized clinical versions of these tasks are under development (Alderman, Evans, Burgess, & Wilson, 1993; Wilson, 1993).

Because there are few standardized measures of planning, planning skills also should be observed and evaluated throughout the assessment. Observation of the patient's approach to visuospatial constructional tasks (e.g., Rey-Osterrieth Complex Figure copy, Block Design, Object Assembly) can provide additional information on nonverbal planning skills. Observing performance and recording response latencies can provide information on impulsivity. Impulsivity also can be noted on continuous performance tests (errors of commission). All of this information can contribute to diagnosis, to understanding breakdown in a patient's functional skils, and to making recommendations for treatment.

Flexibility of thinking of thinking, hypothesis testing, and use of feedback to guide responding are assessed by tasks that require the patient to shift response set on the basis of examiner feedback (Table 11.5). Although the cognitive requirements of these measures differ (Perrine, 1993), each requires the patient to test hypotheses, to determine the correct response principle, and to shift the response principle in use when told to shift explicitly or when told that a response is incorrect. In addition, these measures provide indications of perseverative responding. Flexibility of thinking can also be noted on reasoning measures, such as WAIS-R Similarities and Picture Completion, and perseverative responding can be observed on different verbal and visuospatial tasks, including measures of learning (e.g., CVLT) and constructional skills (e.g., Rey-Osterrieth Complex Figure Test).

Sequencing skills are assessed at different levels throughout evaluation. At a simple level, Part A of the Trail Making Test (Reitan & Wolfson, 1985) examines the ability to sequence numbers in order. Part B of the test introduces a more complex, alternating sequence, and is more sensitive to dysfunction. Nevertheless, on both tasks, it is important to distinguish between slow but accurate performance, which can reflect a deficit in focused or sustained attention, and errors of sequencing, which are more likely to reflect executive deficits. WAIS-R Picture Arrangement requires both reasoning and sequencing skills. The patient must be able to discern the obvious and subtle information in the cartoon pictures, and then use this information to place the pictures in the correct order. By asking the patient to tell the story verbally following completion, as suggested in the WAIS-R as a Neuropsychological Instrument (WAIS-RNI; Kaplan et al., 1991), one can determine whether the patient can provide a viable story for an incorrect sequence or, alternately, provides an incorrect explanation for a correct sequence. The latter can be more indicative of a reasoning deficit. The WAIS-RNI also includes Sentence Arrangement, a measure of verbal sequencing and flexibility of thinking.

Although *organizational skills* are difficult to separate from executive skills described so far, it is important to understand the patient's ability to perceive implicit organization of presented material and to make use of explicit organization to facilitate a response. With respect to verbal organizational skills, one can observe the degree to which an increase in the explicit organization of presented material facilitates the patient's performance. For example, a patient can have difficulty recalling a word list, but can perform within the expected range when recalling semantically organized paragraphs. Similarly, on the CVLT, the extent to which the patient organizes his or her recall by categories, rather than recalling words by rote, can be examined. One can also compare performance using letters on the Controlled Oral Word Association Test (COWAT) to performance using semantic categories (Lezak, 1983; Spreen & Strauss, 1991). Although most individuals generate more words when prompted with a category rather than a letter, a low COWAT performance with letters followed by a relatively better or even normal performance for categories suggests that organizational difficulties are contributing to word search and retrieval deficits (Monsch et al., 1994). In the visuospatial realm, flow-charting the sequence of a patient's performance on the Rey Osterrieth Complex Figure Test (ROCF; Lezak, 1983; Spreen & Strauss, 1991) or WAIS-R Block Design can indicate whether the patient is taking an organized or a piecemeal approach to construction (Kaplan, 1988). A piecemeal approach to design copy on the ROCF can have a substantial effect on subsequent ability to recall the figure. Several systems for quantifying organization have been described (Bennett-Levy, 1984; Kirk & Kelly, 1986; Stern et al., 1994; Waber & Holmes, 1985).

Reasoning abilities, although evaluated separately from executive functions and problem solving, can be influenced by underlying executive skills. Therefore, flexibility of thinking and planning must be considered when evaluating performance on reasoning measures. Performance on measures of verbal reasoning can reveal concreteness or impulsivity. Good performances, however, do not always indicate absence of impairment (Lezak, 1982, 1983). For example, verbal reasoning measures, such as those on the WAIS-R, tend to tap old verbal knowledge rather than novel reasoning skills. As alternatives or adjuncts, tests of verbal analogical reasoning, measures of proverb interpretation, and cognitive estimation tasks can provide information on verbal reasoning. The latter, in particular, are sensitive to reasoning deficits associated with executive dysfunction (Goldstein & Green, this volume; Shallice & Evans, 1978).

There are few pure measures of nonverbal reasoning abilities, perhaps because, in our culture, verbal reasoning skills are emphasized. Luria (1980), for example, has discussed the role of verbal mediation in reasoning and problem solving. Although the purest measure of nonverbal reasoning may be the Raven's Progressive Matrices (Raven, 1960, 1965), performance on that task often can be mediated verbally. This suggests that most nonverbal reasoning tasks are best conceptualized as requiring a combination of verbal and visual skills (Table 11.5).

In summary, *arousal and attention, sensory and motor functions,* and *executive, problem-solving, and reasoning abilities* are the fundamental skills on which higher level skills in the framework depend. These skills are particularly sensitive to disruption by diffuse brain dysfunction (Lezak, 1983), and so also tend to be those affected by mild disorder or early in the course of progressive disease. Thus, a full understanding of the disruption of foundation skills is critical to understanding breakdown in functioning at higher levels of the framework. In contrast to foundation skills, modality-specific skills, discussed next, tend to be disrupted by focal, rather than diffuse, brain dysfunction.

Modality-Specific Skills

Language Functions

As discussed by authors in this volume (Caplan; Glosser & Friedman; Kay & Franklin), advances in the past decade have increased our knowledge about the cognitive neuropsychology of spoken and written language. For routine assessment and particularly in practices where language disorder is infrequent or in which the emphasis may be on diagnosis, however, a complete cognitive neuropsychological assessment may not be necessary or practical. Instead, an approach similar to that described by Albert, Goodglass, Helm, Rubens, and Alexander (1981) is recommended.

Table 11.6 presents the outline for assessment of language, in which language functions are divided into two principal areas: *spoken* and *written language*. Within each of these areas, functions are further divided into those that reflect language *input* and language *output*. Thus, spoken language includes *comprehension* (*single word, syntax*) and *production* (*speech, repetition, naming, single word,* and *discourse*), and written language includes *reading* (*letter and word recognition, comprehension*) and *writing* (*spelling, mechanics, dictation, discourse*). In general, any evaluation should at least screen each of these areas, with more in-depth assessment applied as needed.

Single-word comprehension skills can be assessed in a relatively straightforward manner (Table 11.6). Specific test selection can be influenced by the patient's language production and visuospatial perceptual skills. For example, when speech or language production is impaired, the Peabody Picture Vocabulary Test-Revised (Dunn & Dunn, 1981), which requires only a pointing response, can be useful, but WAIS-R Vocabulary (Wechsler, 1981) is a better choice for a patient with visual difficulties. In contrast to single-word comprehension, assessment of a patient's *comprehension of lengthy and grammatically complex information* (*syntactic comprehension*) is more difficult. Gross impairment can be noted during the interview and following presentation of complex task instructions. The measures that are used typically for more in-depth assessment have certain limitations, however. For example, the Token Test (De Renzi & Vignolo, 1962; Spreen & Strauss, 1991) provides a relatively rapid measure of syntactic comprehension, but it is limited to only one aspect of comprehension and can miss deficits in other areas. Further, patients with attentional disorders can have difficulty attending to the lengthier items. Therefore, when a detailed understanding of syntactic comprehension is necessary, it is better to use cognitive neuropsychological measures (see Caplan, this volume).

Speech production, which refers only to the *motor and prosodic* aspects of language, should be observed throughout the evaluation, noting characteristics including articulation, rate, volume, and prosody. Portions of the Boston Diagnostic Aphasia Examination (BDAE; Goodglass & Kaplan, 1983) can help to assess and to quantify these aspects of speech. Similarly, *language production,* which refers to the *linguistic aspects* of production, is also observed, with particular attention to fluency, grammatic structure, and word finding. Information on language production also can be gleaned from WAIS-R subtests that require a verbal response. For example, Picture Completion

TABLE 11.6. Language Functions

I. Spoken language
 A. Comprehension
  1. Single word
   a. Vocabulary (WAIS-R; Wechsler, 1981)
   b. Peabody Picture Vocabulary Test (Dunn & Dunn, 1981)
  2. Syntax
   a. Token Test (De Renzi & Vignolo, 1962; Spreen & Strauss, 1991)
   b. Complex Ideational Material (BDAE; Goodglass & Kaplan, 1983)
   c. Comprehension of test instructions and conversation
 B. Production
  1. Speech
   a. Fluency Rating (BDAE; Goodglass & Kaplan, 1983)
   b. Observation
  2. Repetition
   a. Sentence Repetition Test (Spreen & Benton, 1977)
   b. Memory for Sentences (WJ-R; Woodcock & Johnson, 1989)
   c. Repetition sections of BDAE (Goodglass & Kaplan, 1983)
  3. Naming—Boston Naming Test (Kaplan, Goodglass, & Weintraub, 1983)
  4. Single word—Controlled Oral Word Association Test (letters, categories; Lezak; 1983; Spreen & Strauss, 1991)
  5. Discourse
   a. Cookie Theft Picture (BDAE; Goodglass & Kaplan, 1983)
   b. Conversation
II. Written language
 A. Reading
  1. Letter and word recognition
   a. Reading (WRAT 3; Wilkinson, 1993)
   b. Letter-Word Identification (WJ-R; Woodcock & Johnson, 1989)
  2. Comprehension
   a. Passage Comprehension (WJ-R; Woodcock & Johnson, 1989)
   b. Nelson-Denny Reading Test (Brown, Fishco, & Hanna, 1993)
   c. Gray Oral Reading Test (Wiederholt & Bryant, 1992)
 B. Writing
  1. Spelling
   a. Spelling (WRAT 3; Wilkinson 1993)
   b. Dictation (WJ-R; Woodcock & Johnson, 1989)
  2. Mechanics: Dictation (WJ-R; Woodcock & Johnson, 1989)
  3. Dictation
   a. Dictation (WJ-R; Woodcock & Johnson, 1989)
   b. Words and Sentences to Dictation (BDAE; Goodglass & Kaplan, 1983)
  4. Discourse
   a. Writing Samples (WJ-R; Woodcock & Johnson, 1989)
   b. Cookie Theft Picture Description (BDAE; Goodglass & Kaplan, 1983)

can reveal word-finding difficulties, because the patient can provide a correct response through pointing or circumlocution, without having to target a specific word.

In addition to observations of speech and language production, it is important to evaluate *repetition* ability. Dissociations between repetition and other aspects of language production can be useful diagnostically (Albert et al., 1981; Goodglass & Kaplan, 1983). Quantitative and qualitative findings on repetition measures can help distinguish between impairment due to attention (e.g., leaving out words but preserving sentence meaning) and impairment due to language disturbance (e.g., paraphasic errors, inability to repeat very short sentences).

Assessment of language production includes evaluation of *naming, single-word,* and *discourse* production. It is important to evaluate confrontation naming, since disorders of naming are among the most common language disturbances. A frequently used measure, the Boston Naming Test (Kaplan, Goodglass, & Weintraub, 1983), includes a large number of items and methods to cue the patient phonemically or semantically. The types of errors produced can be categorized, to provide further information on the characteristics of the language disorder, although Kay and Franklin (this volume) note that differences in errors do not necessarily help to define the particular aphasic syndrome. When a patient initially is unable to name an item, it can be useful to ask, "What do you do with it?" or "Tell me something about it" prior to providing a cue. The patient's response to this question can help to distinguish a naming or word-finding difficulty (e.g., the patient can indicate knowledge of the item but cannot name it) from a visuospatial perceptual difficulty (e.g., the patient describes something else, to which the presented item looks similar).

The ability to generate single words without structure, such as that provided in a naming test, should also be examined. It is important to consider, however, that deficits in executive functions (organized word search and retrieval skills) can limit performance on standardized measures of this skill, such as the COWAT, even when there is no language impairment (Kaplan, 1993, March; Monsch et al., 1994). Thus, qualitative aspects of the patient's production (e.g., paraphasic errors, word finding in conversation versus slow initiation, poor ability to organize verbal information) must be used to determine the source of impaired single-word production.

In contrast to assessment of single-word production, assessment of language production at the level of *discourse* is more difficult. Asking a patient to describe a picture, such as the Cookie Theft Picture on the BDAE (Goodglass & Kaplan, 1983), provides a standard stimulus, but the patient's output must be rated qualitatively. To this author's knowledge, there are no standardized measures of discourse production that include normative data.

Written language can be impaired concomitantly with or independently of spoken language. Disorders of *reading* are described by Glosser and Friedman (this volume), along with detailed assessment methods. Several specific assessment instruments for *letter and word recognition* and *comprehension* are listed in Table 11.6. The Letter–Word Identification subtest of the Woodcock-Johnson Psychoeducational Battery-Revised (WJ-R), which provides information about letter- and word-reading recognition skills, can be used for initial screening. Recording the patient's response verbatim can provide information about the type of breakdown in single-word reading skills. This information can then be used to design a more extensive assessment of single-word reading (see Glosser & Friedman, this volume). Similarly, the WJ-R Passage Comprehension subtest is a useful screen for reading comprehension, but the Comprehension subtest of the Nelson-Denny Reading Test (Brown, Fishco, & Hanna, 1993), which measures both reading rate and comprehension, is a better choice when more ddetailed information is needed. Further, by allowing the patient to continue beyond the standard time limit on this test, information can be obtained regarding the extent to which time constraints reduce comprehension.

Until recently, few standardized measures of *writing* were available, but this is beginning to change. It is now possible to evaluate *spelling, mechanics,* writing to *dictation,* and *discourse* production formally (Table 11.6). For example, on the WJ-R, items on the Dictation subtest are scored strictly for spelling, punctuation, making words plural, and other aspects of mechanics, but those on the Writing Samples subtest are scored based only on whether the patient is able to express his or her thoughts clearly, within the constraints defined by each item. Hence, one can distinguish between mechanical difficulties and the ability of the patient to put his or her thoughts into words. For more detailed evaluation, there are cognitive neuropsychological models and measures of writing analogous to those for reading (McCarthy & Warrington, 1990; Roeltgen, 1985).

Visuospatial Functions

Visuospatial functions, the second area of modality-specific skills, are divided into *perceptual, constructional,* and *spatial awareness skills,* as outlined in Table 11.7. For initial assessment, it is important to have information on each of these areas. If evidence of impairment is found, then more comprehensive assessment, using methods described by Capruso, Hamsher, and Benton (this volume) can be completed.

Visuospatial *perceptual skills* refer to the initial processing of visuospatial information, beyond the basic sensory level and independently of a motor response. Thus, these skills represent aspects of the *input* of visual information. Initial indications of visuospatial perceptual difficulties can be noted on WAIS-R Picture Completion and Picture Arrangement subtests. On the latter, having the patient verbalize the story can help determine if the pictures are being perceived adequately. Similarly, responses on the Boston Naming Test (Kaplan et al., 1983) can be illuminating. Frequent misperceptions include "bus" for *harmonica* or "strawberry" for *acorn.* The way in which a patient approaches visuospatial constructional tasks, such as WAIS-R Block Design or Object Assembly subtests or the ROCF also can provide information on perceptual skills.

When visuospatial perceptual deficits are suggested by general evaluation results, specific perceptual measures can help delineate the nature of the deficit. These measures (Table 11.7) range from simple to complex, with substantial differences in their task demands. Capruso, Hamsher, and Benton (this volume) discuss in detail how

TABLE 11.7. Visuospatial Functions

I. Perceptual skills
  A. Visual Form Discrimination Test (Benton, Hamsher, Varney, & Spreen, 1983)
  B. Judgment of Line Orientation (Benton et al., 1983)
  C. Facial Recognition Test (Benton et al., 1983)
  D. Embedded Figures (Spreen & Strauss, 1991)
  E. Hooper Visual Organization Test (Western Psychological Services, 1983)
II. Constructional skills
  A. Drawing
    1. Rey-Osterrieth or Taylor Complex Figure (Lezak, 1983; Spreen & Strauss, 1991)
    2. Boston Spatial Quantitative Battery figures (Goodglass & Kaplan, 1983)
    3. Visual Reproduction (WMS-R; Wechsler, 1987)
  B. Two- and three-dimensional constructions
    1. Block Design (WAIS-R; Wechsler, 1981)
    2. Object Assembly (WAIS-R; Wechsler, 1981)
    3. Three-Dimensional Block Construction (Benton et al., 1983)
III. Spatial awareness skills
  A. Right–Left Orientation (Benton et al., 1983)
  B. Road Map Test of Direction Sense (Money, 1976)

these and other measures can be used and the specific aspects of perception assessed by each. McCarthy and Warrington (1990) also discuss methods for detailed assessment of visuospatial perception.

Assessment of visuospatial *constructional skills* has long been a key component of neuropsychological evaluation. Perhaps this is because of the richness of information provided by constructional tasks. These tasks are multifactorial and require integration of both *input and output* skills, including basic visual and motor skills, visuospatial perceptual skills, organizational skills, and planning. Thus, the neuropsychologist must review findings from other portions of the evaluation and must consider carefully the reasons why a patient is having difficulties with a constructional task. For example, Kaplan (1993, March) has stated that a patient can fail an item on WAIS-R Block Design for any of the following reasons: (1) a lack of motor skills needed to manipulate the blocks, (2) an inability to see or perceive the model accurately, (3) an inability to plan an organized approach to the task, or (4) an inability to comprehend or to cooperate with the procedure (e.g., the patient eats the blocks or throws them at the examiner). In each instance, the reason for failure is different and can reflect a different type of breakdown in brain functioning.

Kaplan (1988, 1990) also has described how patients with lateralized brain lesions can differ in their approaches to constructional tasks. Specifically, patients with left-hemisphere lesions tend to reproduce the outer contour of presented models (e.g., 2 × 2 or 3 × 3 configuration on Block Design; outer shape of the ROCF), but make errors in the internal details. In contrast, patients with right-hemisphere lesions may attempt to reproduce individual details (e.g., inner pattern on the blocks; diamond or crosses on the ROCF) without integrating the details into an overall configuration. Several recent studies have further demonstrated these types of dissociations among different patient groups (Delis et al., 1992; Kramer, Kaplan, Blusewicz, & Preston, 1991), and also have shown how impairment in different aspects of cognitive and motor functioning can lead to the observed poor performance on constructional tasks (Carlesimo, Fadda, & Caltagirone, 1993).

When administering constructional tasks, observation and tracking of performance are critical to understanding how constructional skills are impaired. Although scores yield valuable information about the performance level, additional information is provided by noting the patient's approach. For example, the examiner can sketch the final solution on WAIS-R Block Design, when it is incorrect. Preferably, the examiner can track the patient's performance block by block via flowchart. Performance on Object Assembly can be similarly tracked by noting how the patient approaches each item (e.g., organized, making full use of contour and details versus no organization, with random placement of pieces and no idea as to what the figure is).

One popular measure of visuospatial constructional skills is the copy portion of the ROCF (Lezak, 1983), for which there are multiple scoring methods. Unfortunately, differences between methods and the associated normative data can lead to different conclusions about performance level (cf., compare methods and normative data in Lezak, 1983, and Spreen & Strauss, 1991). Thus, it is even more important to supplement scoring with qualitative information. Methods for flow-charting the ROCF date from Rey's original recommendation to hand the patient different-colored pencils over the course of copying the figure (Corwin & Bylsma, 1993). Others have adopted a similar approach (Kaplan, 1988; Lezak, 1983; Waber & Holmes, 1985). This method, however, interrupts the drawing process and could change it. Hence, a better method is for the examiner to make a flowchart as the copy is being completed. The direction of each individual line can be indicated by an arrow head, and its sequence can be indicated by a number. In addition to noting the qualitative aspects of the drawing, there are several systems to score the flowchart (Bennett-Levy, 1984; Kirk & Kelly, 1986; Stern et al., 1994; Waber & Holmes, 1985).

Additional constructional measures can be administered as needed. For example, standardized drawings, completed both freely and to copy (e.g., Goodglass & Kaplan, 1983), can be reviewed qualitatively for evidence of planning difficulties, hemi-inattention, inability to reproduce contour or detail, and difficulty with perspective. Several measures provide information on the patient's ability to work in two or three dimensions, reproducing designs freely or from a drawing, photograph, or three-dimensional model (Table 11.7).

A final aspect of visuospatial functions is *spatial awareness,* which includes the patient's awareness of intra- and extrapersonal space. These skills can be disrupted by focal brain dysfunction, and this can have a substantial impact on a patient's functional skills, including following directions and driving. As with constructional skills, these skills reflect both *input* and *output* of visuospatial information. Tests are available to assess discrimination of left and right on self and others (Right–Left Orientation Test; Benton, Hamsher, Varney, & Spreen, 1983) and the ability to track left and right extrapersonally on a map (Standardized Road Map Test of Direction Sense; Money, 1976).

In summary, results from measures of modality-specific skills can help determine whether a patient processes information better in the language or visuospatial domain. Although these skills are generally disrupted by focal brain dysfunction, the clinician must also consider the impact of disorder of foundation skills on the expression of modality-specific skills. Results from assessment of this component have implications for diagnosis, for understanding the best way to present information to a patient, and for planning treatment.

Integrated Skills

As noted earlier, many complex, higher level cognitive skills can be considered as *integrated skills,* since they require interaction, integration, and coordinated functioning of skills at the lower levels of the framework. Thus, general intellectual skills and academic skills could be considered as integrated skills, because of their complex and multifactorial nature. Instead, however, they are placed at the bottom of the framework, because information about these skills provides a context for interpreting performance on more specific measures of cognitive functioning. Similarly, aspects of reasoning and problem solving could be included in this component, but are conceptualized as foundation skills, because they are viewed as integrally related to the executive functions and, as such, are more basic to full expression of functions at the higher levels of the framework. Hence, in this framework, integrated skills are limited to *learning* and *memory,* which, for full expression, require adequate skills at the lower levels of the framework.

Learning and Memory

Because learning and memory impairment is frequent in patients with neurological disorders, a substantial portion of neuropsychological evaluation must be devoted to assessment of learning and memory. Since learning and memory are multifactorial, however, they can be impaired for different reasons (Cohen & Mapou, 1988; Mapou, 1988a). For example, a patient may not learn or may appear to forget information because he or she does not process it initially. That is, the learning or memory impairment can be secondary to a disorder of attention or a disorder in the organizational skills necessary for efficient encoding. Specific disorders of language or visuospatial skills also can contribute to memory difficulties. Finally, there are "pure" disorders of learning and memory seen in patients with amnestic syndromes associated with Korsakoff's disease, herpes encephalitis, or stroke. Thus, thorough assessment of learning and memory must include not only specific learning and memory measures, but measures of most other aspects of cognition.

The outline for assessment of learning and memory is shown in Table 11.8. Complete assessment of learning and memory should include comparison of learning and memory for material presented in the verbal and visual modalities, comparison of single- and multiple-trial learning, and comparison of recall and recognition. To facilitate making these comparisons, learning and memory are divided into *verbal* and

TABLE 11.8. Learning and Memory

I. Verbal
  A. Learning
    1. California Verbal Learning Test (Delis et al., 1987)
    2. Rey Auditory Verbal Learning Test (Lezak, 1983; Spreen & Strauss, 1991)
    3. Selective Reminding Test (Buschke, 1973; Hannay & Levin, 1985; Spreen & Strauss, 1991)
    4. Story Recall (Heaton, Grant, & Matthews, 1991)
  B. Immediate and delayed recall
    1. Logical Memory I and II (WMS-R; Wechsler, 1987)
    2. California Verbal Learning Test (Delis et al., 1987)
    3. Rey Auditory Verbal Learning Test (Lezak, 1983; Spreen & Strauss, 1991)
    4. Selective Reminding Test (Buschke, 1973; Hannay & Levin, 1985; Spreen & Strauss, 1991)
    5. Story Recall (Heaton et al., 1991)
  C. Recognition
    1. Recognition Memory Test (Words; Warrington, 1984)
    2. California Verbal Learning Test (Delis et al., 1987)
    3. Rey Auditory Verbal Learning Test (Lezak, 1983; Spreen & Strauss, 1991)
    4. Boston additions to Logical Memory of the Wechsler Memory Scale (Kaplan, 1988)
II. Visual
  A. Learning
    1. Figure Recall (Heaton et al., 1991)
    2. Nonverbal Selective Reminding Test (Kane & Perrine, 1988)
    3. Continuous Visual Memory Test (Trahan & Larrabee, 1988)
  B. Immediate and delayed recall
    1. Figure Recall (Heaton et al., 1991)
    2. Visual Reproduction I and II (WMS-R; Wechsler, 1987)
    3. Rey-Osterrieth or Taylor Complex Figure Test (Lezak, 1983; Spreen & Strauss, 1991)
  C. Recognition
    1. Nonverbal Selective Reminding Test (Kane & Perrine, 1988)
    2. Continuous Visual Memory Test (Trahan & Larrabee, 1988)
    3. Recognition Memory Test (Faces; Warrington, 1984)
    4. Boston additions to Visual Reproduction of the Wechsler Memory Scale (Kaplan, 1988)

visual areas. Within each of these areas, assessment is divided into *learning, immediate and delayed recall,* and *recognition.* Larrabee and Crook (this volume) have described learning and memory measures in detail. Thus, only general assessment concepts will be discussed here.

One approach to assessment of learning and memory makes use of memory batteries, such as the Wechsler Memory Scale-Revised (WMS-R; Wechsler, 1987). The WMS-R provides information on "global" memory functioning, but also has several weaknesses that limit its use as a tool to understand impairment in specific aspects of learning and memory. First, questions have been raised about both its theoretical and empirical derivation, particularly with respect to how subtests fit with current cognitive psychological knowledge about learning and memory (Loring, 1989). Second, although diagnostically useful information can be obtained from the summary indices, Butters et al. (1988) found that Logical Memory and Visual Reproduction were significantly better than the Verbal and Visual Paired Associates for differentiating demented patients from normal controls. Finally, Butters et al. (1988), Cullum, Butters, Tröster, and Salmon (1990), and Tröster et al. (1993) all have recommended the computation of savings scores on Logical Memory and Visual Reproduction, as these scores appear particularly sensitive to early cognitive decline, as compared to the Memory Indices, and are relatively resistant to normal age-related changes. For these reasons, learning and memory assessment within this framework emphasizes memory measures rather than broad, batteries, such as the WMS-R.

For verbal information, the ability to *learn* material over repeated trials and then retain it during a short delay is usually assessed using word-list learning procedures, such as the CVLT (Delis et al., 1987). There are several other similar list learning tests (Table 11.8), but the CVLT is believed to have several advantages. Although the CVLT and Rey Auditory Verbal Learning Test (RAVLT; Geffen, Moar, O'Hanlon, Clark, & Geffen, 1990; Lezak, 1983; Spreen & Strauss, 1991) have similar formats (in fact, the CVLT was modeled after the RAVLT), the CVLT has a better normative database. More important, because it uses words from four categories, the CVLT facilitates assessment of a patient's organizational encoding strategies. Methods for cued recall and recognition differ widely among RAVLT administrations, and each normative database is tied to a specific administration. In contrast, the CVLT has a single, standardized administration procedure. A final advantage of the CVLT is the availability of an equivalent, alternative form for repeated assessment (Delis et al., 1991). Substantial learning effects have been noted with repeated assessment using the same form on the RAVLT (Crawford, Stewart, & Moore, 1989), and so the availability of an alternate form is an advantage.

The CVLT also has advantages over the Selective Reminding Test (SRT; Buschke, 1973; Hannay & Levin, 1985; Spreen & Strauss, 1991). Loring and Papanicolaou (1987), for example, have argued that SRT indices cannot be directly associated with current cognitive psychological knowledge regarding how verbal information is learned, retained, and subsequently remembered. In contrast, they note that the CVLT method and indices are derived from cognitive psychological research, summarized by Delis et al. (1987).

The CVLT provides information on *verbal learning, immediate and delayed recall,* and *recognition.* During initial learning of List A, several specific questions can be asked. First, does the patient learn the additional, expected amount of information over each trial or, instead, does he or she show a flattened learning curve or even a reduction in learning toward the end of the trials? The latter can reflect proactive interference. Second, when learning the list, does the patient attempt to use the categories to facilitate recall, or does he or she attempt to recall the list by rote? Third, are recalled words distributed as expected over the beginning, middle, and end of the list, or is there a bias toward recalling words at one end of the list? These characteristics can all be observed, quantified, and compared with normative data.

Proactive interference during initial learning of List A can be measured by noting whether release from proactive interference occurs during recall of List B (i.e., better recall of words from unshared than from shared categories; Butters & Cermak, 1980), presented immediately after initial List A learning. Reduction in performance on short-delay free recall of List A, as compared to Trial 5, can indicate retroactive interference from List B. Relative to free recall, improvement on short-delay cued recall can indicate that impaired initial learning and recall reflect difficulty with retrieval of words due to passive encoding, rather than a lack of encoding. Alternately, equally poor free and cued recall can reflect attentional difficulties or lack of awareness of categories; if the words were not encoded by category at all, then cuing by category will not facilitate recall.

Information on retention is provided by long-delay free recall, cued recall, and recognition. The recognition trial, in particular, provides information on storage as compared to retrieval processes. Information processing indices can also be computed. A computerized scoring program facilitates computation of the different indices (Fridlund & Delis, 1987).

As illustrated, the CVLT provides much information about a number of different aspects of verbal learning and memory and can help distinguish among difficulties in initial learning, recall, and recognition. It reflects, however, only one type of material (word list), and it is important to examine verbal learning, recall, and recognition using other types of material, specifically, discourse or short paragraphs. In comparison to a word list, a paragraph is explicitly organized and provides contextual information. Thus, an improvement in recall using paragraphs, as comapred to a word list, can indicate an ability to benefit from increased organization and context of material (Cohen & Mapou, 1988; Mapou, 1988a). When administering measures of paragraph recall, additional data can be obtained by recording the patient's production verbatim. Elements of the story can then be numbered, to indicate the extent to which story order is preserved and whether organizational difficulties are influencing recall. By computing a savings score, the extent to which initially encoded information is retained can be measured, which will help distinguish between attentional difficulties and loss of information over time.

Most paragraph recall measures provide information only on immediate and delayed recall, but not on learning and recognition. Although it is useful to compare single-trial learning on paragraph recall to multiple-trial learning on list-learning procedures, format differences between these measures can contribute to observed performance differences. To address these difficulties, Heaton has developed a Story Memory Test, which includes measures of learning, immediate, and delayed recall (Heaton et al., 1991). Similar to other paragraph recall measures, however, Story Memory does not include a recognition trial.

For some patients with significant speech and language difficulties, it may not be possible to assess learning or free recall. In these instances, it may be necessary to test verbal learning and memory with a pure recognition memory procedure, such as the Recognition Memory Test (Warrington, 1984), which has no requirement for word production (a pointing response can suffice). It is important to note, however, that patients with significant attentional difficulties can have problems completing the task successfully.

Finally, for very impaired patients, it may be necessary to use simpler procedures to assess rudimentary learning and memory skills. Verbal Paired Associates, from the

WMS-R (Wechsler, 1987), can provide some useful information on learning and recall, but because of its many limitations, it should never be used in isolation.

As noted, it is important to evaluate *visual* learning and memory. Although Heilbronner (1992) has questioned whether there is a "pure" visual memory test and whether visual memory task performance is relevant to everyday functioning, comparison of performances on verbal and visual (or, perhaps, less verbal) learning and memory measures can highlight a particular strength or weakness, can help identify the best way in which a patient processes information, and can contribute to diagnosis. In addition, many visual memory tasks provide information on attention, encoding, organizational strategies, and general visuospatial skills.

As in the verbal realm, it is important to examine learning, recall, and recognition. There are few standardized measures of visual learning that use multiple trials. Heaton developed the Figure Memory Test (Heaton et al., 1991), a visual analogue to his Story Memory Test, which includes measures of learning, immediate, and delayed recall. Some information on visual learning can be obtained from the Continuous Visual Memory Test (CVMT; Trahan & Larrabee, 1988), in which seven of the target stimuli are presented six times.

Most visual learning and memory tasks use single-exposure trials, with intentional or incidental recall usually immediately or shortly after presentation and, again, following a delay. This allows the examiner to distinguish between what has been processed immediately after presentation, which reflects the impact of attentional or organizational difficulties, and what is retained after a delay, which reflects the effects of memory impairment. Often, patients with initial encoding difficulties will show reductions in immediate recall, but the same amount of material is recalled following a delay. Free recall alone, without recognition, however, does not make it possible to determine if the patient has processed and retained the information, but is unable to retrieve it. Since few of these measures assess recognition memory, additional, pure recognition tests may be needed, especially when a patient has poor recall or when motor difficulties interfere with task completion. Several visual recognition memory procedures are listed in Table 11.8.

In summary, when measures of verbal and visual learning and memory are used in combination with measures of attention and executive function, the examiner can distinguish among problems in attention, encoding, storage, and retrieval. Differences in learning as a function of single- versus multiple-trial presentation also can be examined. Finally, differences in performance on verbal versus visual measures can reveal differences in processing styles. From the pattern of performance on learning and memory measures, the clinician can then make decisions about diagnosis and treatment.

Personality and Emotional Functioning

Understanding a patient's general personality style and his or her emotional status is essential to interpretation of neuropsychological findings. Within the current framework, *personality style* refers to the patient's long-standing coping patterns and interpersonal style, and *emotional functioning* refers to his or her affective status at the time of evaluation. In many instances, clinical interview will provide sufficient information, and standardized testing will not be necessary. Some patients with neurological disorders will be unable to complete formal personality measures, and obtaining information from family and significant others is especially important.

For patients who are more intact cognitively, objective measures, such as the Minnesota Multiphasic Personality Inventory (MMPI; Hathaway & McKinley, 1967) or MMPI-2 (Butcher, Dahlstrom, Graham, Tellegen, & Kaemer, 1989), can provide useful information about a patient's current level of distress, coping mechanisms, and personality style. Personality profiles on these measures, however, should be interpreted with caution for patients with neurological disorders, as neurological symptoms can elevate a number of MMPI or MMPI-2 scales (Alfano, Neilson, & Paniak, 1992; Bornstein & Kozora, 1990; Cripe, Maxwell, & Hill, 1991; Gass & Russell, 1986; Wooten, 1983). There are similar considerations when using the MMPI/MMPI-2 with patients with general medical illness. Hence, the "traditional" interpretation of a particular profile may not apply. Although attempts have been made to define specific MMPI patterns associated with neurological disease and trauma, these attempts have been unsuccessful, due to the diverse effects of neurological disorder (Mack, 1979). Instead, results on the MMPI or MMPI-2 appear most useful to indicate how the patient is experiencing his or her condition, rather than as an indicator of specific psychiatric disorder (Mack, 1979). Shorter inventories, such as the SCL-90 (Derogatis, 1992), or more specific inventories, such as the Beck Depression Inventory (Beck & Steer, 1987) or the Spielberger State-Trait Anxiety Inventory (Spielberger, Gorsuch, Lushene, Vagg, & Jacobs, 1983), can also be useful.

Projective measures, such as the Rorschach (Exner, 1974), must be used with caution in patients with neurobehavioral disturbance. Language, visuospatial, and executive disorders all can affect a patient's responses to stimuli and render his or her responses invalid as indicators of psychopathology. Provided these issues are taken into consideration, however, projective measures can provide information about the patient's processing of ambiguous material and can supplement results from objective personality measures.

SUMMARY

The proposed framework provides a systematic method for selecting tests and for reviewing neuropsychological findings. Once the patient's overall *global functioning* has been established, the neuropsychologist can review results of measures of *foundation skills*, which include *attention, sensory and motor skills*, and *executive, problem-solving, and reasoning abilities*. Information from these components can indicate why a patient's higher level processing is breaking down. Similarly, review of *modality-specific skills* can indicate more specific processing strengths or weaknesses in *language* and *visuospatial functions*. Once functioning in all of these areas is understood, the neuropsychologist can complete the review with an examination of the *in-*

tegrated skills of *learning* and *memory*. Finally, by understanding the patient's *personality* and *emotional functioning*, possible mediating factors can be considered when coming to final conclusions regarding diagnosis and when making recommendations for intervention.

CASE ILLUSTRATION

The following case illustrates the application of the framework to assessment. It may be helpful to refer back to Figure 11.1, to see how each portion of the evaluation fits into the framework.

History

A.D. was a 57-year-old, right-handed, married, white male who had undergone successful irradiation of a left-hemisphere Grade II astrocytoma 8 years prior to this evaluation. His referral was prompted by recurrence of seizures and by increasing cognitive difficulties in his work as a government regulator. An initial neuropsychological screening elsewhere had revealed significant impairment in attention and memory. He was then referred for more detailed evaluation to help diagnose the basis for his increased cognitive difficulty and to make recommendations for intervention.

Although seizures had been the presenting sign of his tumor, they had resolved following irradiation, and he had been tapered from anticonvulsant medication. For many years following initial treatment, he worked without difficulty and was able to drive. Nine months prior to this evaluation, he experienced a generalized seizure and was placed back on anticonvulsant medication. Establishing a therapeutic dosage had been extremely difficult, and his regimen of Dilantin and phenobarbital at the time of evaluation left him feeling sedated and fatigued much of the time. Neurodiagnostic evaluation, including magnetic resonance imaging (MRI) and positron emission tomography (PET) scans, failed to reveal any evidence of new tumor growth, when results were compared with prior findings. On MRI scans, with and without gadolinium enhancement, extensive signal abnormalities were noted in the medial aspects of the left frontoparietal and occipital lobes, with possible involvement of the right frontal lobe, and were judged to be "compatible with glioma." In addition, periventricular leukomalacia was noted and was thought to be due to the effects of irradiation. On PET scan, there were no focal regions of increased glucose use.

In addition to the recent generalized seizure, A.D. had been experiencing increasing cognitive difficulties, which predated the seizure by 12 to 18 months. He reported difficulties in attention, memory, problem-solving abilities, and word finding, and these difficulties were confirmed by his supervisor at work and by his wife at home. For example, at work, he had difficulty identifying the steps needed to complete tasks that he had performed previously without difficulty. He also had episodes of forgetfulness. Providing cues helped him to complete his work, but because of the high level of his position, his work was deteriorating to the point of placing him at risk for losing his job; a medical retirement was being considered.

Aside from the tumor and seizures, A.D.'s premorbid neurological, psychiatric, and psychosocial history was unremarkable. He had been an excellent student and had completed an M.S. degree in biochemistry. He had worked for the government for more than 20 years, had been promoted over the years, and had been working for the last several years heading a regulatory branch required to respond rapidly to emergency situations in scientific laboratories. He had supervisory responsibility for a staff of 50. With the exception of the initial problems from the tumor and the difficulties that prompted this evaluation, his illness had not interfered significantly with his work performance. He had become increasingly dissatisfied with his work, however, and so for the past 3 years, he had been enrolled in a Master's counseling program. Following completion of the program, he intended to retire from his government job and to work in the counseling field.

During evaluation, A.D. was very cooperative and worked hard at all tasks. He described his mood as "variable" and reported recent increased anxiety. He indicated that he had sought neuropsychological evaluation to determine how his cognitive difficulties might be affecting work and school and to help him make decisions regarding his future. He was particularly concerned about whether he would be able to continue his counseling work.

Neuropsychological data are shown in Table 11.9. Normative data were obtained from Heaton et al. (1991), from Spreen and Strauss (1991), and from associated test manuals (see also Mirsky, Fantie, and Tatman, this volume).

Global Functioning

A.D.'s Global Functioning (WAIS-R) was at the upper end of the average range for Verbal skills (Verbal IQ) and at the upper end of the low average range for Performance skills (Performance IQ). Access to old knowledge was well preserved (Information, Vocabulary, Similarities), but scores on measures of attention (Digit Span, Arithmetic, Digit Symbol) and timed visuospatial skills (Picture Completion, Picture Arrangement, Block Design) were below expectations of high average to superior performance, based on his background and his performance on crystallized intellectual measures.

Foundation Skills

Arousal and Attention

Impairment was noted in deployment of attention. Decreased arousal and fatigue were observed during the neuropsychological screening. Although focused attentional skills were mildly impaired (Digit Symbol, Trail Making Test, Stroop Interference Test), reflected predominantly by slowness, sustained attentional skills were severely impaired, reflected in both slowness and inaccuracy (Continuous Performance Tasks).

Attentional capacity/encoding also was impaired. His span of attention was low average to average for digits (Digit Span-Forwards), but poorer for a long word list (CVLT: Trial 1). A.D. also showed slight decline in task performance as information

TABLE 11.9. Case A.D.: Neuropsychological Data

Domain/test	Raw score	Normative score
Global functioning: General intellectual		
Full Scale IQ (Pro-rated)		99
Verbal IQ (Pro-rated)		108
Information		13
Digit Span		10
Vocabulary		14
Arithmetic		9
Similarities		13
Performance IQ (Pro-rated)		89
Picture Completion		11
Picture Arrangement		8
Block Design		7
Digit Symbol		8
Arousal and attention		
Trail Making Test		
Part A	40 sec.	T = 36
Part B	95 sec.	T = 32
Stroop Interference Test		
Words	72	T = 36
Colors	54	T = 36
Color/Word	30	T = 40
Interference	−1	T = 50
Continuous performance tasks		
X Task—Accuracy	49%	z<<−3.0
X Task—Reaction Time	600 ms	z<<−3.0
AX Task—Accuracy	38%	z<<−3.0
AX Task—Reaction Time	800 ms	z<<−3.0
Consonant Trigrams	26/42	z = −1.6
Motor functions		
Finger Tapping Test		
Dominant	26.8	T = 24
Nondominant	33.6	T = 37
Grooved Pegboard Test		
Dominant	146	T = 14
Nondominant	144	T = 22
Executive, reasoning, and problem-solving abilities		
Wisconsin Card Sorting Test		
Categories Achieved	2	z = −3.3
Total Errors	67	z = −3.6
Perseverative Errors	43	z<<−3.0
Failure to Maintain Set	1	z = −0.2
Rule Governed Drawing	12/12	z = +0.5
Porteus Maze Test—Test Age	9.5	z<<−3.0
Language functions		
Sentence Repetition Test	15	40th percentile
Boston Naming Test	55/60	z = −0.3
Controlled Oral Word Association Test		
F, A, S Total	28	z = −1.2
Animals	15	z = −1.2

TABLE 11.9. (Continued)

Domain/test	Raw score	Normative score
Controlled Oral Word Association Test (continued)		
Fruits and Vegetables	20	
First Names	24	
Boston Diagnostic Aphasia Examination		
Cookie Theft Picture Written Description	No errors	
Visuospatial functions		
Rey-Osterrieth Complex Figure—Copy	29/36	z<< −3.0
Learning and memory		
Wechsler Memory Scale-Revised		
Verbal Memory Index		86
Visual Memory Index		98
General Memory Index		103
Attention/Concentration Index		92
Delayed Recall Index		87
Logical Memory I	19	29th percentile
Logical Memory II	6	6th percentile
Logical Memory Savings	32%	
Visual Reproduction I	36	88th percentile
Visual Reproduction II	21	20th percentile
Visual Reproduction Savings	58%	
California Verbal Learning Test		
Total Words Trials 1 to 5	37	T = 21
Trial 1	6	z = −1
List B	7	z = 0
Short-Delay Free Recall	4	z = −3
Short-Delay Cued Recall	6	z = −3
Long-Delay Free Recall	5	z = −3
Long-Delay Cued Recall	6	z = −3
Long-Delay Recognition	12	z = −2
False Positives	1	z = 0
Total Perseverations	5	z = 0
Intrusions—Free Recall	1	z = 0
Intrusions—Cued Recall	6	z = +4
Semantic Cluster Ratio	0.7	z = −2
Serial Cluster Ratio	5.5	z = +2
Increment in Words Recalled/Trial	+0.7	z = −1
Percent Recall Consistency across Trials 1–5	71%	z = −2
Rey-Osterrieth Complex Figure		
30-minute Delayed Recall	6/36	z = −1.7
Personality and emotional functioning		
MMPI-2 Three-Point Code	3-2-7	

increased from the sentence (Sentence Repetition Test) to the paragraph (Logical Memory I) level. Thus, A.D. showed poorer encoding when the organization of material was not immediately obvious to him, but was better able to encode more organized material. Yet, he showed a tendency to overload as the amount of information presented increased. Resistance to interference was mildly to moderately impaired

(Consonant Trigrams), but mental manipulation skills were average (Digit Span-Backwards, Arithmetic, WMS-R Attention/Concentration Index).

Sensory and Motor Functions

Sensory functions were grossly intact. A.D.'s performances on motor measures were consistently poorer with his right, dominant hand, although performances were reduced bilaterally (Finger Tapping Test, Grooved Pegboard Test). This, perhaps, contributed to his slowness on other tasks with a motor component.

Executive, Problem-Solving, and Reasoning Abilities

Particularly severe impairment was noted in this component. A.D. had difficulty with awareness of problem-solving alternatives, shifting his thinking as required by tasks, and using feedback to guide his responses (Wisconsin Card Sorting Test, observation). Frequently, he became stuck and focused on incorrect details, leading to poor performances on a number of measures. Although verbal planning skills were within normal limits (Rule Governed Drawing), nonverbal planning skills were severely impaired and were marked by impulsivity and an inability to learn from his errors, *despite awareness of the errors* (Porteus Maze Test, observation).

Organizational skills were poor. On Block Design, for example, he took a trial-and-error approach, rather than an organized step-by-step strategy when attempting to construct the details of the designs. Even when the examiner gave him a systematic strategy to apply to the item on which he was working, he was unable to apply the strategy to subsequent items. On the CVLT, he made little use of the categories to facilitate his recall (CVLT: Semantic Cluster Ratio), and instead attempted to recall words by rote (CVLT: Serial Cluster Ratio); recall consistency across trials was poor (CVLT: Percent Recall Consistency across Trials 1–5).

Reasoning skills were variable. A.D. did best with reasoning tasks that tapped old verbal knowledge (Similarities). He did more poorly, however, on tasks with verbal and visuospatial demands. On Picture Completion, this was due mainly to slowness, as he completed several items correctly when time limits were suspended. On Picture Arrangement, however, he had more difficulty. A.D. was unable to complete many of the items, and his oral descriptions indicated that he failed to appreciate some of the subtle details in the pictures. His most notable difficulty was on a novel conceptual thinking task (Cohen-Freides Conceptual Thinking Test; data not shown), which required him to sort eight cards, with one word on each, into two categories of four, and then to sort them, repeatedly, using different criteria. Because the words differed on two semantic dimensions, the cards differed in size, and the letters differed in position, size, and color, a total of six sorts were possible. There were two sets of cards: an initial, learning set, and a second, transfer set. On the first set, he required demonstrations of most of the sorts. On the second set, he successfully completed three of the four previously presented categories and one of the two new categories, but was unable to complete the second of the two new categories. Instead, he perseverated on previously completed categories.

Modality-Specific Skills

Language Functions

Comprehension and production of spoken language were within the expected range (Vocabulary, Boston Naming Test, observation), with the exception of production of single words beginning with specific letters and from one category, which was mildly impaired (COWAT: F,A,S Total, Animals Total). This appeared to reflect the contribution of impaired organizational skills, rather than being a frank language deficit, since his performance improved substantially with the structure of two other semantic categories (COWAT: Fruits and Vegetables, First Names). A.D. also showed some word-finding difficulties on reasoning tasks (Similarities, Picture Completion). His ability to produce a writing sample was within expectations (Boston Diagnostic Aphasia Examination: Cookie Theft Picture Written Description).

Visuospatial Functions

There was no gross evidence of visuospatial perceptual impairment (Boston Naming Test, Picture Completion, observation). In contrast, A.D.'s visuospatial constructional skills were impaired, due to his difficulties with organizing an approach to his constructions (Block Design, Rey-Osterrieth Complex Figure Test-Copy).

Integrated Skills: Learning and Memory

Overall memory skills on the WMS-R were in the low average to average range (General Memory Index). On the CVLT, in addition to organizational difficulties, A.D. showed minimal improvement over the five learning trials (Total Words Trials 1 to 5; Increment in Words Recalled/Trial). Immediate (Short-Delay Free Recall) and 20-minute (Long-Delay Free Recall) delayed recall were both severely impaired, and delayed recognition (Long-Delay Recognition) was only slightly better, indicating that A.D.'s difficulties on the CVLT were due to problems with initial encoding. Although immediate recall of paragraphs was in the average range (Logical Memory I), A.D. lost much information over the 30-minute delay (32% savings), and his delayed recall was moderately impaired (Logical Memory II).

Performances on visual memory tasks were similar. Recall of simple visual designs was in the high average range (Visual Reproduction I), but A.D. lost considerable information during the delay (58% savings), and his delayed recall was at the low end of the average range (Visual Reproduction II). With increased complexity, his recall of visual information was severely impaired following a 30-minute delay (Rey-Osterrieth Complex Figure).

Personality and Emotional Functioning

A.D. completed the MMPI-2 in an honest manner, although he showed a slight tendency to gloss over and minimize his difficulties. The following symptoms and personality characteristics were noted in his profile (327-point code, review of other scales and critical items). A.D. reported a significant degree of depression, anxiety, and fatigue. He was experiencing difficulties concentrating, decreased interest in most activities, and reduced energy and efficiency in work-related activities. Somatic complaints were also evident. Interpersonally, A.D. presented as someone who tended to depend on others and to elicit nurturing support from those around him. At the same time, his positive characteristics of competitiveness and industriousness were evident, although his current state was limiting their expression. A.D. presented a strong veneer and frequently attempted to cover expression of his inner feelings. This defense, however, was not always successful, leading to feelings of anxiety and guilt about his situation. Finally, there was evidence in the profile that A.D., in general, tended to be very outgoing, social, personable, and well liked by others, although, again, these characteristics were being limited by his current depression and anxiety.

Summary and Recommendations

The evaluation revealed impairment in many aspects of A.D.'s cognitive and motor functioning, and these were consistent with his complaints, the observations of others, and the locus of structural brain damage noted on MRI scans. Although many skills were within the low average to average range, these were substantially below expectations, given his background. Particularly notable were his impairments in sustained attention, executive functions, and learning and memory. Learning and memory were reduced due to poor initial encoding, failure to use organization to facilitate recall, and loss of information over a delay. In contrast to areas of deficit, old verbal knowledge, language skills, and visuospatial skills were relatively well preserved. Interpersonal skills also remained an area of strength, and A.D. was fairly aware of his deficits and limitations. Despite awareness, however, he was usually unable to take steps needed to compensate for his difficulties, without guidance from others. A.D. was appropriately distressed about his situation. Nevertheless, this distress was insufficient to explain the degree of deficit.

Based on these findings, a number of recommendations were made. First, given his attentional impairments, it was recommended that his anticonvulsant medication regimen be reviewed for possible modification, since it was thought that these medications could be further reducing A.D.'s level of arousal and his attentional abilities. Second, it was recommended that he be provided with a supported work environment, including the use of a job coach. It was thought that a job coach might be able to help him to develop and apply compensatory strategies needed to continue working on the job. For example, it was suggested that using written instruction sheets might help A.D. cue himself to complete steps of common tasks. It was recognized, however, that the constraints of his work environment might not make this type of intervention possible.

A combined program of psychotherapy and cognitive remediation was also recommended. The focus of the program was to be on (1) helping him identify when he was having difficulties with a particular task, (2) breaking down the task into its component steps, and then (3) completing these steps in a consistent, organized manner.

It was thought that psychotherapy might help him identify more consistently when his problems occurred and might also help him integrate compensatory strategies into his life. Group psychotherapy, with high-level professionals who had suffered traumatic brain injury or similar types of neurological disorder, was recommended. It was thought that this could help A.D. with adjustment issues and could help him learn how others had coped with similar difficulties.

There were ethical concerns about A.D.'s ability to continue in his counseling program and to work effectively with his counseling clients. The examiner contacted A.D.'s supervisor and asked her to review his performance carefully using tape recordings from his counseling sessions. His counseling supervisor reported no decrements in A.D.'s counseling work. Notably, she stated that A.D. had successfully dealt with several difficult clients in the weeks around the neuropsychological evaluation. Review of the task demands indicated that A.D. was able to capitalize on his well-preserved verbal and interpersonal skills in the counseling sessions. He compensated for memory difficulties by taking notes. Since he was continuing to be supervised closely, it was believed that problems would be noticed and addressed, if and when they occurred. Because this was a significant part of A.D.'s life, the examiner was concerned about taking this away from him. Hence, it was recommended that his progress continue to be monitored carefully by audiotape, that he continue to take notes in sessions, and that he be provided with continuous feedback on his progress. A.D. was agreeable to these recommendations and recognized that he might have to give up the counseling work if it became apaprent to his supervisor that his performance was deteriorating.

The final recommendation was for neuropsychological reevaluation in 9 to 12 months. It was believed that this would help track any progression of his difficulties and would provide further information that would help with career decision making.

A.D. was seen for follow-up neuropsychological evaluation approximately 1 year later by a different examiner. Findings were consistent with the initial evaluation and showed no evidence of progressive decline in functioning. Within the year since the first evaluation, A.D.'s wife had died suddenly. He had sought counseling to deal with her death, but had not yet made a decision regarding his government job. The neuropsychologist evaluating him did not believe that A.D. would be capable of functioning as an independent counseling practitioner. He referred A.D. for a short period of speech/language therapy, to help him develop compensatory strategies. Although A.D. was referred for group psychotherapy as originally recommended, he was unable to follow through on this, due to his inability to drive independently.

CONCLUSIONS

This chapter has presented a framework for neuropsychological assessment. Although not strictly a cognitive neuropsychological model, the framework provides a method for selecting tests and for reviewing and integrating neuropsychological findings systematically. The framework also can be used with widely available clinical instruments, and incorporates both quantitative and qualitative information. It is believed that results of neuropsychological assessment must be conceptualized within this type of framework, based on knowledge of brain–behavior relationships. The failure to review findings systematically and comprehensively, similar to the way in which a physician reviews findings from a physical examination, can lead to missing important information. Further, use of a framework such as this can facilitate treatment planning. It also can facilitate explaining findings to the patient, always an important part of the assessment enterprise.

ACKNOWLEDGMENTS

The author would like to thank Daisy Pascualvaca, Ph.D., for providing data from the initial neuropsychological screening of A.D., and William Garmoe, Ph.D., for providing a summary of A.D.'s follow-up evaluation. The author would also like to thank Wendy A. Law, Ph.D., for her helpful comments during preparation of this chapter.

REFERENCES

Albert, M. L., Goodglass, H., Helm, N. A., Rubens, A. B., & Alexander, M. P. (1981). *Clinical aspects of dysphasia*. Vienna: Springer-Verlag.

Alderman, N., Evans, J. J., Burgess, P., & Wilson, B. A. (1993). Behavioural assessment of the dysexecutive syndrome. *Journal of Clinical and Experimental Neuropsychology, 15*, 69–70.

Alfano, D. P., Neilson, P. M., & Paniak, C. E. (1992). The MMPI and closed-head injury. *The Clinical Neuropsychologist, 6*, 134–142.

Baddeley, A., Emslie, H., & Nimmo-Smith, I. (1992). *Speed and Capacity of Language-Processing Test*. Bury St. Edmunds, England: Thames Valley Test Co.

Barkley, R. A. (1988). Attention. In M. G. Tramontana & S. R. Hooper (Eds.), *Assessment issues in child neuropsychology* (pp. 145–176). New York: Plenum Press.

Barona, A., Reynolds, C. R., & Chastain, R. (1984). A demographically-based index of premorbid intelligence for the WAIS-R. *Journal of Consulting and Clinical Psychology, 52*, 885–887.

Beck, A. T., & Steer, R. A. (1987). *Beck Depression Inventory manual*. San Antonio: Psychological Corporation.

Bennett-Levy, J. (1984). Determinants of performance on the Rey-Osterrieth Complex Figure Test: An analysis, and a new technique for single-case assessment. *British Journal of Clinical Psychology, 23*, 109–119.

Benton, A. L., Hamsher, K. deS., Varney, N. R., & Spreen, O. (1983). *Contributions to neuropsychological assessment*. New York: Oxford University Press.

Bornstein, R. A. (1986a). Consistency of intermanual discrepancies in normal and unilateral brain lesion patients. *Journal of Consulting and Clinical Psychology, 54*, 719–723.

Bornstein, R. A. (1986b). Normative data on intermanual differences on three tests of motor performance. *Journal of Clinical and Experimental Neuropsychology, 8*, 12–20.

Bornstein, R. A., & Kozora, E. (1990). Content bias of the MMPI Sc scale in neurological patients. *Neuropsychiatry, Neuropsychology, and Behavioral Neurology, 3*, 200–205.

Briggs, G. G., & Nebes, R. D. (1975). Patterns of hand preference in a student population. *Cortex, 11*, 230–238.

Brown, J. (1958). Some tests of the decay theory of immediate memory. *Quarterly Journal of Experimental Psychology, 10*, 12–21.

Brown, J. I., Fishco, V. V., & Hanna, G. (1993). *The Nelson-Denny Reading Test.* Chicago: Riverside Publishing Co.

Buschke, H. (1973). Selective reminding for analysis of memory and learning. *Journal of Verbal Learning and Verbal Behavior, 12,* 543–550.

Butcher, J. N., Dahlstrom, W. G., Graham, J. R., Tellegen, A., & Kaemer, B. (1989). *Manual for administration and scoring. Minnesota Multiphasic Personality Inventory-2: MMPI-2.* Minneapolis: University of Minnesota Press.

Butters, N. (1993). Some comments on the goals and direction of *Neuropsychology. Neuropsychology, 7,* 3–4.

Butters, N., & Cermak, L. S. (1980). *Alcoholic Korsakoff's syndrome: An information processing approach to amnesia.* New York: Academic Press.

Butters, N., Salmon, D. P., Cullum, C. M., Cairns, P., Tröster, A. I., & Jacobs, D. (1988). Differentiation of amnesic and demented patients with the Wechsler Memory Scale-Revised. *The Clinical Neuropsychologist, 2,* 133–148.

Carlesimo, G. A., Fadda, L., & Caltagirone, C. (1993). Basic mechanisms of constructional apraxia in unilateral brain-damaged patients: Role of visuo-perceptual and executive disorders. *Journal of Clinical and Experimental Neuropsychology, 15,* 342–358.

Cohen, R. F., & Mapou, R. L. (1988). Neuropsychological assessment for treatment planning: A hypothesis testing approach. *Journal of Head Trauma Rehabilitation, 3*(1), 12–23.

Corwin, J., & Bylsma, F. W. (1993). Translations of excerpts from Andre Rey's "Psychological examination of traumatic encephalopathy" and P. A. Osterrieth's "The Complex Figure Copy Test." *The Clinical Neuropsychologist, 7,* 3–21.

Crawford, J. R., Stewart, L. E., & Moore, J. W. (1989). Demonstration of savings on the AVLT and development of a parallel form. *Journal of Clinical and Experimental Neuropsychology, 11,* 975–981.

Cripe, L. I., Maxwell, J., & Hill, E. L. (1991). Discrimination of neurologic, pain, and psychiatric patients with MMPI variables. *The Clinical Neuropsychologist, 5,* 278.

Cullum, C. M., Butters, N., Tröster, A. I., & Salmon, D. P. (1990). Normal aging and forgetting rates on the Wechsler Memory Scale-Revised. *Archives of Clinical Neuropsychology, 5,* 23–30.

Delis, D., Kramer, J. H., Kaplan, E., & Ober, B. A. (1987). *California Verbal Learning Test* (Research ed.). San Antonio: Psychological Corporation.

Delis, D. C., Massman, P. J., Butters, N., Salmon, D. P., Shear, P. K., Demadura, T., & Filoteo, J. V. (1992). Spatial cognition in Alzheimer's disease: Subtypes of global–local impairment. *Journal of Clinical and Experimental Neuropsychology, 14,* 463–477.

Delis, D. C., McKee, R., Massman, P. J., Kramer, J. H., Kaplan, E., & Gettman, D. (1991). Alternate form of the California Verbal Learning Test: Development and reliability. *The Clinical Neuropsychologist, 5,* 154–162.

De Renzi, E., & Vignolo, L. (1962). The Token Test: A sensitive test to detect receptive disturbances in aphasics. *Brain, 85,* 665–678.

Derogatis, L. R. (1992). *SCL-90-R administration, scoring, and procedure manual* (2nd ed.). Minneapolis, MN: National Computer Systems.

Dodrill, C. B., & Thoreson, N. S. (1993). Reliability of the Lateral Dominance Examination. *Journal of Clinical and Experimental Neuropsychology, 15,* 183–190.

Dunn, L. M., & Dunn, L. M. (1981). *Peabody Picture Vocabulary Test-Revised.* Circle Pines, MN: American Guidance Services.

Eppinger, M. G., Craig, P. L., Adams, R. L., & Parsons, O. A. (1987). The WAIS-R index for estimating premorbid intelligence: Cross-validation and clinical utility. *Journal of Consulting and Clinical Psychology, 55,* 86–90.

Eslinger, P. J., & Damasio, A. R. (1985). Severe disturbance of higher cognition after bilateral frontal lobe ablation: Patient EVR. *Neurology, 35,* 1731–1741.

Exner, J. E. (1974). *The Rorschach: A comprehensive system.* New York: Wiley & Sons.

Feldman, M. J., & Drasgow, J. (1981). *Visual-Verbal Test.* Los Angeles: Western Psychological Services.

Fridlund, A. J., & Delis, D. C. (1987). *California Verbal Learning Test research edition: IBM user's guide*. San Antonio: Psychological Corporation.

Gass, C. S., & Russell, E. W. (1986). Minnesota Multiphasic Personality Inventory correlates of lateralized cerebral lesions and aphasic deficits. *Journal of Consulting and Clinical Psychology, 54*, 359–363.

Geffen, G., Moar, K. J., O'Hanlon, A. P., Clark, C. R., & Geffen, L. B. (1990). Performance measures of 16- to 86-year-old males and females on the Auditory Verbal Learning Test. *The Clinical Neuropsychologist, 4*, 45–63.

Geschwind, N., & Behan, P. O. (1984). Laterality, hormones, and immunity. In N. Geschwind & A. M. Galaburda (Eds.), *Cerebral dominance* (pp. 211–224). Cambridge, MA: Harvard University Press.

Geschwind, N., & Galaburda, A. M. (1987). *Cerebral lateralization*. Cambridge, MA: MIT Press.

Golden, C. J. (1978). *Stroop Color and Word Test: A manual for clinical and experimental uses*. Chicago: Stoelting.

Goodglass, H., & Kaplan, E. (1983). *The assessment of aphasia and related disorders*. Philadelphia: Lea & Febiger.

Gordon, M. (1989). *The Gordon Diagnostic System*. Dewitt, NY: Gordon Systems, Inc.

Gorham, D. R. (1956). A proverbs test for clinical and experimental use. *Psychological Reports, 1*, 1–12.

Grober, E., & Sliwinski, M. (1991). Development and validation of a model for estimating pre-morbid verbal intelligence in the elderly. *Journal of Clinical and Experimental Neuropsychology, 13*, 933–949.

Gronwall, D. M. A. (1977). Paced auditory serial-addition test: A measure of recovery from concussion. *Perceptual and Motor Skills, 44*, 367–373.

Hannay, H. J., & Levin, H. S. (1985). Selective Reminding Test: An examination of the equivalence of four forms. *Journal of Clinical and Experimental Neuropsychology, 7*, 251–263.

Hartman, D. E. (1991). Reply to Reitan: Unexamined premises and the evolution of clinical neuropsychology. *Archives of Clinical Neuropsychology, 6*, 147–165.

Hathaway, S. R., & McKinley, J. C. (1967). *Minnesota Multiphasic Personality Inventory manual* (rev. ed.). New York: Psychological Corporation.

Heaton, R. K., Chelune, G. J., Talley, J. L., Kay, G. G., & Curtiss, G. (1993). *Wisconsin Card Sorting Test Manual-Revised and Expanded*. Odessa, FL: Psychological Assessment Resources.

Heaton, R. K., Grant, I., & Matthews, C. G. (1991). *Comprehensive norms for an expanded Halstead-Reitan Battery*. Odeassa, FL: Psychological Assessment Resources.

Heilbronner, R. L. (1992). The search for a "pure" visual memory test: Pursuit of perfection? *The Clinical Neuropsychologist, 6*, 105–112.

Heilman, K. M., Watson, R. T., & Valenstein, E. (1985). Neglect and related disorders. In K. M. Heilman & E. Valenstein (Eds.), *Clinical neuropsychology* (pp. 243–293). New York: Oxford University Press.

Kane, R. L., & Perrine, K. R. (1988). Construct validity of a nonverbal analogue to the selective reminding verbal learning test. *Journal of Clinical and Experimental Neuropsychology, 10*, 85.

Kaplan, E. (1988). A process approach to neuropsychological assessment. In T. Boll & B. K. Bryant (Eds.), *Clinical neuropsychology and brain function: Research, measurement, and practice* (pp. 129–167). Washington, DC: American Psychological Association.

Kaplan, E. (1990). The process approach to neuropsychological assessment of psychiatric patients. *Journal of Neuropsychiatry and Clinical Neurosciences, 2*, 72–87.

Kaplan, E. (1993, March). *The Boston Process Approach to neuropsychological assessment*. Workshop held at Walter Reed Army Medical Center, Washington, DC.

Kaplan, E., Fein, D., Morris, R., & Delis, D. C. (1991). *The WAIS-R as a neuropsychological instrument*. San Antono: Psychological Corporation.

Kaplan, E., Goodglass, H., & Weintraub, S. (1983). *Boston Naming Test*. Philadelphia: Lea & Febiger.

Kirk, U., & Kelly, M. S. (1986). *Scoring scale for the Rey-Osterrieth Complex Figure*. New York: Columbia University.

Kramer, J. H., Kaplan, E., Blusewicz, M. J., & Preston, K. A. (1991). Visual hierarchical analysis of Block Design configural errors. *Journal of Clinical and Experimental Neuropsychology, 13,* 455–465.

Leckliter, I. N., & Matarazzo, J. D. (1989). The influence of age, education, IQ, gender, and alcohol abuse on Halstead-Reitan Neuropsychological Test Battery performance. *Journal of Clinical Psychology, 45,* 484–511.

Leonberger, F. T. (1989). The question of organicity: Is it still functional? *Professional Psychology: Research and Practice, 20,* 411–414.

Lezak, M. D. (1982). The problem of assessing executive functions. *International Journal of Psychology, 17,* 281–297.

Lezak, M. D. (1983). *Neuropsychological assessment* (2nd ed.). New York: Oxford University Press.

Lezak, M. D. (1988). IQ: R. I. P. *Journal of Clinical and Experimental Neuropsychology, 10,* 351–361.

Loring, D. W. (1989). The Wechsler Memory Scale-Revised, or the Wechsler Memory Scale-Revisited? *The Clinical Neuropsychologist, 3,* 59–69.

Loring, D. W., & Papanicolaou, A. C. (1987). Memory assessment in neuropsychology: Theoretical considerations and practical utility. *Journal of Clinical and Experimental Neuropsychology, 9,* 340–358.

Luria, A. R. (1980). *Higher cortical functions in man* (2nd ed.). New York: Basic Books.

Mack, J. L. (1979). The MMPI and neurological dysfunction. In C. S. Newmark (Ed.), *MMPI: Clinical and research trends* (pp. 53–79). New York: Praeger.

Mapou, R. L. (1988a). An integrated approach to the neuropsychological assessment of cognitive function. In J. M. Williams & C. J. Long (Eds.), *Cognitive approaches to neuropsychology* (pp. 101–122). New York: Plenum Press.

Mapou, R. L. (1988b). Testing to detect brain damage: An alternative to what may no longer be useful. *Journal of Clinical and Experimental Neuropsychology, 10,* 271–278.

Matarazzo, J. D. (1990). Psychological assessment versus psychological testing. *American Psychologist, 45,* 999–1017.

Matthews, C. G., & Kløve, H. (1964). *Instruction manual for the Adult Neuropsychology Test Battery.* Madison, WI: University of Wisconsin Medical School.

McCarney, D., & Greenberg, L. M. (1990). *Test of Variables of Attention Computer Program Version 5.01 for IBM PC or IBM Compatibles. TOVA manual.* Minneapolis: University of Minnesota Press.

McCarthy, R. A., & Warrington, E. K. (1990). *Cognitive neuropsychology: A clinical introduction.* San Diego: Academic Press.

Money, J. (1976). *A Standardized Road-Map Test of Directional Sense.* San Rafael, CA: Academic Therapy Publications.

Monsch, A. U., Bondi, M. W., Butters, N., Paulsen, J. S., Salmon, D. P., Brugger, P., & Swensen, M. R. (1994). A comparison of category and letter fluency in Alzheimer's disease and Huntington's disease. *Neuropsychology, 8,* 25–30.

Nelson, H. E., & O'Connell, A. (1978). Dementia: The estimation of premorbid intelligence levels using the New Adult Reading Test. *Cortex, 14,* 234–244.

Oldfield, R. C. (1971). The assessment and analysis of handedness: The Edinburgh inventory. *Neuropsychologia, 9,* 97–113.

Parasuraman, R. (1984). Sustained attention in detection and discrimination. In R. Parasuraman & D. R. Davies (Eds.), *Varieties of attention* (pp. 243–271). Orlando, FL: Academic Press.

Perrine, K. (1993). Differential aspects of conceptual processing in the Category Test and Wisconsin Card Sorting Test. *Journal of Clinical and Experimental Neuropsychology, 15,* 461–473.

Peterson, L. R., & Peterson, M. J. (1959). Short-term retention of individual verbal items. *Journal of Experimental Psychology, 58,* 193–198.

Porteus, S. D. (1965). *Porteus Maze Test: Fifty years' application.* New York: Psychological Corporation.

Purdue Research Foundation. (1948). *Examiner's manual for the Purdue Pegboard.* Chicago: Science Research Associates.

Raven, J. C. (1960). *Guide to the Standard Progressive Matrices.* London: H. K. Lewis.

Raven, J. C. (1965). *Guide to using the Coloured Progressive Matrices*. London: H. K. Lewis.

Reitan, R. M., & Davison, L. A. (Eds.). (1974). *Clinical neuropsychology: Current status and applications*. Washington, DC: V. H. Winston & Sons.

Reitan, R. M., & Wolfson, D. (1985). *The Halstead-Reitan Neuropsychological Test Battery: Theory and clinical interpretation*. Tucson: Neuropsychology Press.

Roeltgen, D. (1985). Agraphia. In K. M. Heilman & E. Valenstein (Eds.), *Clinical neuropsychology* (pp. 75–96). New York: Oxford University Press.

Rosvold, H. E., Mirsky, A. F., Sarason, I., Bransome, E. D., & Beck, L. H. (1956). A continuous performance test of brain damage. *Journal of Consulting Psychology, 20*, 343–350.

Shallice, T., & Burgess, P. (1991). Deficits in strategy application following frontal lobe damage. *Brain, 114*, 727–741.

Shallice, T., & Evans, M. E. (1978). The involvement of the frontal lobes in cognitive estimation. *Cortex, 14*, 294–303.

Shum, D. H. K., McFarland, K. A., & Bain, J. D. (1990). Construct validity of eight tests of attention: Comparison of normal and closed head injured subjects. *The Clinical Neuropsychologist, 4*, 151–162.

Sohlberg, M. M., & Mateer, C. A. (1989). *Introduction to cognitive rehabilitation*. New York: Guilford Press.

Spielberger, C. D., Gorsuch, R. L., Lushene, R., Vagg, P. R., & Jacobs, G. A. (1983). *Manual for the State-Trait Anxiety Inventory (Form Y)*. Palo Alto: Consulting Psychologists Press.

Spreen, O., & Benton, A. L. (1977). *Neurosensory Center Comprehensive Examination for Aphasia*. Victoria, B. C.: University of Victoria, Neuropsychology Laboratory.

Spreen, O., & Strauss, E. (1991). *A compendium of neuropsychological tests*. New York: Oxford University Press.

Squire, L. S., & Butters, N. (Eds.). (1992). *The neuropsychology of memory* (2nd ed.). New York: Guilford Press.

Stebbins, G. T., Gilley, D. W., Wilson, R. S., Bernard, A., & Fox, H. (1990). Effects of language disturbances on premorbid estimates of IQ in mild dementia. *The Clinical Neuropsychologist, 4*, 64–68.

Stebbins, G. T., Wilson, R. S., Gilley, D. W., Bernard, D. A., & Fox, H. (1990). Use of the National Adult Reading Test to estimate premorbid IQ in dementia. *The Clinical Neuropsychologist, 4*, 18–24.

Stern, R. A., Singer, E. A., Duke, L. M., Singer, N. G., Morey, C. E., Daughtrey, E. W., & Kaplan, E. (1994). The Boston Qualitative Scoring System for the Rey-Osterrieth Complex Figure: Description and interrater reliability. *The Clinical Neuropsychologist, 8*, 309–322.

Stuss, D. T., Stethem, L. L., Hugenholtz, H., & Richard, M. T. (1989). Traumatic brain injury: A comparison of three clinical tests, and analysis of recovery. *The Clinical Neuropsychologist, 3*, 145–156.

Stuss, D. T., Stethem, L. L., & Poirier, C. A. (1987). Comparison of three tests of attention and rapid information processing across six age groups. *The Clinical Neuropsychologist, 1*, 139–152.

Thorndike, R. L., Hagen, E. R., & Sattler, J. M. (1986). *Stanford-Binet Intelligence Scale* (4th ed.). Chicago: Riverside Publishing Co.

Trahan, D. E., & Larrabee, G. J. (1988). *Professional manual: Continuous Visual Memory Test*. Odessa, FL: Psychological Assessment Resources.

Tröster, A. I., Butters, N., Salmon, D. P., Cullum, C. M., Jacobs, D., Brandt, J., & White, R. F. (1993). The diagnostic utility of savings scores: Differentiating Alzheimer's and Huntington's diseases with the Logical Memory and Visual Reproduction tests. *Journal of Clinical and Experimental Neuropsychology, 15*, 773–788.

Waber, D. P., & Holmes, J. M. (1985). Assessing children's copy productions of the Rey-Osterrieth Complex Figure. *Journal of Clinical and Experimental Neuropsychology, 7*, 264–280.

Warrington, E. K. (1982). The double dissociation of short and long-term memory deficits. In L. S. Cermak (Ed.), *Human memory and amnesia* (pp. 61–76). Hillsdale, NJ: Lawrence Erlbaum.

Warrington, E. K. (1984). *Recognition Memory Test*. Windsor, England: NFER-Nelson.

Warrington, E. K., & James, M. (1991). *Visual Object and Space Perception Battery*. Bury St. Edmunds, England: Thames Valley Test Co.

Wechsler, D. (1981). *Wechsler Adult Intelligence Scale-Revised manual*. San Antonio: Psychological Corporation.

Wechsler, D. (1987). *Wechsler Memory Scale-Revised*. San Antono: Psychological Corporation.

Western Psychological Services. (1983). *Hooper Visual Organization Test manual*. Los Angeles: Author.

Whyte, J. (1992a). Attention and arousal: Basic science aspects. *Archives of Physical Medicine and Rehabilitation, 73*, 940–949.

Whyte, J. (1992b). Neurologic disorders of attention and arousal: Assessment and treatment. *Archives of Physical Medicine and Rehabilitation, 73*, 1094–1103.

Wiederholt, J. L., & Bryant, B. R. (1992). *Gray Oral Reading Tests* (3rd ed.). Austin: Pro-Ed.

Wilkinson, G. S. (1993). *Wide Range Achievement Test 3*. Wilmington, DE: Jastak Associates.

Wilson, B. A. (1993). Ecological validity of neuropsychological assessment: Do neuropsychological indexes predict performance in everyday activities? *Applied and Preventive Psychology, 2*, 209–216.

Woodcock, R. W., & Johnson, M. B. (1989). *Woodcock-Johnson Psychoeducational Battery-Revised*. Chicago: Riverside Publishing Co.

Wooten, A. (1983). MMPI profiles among neuropsychology patients. *Journal of Clinical Psychology, 39*, 392–406.

12

Integrating Cognitive and Clinical Neuropsychology

Current Issues and Future Directions

JACK SPECTOR

INTRODUCTION

This volume was designed to describe the application of cognitively based neuropsychological methods to clinical practice. What the present chapters have in common is neither a specific set of procedures nor a particular theoretical model, but rather an endorsement of cognitively based neuropsychological assessment methods. These methods emphasize the assessment of individual cognitive processes, in order to understand the nature of brain–behavior relationships in persons with known or suspected brain impairment (Margolin, 1991). In addition, most chapters discuss comparison of performance on standardized tests to normative data, as part of developing an understanding of the nature of an individual patient's deficits. Thus, cognitively based assessment represents an approach that incorporates contributions from both cognitive and clinical neuropsychology.

It is relatively easy to define what cognitively based neuropsychological assessment typically does *not* involve. Standardized testing, strict scoring of responses, and referencing performance to normative data are not the only or most important goals in cognitively based neuropsychological evaluation (cf. Coltheart, 1985; McCarthy & Warrington, 1990). What these approaches *do* involve is somewhat more difficult to define, but includes, first, a breakdown of cognitive functioning into distinct functional domains (e.g., attention, memory, language), with the assumption that each cognitive domain is mediated by a number of functionally distinct, underlying processing com-

JACK SPECTOR • Division of Neurosurgery and Department of Psychology, Walter Reed Army Medical Center, Washington, DC 20307-5001.

Clinical Neuropsychological Assessment: A Cognitive Approach, edited by Robert L. Mapou and Jack Spector. Plenum Press, New York, 1995.

ponents. Paralleling the cognitive neuropsychological methods, these components, or modules (Fodor, 1983), are believed to interact, and can be understood or recognized only by applying a hierarchical model of cognitive functioning and by testing limits methodically and specifically (Coltheart, 1985; Shallice, 1979). For example, Mirsky, Fantie, and Tatman (Chapter 2, this volume) have illustrated the application of a multicomponent model of attention to clinical assessment. Similarly, Glosser and Friedman (Chapter 5, this volume) have shown how a cognitive neuropsychological model of reading, in which several routes of single-word reading are hypothesized, can be used to understand clinical disorders of reading.

A second aspect of cognitively based assessment is an appreciation of the single-case study as a means for understanding the various interactions within and among cognitive processing components and domains that, in combination, determine the final, observed test performance (Marshall & Newcombe, 1984; Robertson, Knight, Rafal, & Shimamura, 1993). This, again, reflects contributions from cognitive neuropsychology, in that the single-case study can illustrate the specific interactions between cognitive processing components and domains that, in combination, determine that individual's unique cognitive capacities. In fact, some cognitive neuropsychologists, the so-called "radical neuropsychologists" (McCloskey, 1993; Robertson et al., 1993), believe that the cognitive processing differences between similarly diagnosed patients are so great that important sources of variance are lost when these patients are grouped together under a single, encompassing diagnosis (Bub & Bub, 1988; Caramazza & Badecker, 1989). Therefore, for the radical neuropsychologists, the single-case study may be the only legitimate means to investigate and understand cognition.

Finally, in cognitively based assessment approaches, there is an emphasis on understanding the process by which a patient solves a neuropsychological task, through observing performance and analyzing errors, in addition to noting the final outcome or summary score. Thus, cognitively based assessment emphasizes both "process and achievement" aspects of individual performance on neuropsychological tests, reflecting influences of both cognitive and clinical neuropsychology.

Several definitions are necessary before proceeding to examine the complementary contributions of cognitive and clinical neuropsychology to the assessment methods described in this volume. For the purposes of clarity, the term *cognitive neuropsychology* will be used to refer specifically to the types of approaches described by Coltheart (1985), McCarthy and Warrington (1990), and others, in which the performance of neurologically compromised individuals is of interest primarily for developing and evaluating theoretical models of normal cognitive function. In contrast, the term *clinical neuropsychology* will be used to refer to the more familiar, psychometrically based clinical assessment approaches designed to identify specific cognitive strengths and weaknesses in neurologically compromised individuals, by using more quantitative and actuarial methods of interpretation. Finally, the term *cognitively based assessment* will be used to refer to the types of approaches described in this volume that emphasize relating the pattern and level of cognitive performance to specific types of brain disorder. That is, the patient's particular pattern of cognitive strengths and deficits is used to (1) diagnose the neurological or psychiatric disorder and (2) make recommendations for treatment. Therefore, cognitively based assessment incorporates elements of both clinical and cognitive neuropsychology (see, for example, Mapou, 1988a, and Chapter 11, this volume), in that (1) there is an emphasis on cognition and understanding the process by which a patient accomplishes a task, and (2) the importance of referencing results to normative data is not completely discarded.

This chapter will discuss some of the origins, issues, and advantages of cognitively based neuropsychological assessment. Several of the common influences on cognitive and clinical neuropsychology will be discussed first. It will be shown that these two approaches have much in common historically and that integration of these common elements form the foundation of cognitively based assessment. Next, issues regarding selection of appropriate psychometric measures will be discussed, with particular emphasis on single-case versus group-based research designs and the necessity of developing new testing methodologies. In the following section, the relative importance of neural models will be considered, after which the advantages of cognitively based assessment for evaluation of complex clinical problems, including psychiatric and psychosocial aspects of neurological disorder, will be addressed. The chapter will conclude with discussion of the contributions of these methods to the development of treatment interventions.

COMMON INFLUENCES ON COGNITIVE AND CLINICAL NEUROPSYCHOLOGY

Despite differences in their emphases, cognitive and clinical neuropsychology draw from a number of related disciplines for their terminology, methods, and objectives. According to Margolin (1991), the first forays into detailed description of higher cognitive processes and their clinical correlation appear in the literature on aphasia. In fact, many of the terms now used to describe cognitive functioning in different domains, such as fluency, depth of processing, pragmatics, and context, were originally used with respect to language and language-related functions (Lesser, 1987). In clinical neuropsychology, the use of test batteries and multiple, complementary instruments permitted assessment of language functions for the purpose of aphasia subtyping, and formed the basis for diagnostic strategies involving other cognitive processes (Luria, 1980). In cognitive neuropsychology, critiques of aphasia subtyping led to a rejection of these strongly localizationistic models of language and to the development of modular, cognitive processing models. Similar types of models were developed in turn for other realms of cognitive functioning (McCarthy & Warrington, 1990).

In addition to terminology and models, a number of the methods for assessment and clinical description that form the basis of both cognitive and clinical neuropsychology owe much to the study of brain and language (Lesser, 1987; Margolin, 1991). Even as the first efforts at defining a neuropsychology of language fell into a tradition of localization and syndrome analysis, ironically the first rejections of the localizationistic model appear in the area of language as well (Caramazza, 1984). This became an important foundation of cognitive neuropsychology, with its emphasis on the unique aspects of information processing within each individual, combined with the rejection of group normative performance. Similarly, Caplan (Chapter 4, this volume) and Glosser and Friedman (Chapter 5, this volume) note that modern aphasiology also provided clinical neuropsychology with a rejection of traditional localizationistic models, as well as a diverse literature, a multidisciplinary tradition, and a well-established appreciation for variations in normal functioning. Thus, both cognitive and clinical neuropsychology share a long and close relationship with aphasiology and psycholinguistics (Margolin, 1991).

A second common influence on cognitive and clinical neuropsychology is the work of A. R. Luria. Jørgensen and Christensen (Chapter 8, this volume) suggest that Luria's contributions to cognitively based assessment include an emphasis on the dynamic and integrated nature of higher cognitive processes within individuals, across persons, and across stimulus and response modalities. As specific examples, McCarthy and Warrington (1990) detailed Luria's influence on cognitive neuropsychological descriptions of motor performance, acoustic analysis, aphasia subtyping, verbal comprehension, and short-term memory. Similarly, Luria advocated the intentional deemphasis of group data and normatively based testing, and the idea that standardization and reproducibility are the only paths to establishing the usefulness of evaluation efforts (see Jørgensen & Christensen, Chapter 8, this volume). Thus, Luria's approach contributed to an emphasis on the single-case study as a means to understanding brain functioning in clinical settings.

Within clinical neuropsychology, the concept of interrelated functional systems, the futility of localization within such an integrated system, and the value of double dissociation to elucidate brain function also can be traced to Luria (1973, 1980). Many practicing clinical neuropsychologists today use aspects of Luria's model to conceptualize brain functioning and to guide clinical assessment (Mapou, Spector, & Kay, in press).

A third influence on both cognitive and clinical neuropsychology is the work of Teuber (McCarthy & Warrington, 1990). In a series of studies, Teuber and Rudel (1962) constructed a set of tasks designed to systematically identify discrete components of spatial, perceptual, and attentional skills, laying the groundwork for many cognitive neuropsychological methods. In addition, Teuber went on to detail the ways that cognitive processes were differentially affected in acute and chronic brain disease and at different points in the lifespan, providing contributions to clinical neuropsychology, as well. Thus, Teuber's application of experimental rigor and laboratory standards of control to test models of brain and behavior established a standard and methodology for cognitive neuropsychology, and also helped shape the careers of a number of clinical neuropsychologists who followed.

A final influence on cognitive and clinical neuropsychology, although more so on the former than the latter, is the work of the "radical" cognitive neuropsychologists. As noted, the radical position holds that research designs that group individual patients into diagnostic categories in an attempt to identify common cognitive deficits are flawed, in that they typically collapse data over meaningful qualities of individual patient behavior. These group approaches are seen as problematic, because they often attribute genuine differences in the effects of brain damage identified between similarly diagnosed individuals to error variance (Bub & Bub, 1988; Caramazza & Badecker, 1989; Shallice, 1979). For the radical cognitive neuropsychologist, the range of cognitive activities of which humans are capable is reflected in the variability that can be identified between different patients with similar diagnoses. Therefore, the radical cognitive neuropsychological position asserts that single-case methods are the only way to understand brain–behavior relationships, and that the goal of such investigations is an improved understanding of normal brain functioning (Caramazza & McCloskey, 1988; McCloskey, 1993; Whitaker & Slotnick, 1988). Thus, description of the range of cognitive activities identified through single-case studies is the hallmark of radical cognitive neuropsychology, as is the emphasis on modularity (Fodor, 1983), the belief that cognitive functions are organized into discrete operational modules, and that through the assessment of such modules, the nature of relationships among modules can be tested. These principles reflect some of the integral foundations of current methods used in both cognitive and clinical neuropsychological investigation.

In summary, both cognitive and clinical neuropsychology have been shaped by a number of common influences, including aphasiology and linguistics, Luria's model of brain functioning, Teuber's research on discrete cognitive skills and his method of controlled evaluation of cognitive models, and single-subject experimental methodologies. Radical approaches to cognitive neuropsychology, in particular, established a justification for the single-case investigation as a way to understand cognitive functioning in normal and brain-impaired patients, and led to the development of highly individualized assessment methods. These influences are reflected in the work of many of the contributors to this volume.

ISSUES OF STANDARDIZATION, LOCALIZATION, AND HIGHER ORDER FUNCTIONING

What Should Be the Role of Psychometrics in Cognitively Based Assessment?

The approaches described in this volume vary in the amount of emphasis placed on psychometric rigor and normative data. Some process-oriented neuropsychologists use standardized instruments as a starting point for clinical investigation (cf. Kaplan, 1988; Lezak, 1983; Walsh, Chapter 10, this volume), and most contributors to this volume use normative data for interpretation. However, several contributors (see, for example, Jørgensen & Christensen, Chapter 8; and Kay & Franklin, Chapter 9) place substantially less emphasis on such strategies from the start. Similarly, although some of the theoretical models that have been developed to describe cognitive functioning are derived directly from the results of research using familiar, normatively based tests (see Mirsky, Fantie, and Tatman, Chapter 2, this volume), others use only nonstandardized measures (see Caplan, Chapter 4, this volume; Caramazza, 1986).

Based on what has been discussed previously, it might appear, at first, that standardized, normatively based tests would be antithetical to cognitively based assessment approaches. In fact, it could be argued that in clinical practice, such instruments promote the loss of meaningful data by overly structuring the assessment process. This could prevent identification of an individual patient's unique pattern of cognitive strengths and weaknesses, by failing to test limits and by failing to recognize that a final score on a test can reflect vastly different approaches to the solution.

On the other hand, if group or normatively based data are accepted as an important source of information from which valid generalizations can be made (Kane, Goldstein, & Parsons, 1989; Reitan, 1989), conclusions can be drawn regarding larger groups of patients or wider ranges of skills, and predictions can be tested. Therefore, the psychometric tradition provides standardization, diagnostic utility, relatively easy scoring of data, and a more atheoretical stance regarding the structure of human cognition (Kane, 1991). The latter point is particularly important, because it permits the relationships between the modules of cognitive behavior to declare themselves without the imposition of a direct theoretical framework. Ironically, this is a goal of the cognitive neuropsychological method, as well (Caramazza, 1992). Finally, standardized measures are readily available, are accompanied by normative data and guidelines for interpretation, are more easily accessed, and in principle, ensure standardization of administration and interpretation across clinical settings and examiners. For these reasons, standardized measures offer a number of important features that facilitate clinical assessment.

In contrast to these features, there are several disadvantages of cognitive neuropsychological measures. For example, Mapou (1988a, and Chapter 11, this volume) notes that most cognitive neuropsychological instruments are unavailable to clinical neuropsychologists and are not easily applied to clinical practice. Unpublished, modified, or overly flexible instruments commonly used in cognitive neuropsychology are not easily taught, transferred between settings, or applied to different clinical samples. Moreover, clinical interpretation requires considerable experience with the specific tests. Based on these difficulties, it can be argued, therefore, that the techniques and procedures of cognitive neuropsychology have the most meaningful effects on mainstream clinical practice only after assessment measures have been demonstrated to possess psychometrically useful levels of reliability and validity. Examples of such measures include the California Verbal Learning Test (Delis, Kramer, Kaplan, & Ober, 1987) and cognitive neuropsychological methods that recently have been standardized and published (see Mapou, Chapter 11, this volume, for a brief discussion).

Thus, there are many advantages of using psychometrically derived instruments for cognitively based assessment in clinical practice. However, there are questions as to whether traditional psychometric standards can be, or even should be, applied to certain aspects of cognitively based assessment. For example, reliability and validity imply standards for instruments and test behavior that may not be meaningful for the cognitive neuropsychological investigation (Bates, Appelbaum, & Allard, 1991; Caramazza & Badecker, 1989; Jørgensen & Christensen, Chapter 8, this volume). Similarly, statistical power (a test's sensitivity to "true" differences between subjects) and its relationship to the null hypothesis imply a dichotomy between normal and abnormal cognitive activity rather than a continuum of function. Consequently, psychometric power frequently requires the sacrifice of the rare, marginal, complex, or subclinical case (McCloskey, 1993). As a developing science, cognitive neuropsychology is dependent on relatively rare syndromes and clinical subtypes in order to develop and test models of brain and behavior. Because of this, cognitive neuropsychologists have argued that they cannot afford to lose data to a false negative error, as may occur with psychometrically driven measurements (Caramazza, 1992). Consequently, the dichotomy between intact and impaired performance, and the associated need for psychometric rigor, is rejected by many strict cognitive neuropsychologists (Caplan, 1988; Newcombe & Marshall, 1988).

In view of these diverse and equally valid psychometric issues, cognitively based assessment methods may require an independent set of metrics that differ from, or perhaps complement, traditional measures of reliability and validity. For example, measures of dynamic change, such as sensitivity and stability, may be more appropriate to these methods (Hoffman, Jacobs, & Gerras, 1992). In addition to new data analysis techniques, data collection methods are needed that can more easily capture qualitative aspects of patient performance, along with more traditional quantitative final outcome data. Thus, these methods might benefit from measures of response efficiency, such as reaction time (Benton, 1986; Thorne, Genser, Sing, & Hegge, 1988).

To facilitate these types of data collection and analyses, there is an increasingly accessible technology of single-subject and time-series statistical designs. For example, cross-sectional time-series (Simonton, 1977) and path-analytic models (Algina & Swaminathan, 1979) may be particularly useful in testing cognitive models within a single patient. Similarly, microcomputer technology offers particular promise for this type of data collection, because this technology facilitates repeatable neuropsychological procedures, portable test materials, task modification, real-time data analysis, and millisecond timing accuracy (Kane & Kay, 1992).

Coincidentally, the increase in computer-based testing comes at a time when there has been a renewed interest in reaction time and efficiency measures in clinical neuropsychology (Benton, 1986). It has been demonstrated that individual performance variability, as can be captured in reaction time tasks, may be a more sensitive index of brain-related impairment than summary scores such as response accuracy or speed. However, computation of means and standard deviations of response times can be facilitated by computerization and very rapid data access (Kane & Kay, 1992). As reaction time measures become more relevant to clinical assessment, task demands may eventually outstrip the capabilities of the paper-and-pencil clinical examination and may necessitate a clinical neuropsychological laboratory that is mobile and computer dependent (Kennedy, Wilkes. Dunlop, & Kuntz, 1987).

To summarize, part of what defines cognitively based assessment resists traditional standardization. However, what can be systematized is a cognitive *approach* to clinical problems. This approach is a decision-making and assessment algorithm that is based on a model of cognition, rather than being based on the procedures or instruments themselves (see, for example, Mapcu, Chapter 11, this volume). In other words, modularity, or the division of cognitive function into distinct cognitive domains, combined with the generation, testing, and modification of cognitive models and the use of single-case or multiple-baseline research designs, can be integrated into clinical practice.

Does Cognitively Based Assessment Require Neural Correlation?

Within cognitive neuropsychology, there is disagreement as to whether the development of theoretical models for understanding cognition and behavior must be linked directly to normal or abnormal brain function. The radical cognitive neuropsychologists have suggested that this places unrealistic constraints on the development of models governing the relation of cognitive activities to each other and that a theoretically required relation between brain and behavior may be neither necessary nor useful (Caramazza, 1992). Sokol, McCloskey, Cohen, and Alimonosa (1991) argued that the radical position is most interested in the interrelation among different cognitive operations and that the relation of cognition to brain structure or function is by no means required. In contrast, in their volume on cognitive neuropsychology, McCarthy and Warrington (1990) consistently discussed the relation between cognitive disorders and neuropathology. Similarly, Robertson et al. (1993) have taken issue with Sokol and other proponents of the radical neuropsychological position that "the neural correlates of cognitive deficits are deemed to be virtually irrelevant" (p. 710). Robertson et al. (1993) asserted, instead, that the purpose of neuropsychology is to address brain–behavior relations, and, therefore, it must relate observed behavior to changes in brain structure or function. In addition to disagreement on the importance of neural correlation, Robertson et al. (1993) and others (Zurif, Gardner, & Brownell, 1989; Zurif, Swinney, & Fodor, 1991) also have raised serious doubts about whether brain–behavior relations can be elucidated using only the single-case method.

The question, therefore, with regard to cognitively based assessment, is whether rejecting a strict localizationalist/connectionist model necessitates rejecting a relationship between neural structure and cognitive functioning. Furthermore, despite its emphasis on normal functioning, it appears that cognitive neuropsychology remains lesion and syndrome dependent, if on a case-by-case basis (Caramazza & Badecker, 1991). Taking a more moderate position, many cognitively based, process-oriented, or Luria-influenced neuropsychologists believe that few cognitive functions lateralize or localize to discrete brain regions (Caramazza, 1984; Margolin, 1991). Nevertheless, the brain is not irrelevant, and cognitive functioning is viewed as requiring the integrated functioning of different brain systems (cf. Luria, 1980). For this reason, among others, Mapou (1988b) has argued that using neuropsychological testing to localize or lateralize brain function is no longer a necessary enterprise and that instruments should be evaluated based on their sensitivity to changes in specific aspects of cognitive function, rather than their sensitivity to brain damage per se.

In response to these more moderate positions, Kane, Goldstein, and Parsons (1989) and Reitan (1989), from a psychometric perspective, have suggested that sensitivity, localization, and lateralization remain the ultimate tests of an instrument's validity. They noted that it is precisely the sensitivity of a measure to brain dysfunction that defines it as a neuropsychological test and that distinguishes it from measures designed primarily to assess cognition. For example, the Woodcock-Johnson Psycho-educational Test Battery-Revised (Woodcock & Johnson, 1989) includes many excellent measures of cognitive function, derived from the work of Cattell and others on human intelligence. Although it is being used increasingly in neuropsychological practice, studies of its sensitivity to brain dysfunction are only beginning (Woodcock, personal communication). Therefore, it cannot yet be truly classified as a neuropsychological measure, although, based on knowledge of brain–behavior relationships, hypotheses about the relation of different tests to brain functioning can be made.

Regardless of the strict theoretical position one adopts, it is clear that brain functioning cannot be ignored when the attempt to understand cognition is geared toward identification of relative cognitive strengths and weaknesses in neurologically compromised individuals. Furthermore, the ability to relate neural function and cognition has been advanced greatly in recent years, through the development of procedures that permit access to information regarding central nervous system (CNS) structure or function while an individual is engaging in specific cognitive tasks. Positron emission tomography (LeBerge, 1990; LeBerge & Buschbaum, 1990), single photon emission computed tomography (Grady et al., 1990), regional cerebral blood flow (Gur, Jaggi, Ragland, & Resnick, 1993), and other dynamic imaging techniques have been used to evaluate the relation between specific cognitive functions and cortical activity in neurologically intact individuals. Cognitive functions also can be localized when these techniques are used during neurosurgical procedures, such as ablation (Burchiel, Clarke, Ojemann, Dacey, & Winn, 1989), intraoperative stimulation (Lee, Loring, Flanigin, Smith, & Meador, 1988), extraoperative mapping (Luders et al., 1991), or selective cerebral vascular occlusion (Spector, Kay, Geyer, Deveikes, & Sullivan, 1990). Similarly, topographic EEG and cognitive event-related potentials have been shown to be sensitive to subtle manipulations of language and visuospatial stimuli in patients with known brain lesions (Bashore, 1990; Starbuck, Kay, & Robinson, 1993). By combining cognitive neuropsychological methods with dynamic neuroimaging technology, it is becoming possible to establish the neural substrates underlying specific cognitive operations that occur during actual test performance. This, in turn, will strengthen the brain–behavior basis of neuropsychological assessment, without detracting from the goal of understanding cognition.

Can Cognitively Based Assessment Be Applied to Psychiatric and Psychosocial Dysfunction Following Neurological Insult?

For the most part, the emphasis of cognitively based assessment in the present volume has been on clinical evaluation of discrete information processing skills. However, it is well known that brain damage often asserts itself in more obvious ways, such as, for example, by what Goldstein defined as the loss of the "abstract attitude" (Goldstein, 1942), by a loss of insight, or by difficulties in psychosocial or adaptive functioning. In such instances, neurologically impaired patients may be categorized by their specific cognitive deficits, but their actual disabilities are defined by limitations in other areas, including loss of insight, egocentricity, stimulus-bound behavior, mental inflexibility, and impulsivity, all of which can have a significant impact on everyday functioning (Lezak, 1978).

At present, predicting impairment in everyday functioning from neuropsychological deficits is an imperfect science. For example, difficulties shifting a decision rule from color to form on a sorting task may or may not predict difficulties recognizing when a job requirement or relationship has changed, when an alternate automobile route is needed, or when a checkbook balance or restaurant bill should be scrutinized. Much more effort has gone into establishing the relationship between neuropsychological tests and the functions they purport to measure than into investigating the relationship between those functions and their real-world counterparts. Thus, although some initial work has been done (Heaton & Pendleton, 1981; Naugle & Chelune, 1990), the ecological validity of most neuropsychological measures remains uncertain.

Emphasis on the cognitive aspects of assessment, however, may contribute to better understanding the relation between neuropsychological performance and everyday functioning. For example, there have been a few cognitive neuropsychological examinations of selected higher order skills, each representing an ecologically valid extension of the specific cognitive domain under investigation: language and humor (Bihrle, Brownell, Powelson, & Gardner, 1986) and attention, reaction time, and driving (Stokx & Gaillard, 1986). Perhaps the most impressive studies of the potential application of cognitively based approaches to real-life, psychosocial situations have been in the area of insight and awareness. Within these larger realms, evaluations of the relationships between specific cognitive domains and their respective real-life equivalents have included studies of memory and metamemory (Zelinski, Gilewski, & Thompson, 1980), language and self-awareness of aphasia (Marshall & Tompkins, 1982), and awareness of impairment or disability as a whole (Prigatano & Schacter, 1991; Schacter, 1990). In particular, explorations of the cognitive basis for the self-awareness of disability have been ongoing for some decades. Weinstein and Cole (1963) were among the first to detail the behavioral neurology of anosognosia, influencing the later work of Schacter (1990), who proposed a modular system to address the structure of the specific cognitive elements of anosognosia and self-appraisal.

In another area of application, the nature of impulsivity and self-control has been examined in a series of experiments by Lhermitte (1986; Lhermitte, Pillon, & Serdaru, 1986). These studies explored the nature of utilization behavior in patients with frontal and parietal lobe lesions. In such patients, the absence of frontal control was believed to leave them particularly susceptible to the "press" of an object or circumstance, regardless of actual environmental context. The nature of impulsivity, of stimulus-bound behavior, and by implication, the nature of autonomy in such patients was investigated using a single-case method to establish and test a modular model of higher order functioning.

A third, but by no means final, area of application of cognitively based assessment methods to everyday functioning is differentiating feigned deficit from actual deficit resulting from brain injury. In this regard, there are a number of approaches that commonly are used to identify persons who are motivated to perform poorly, based on research about the response tendencies of such individuals (Wiggins & Brandt, 1988). For example, when presented with lengthy verbal information, in either list or paragraph form, most normal and brain-injured persons remember items from the beginning and end about equally well, and from the middle of the array less efficiently, if at all. This well-known "serial position" effect is one of the early, well-established cognitive findings from experimental psychology. In contrast to expectations, it has been demonstrated that individuals instructed to malinger fail to demonstrate the expected serial position effect. Instead, they recall information from the middle and from the end of the information set about equally well, and from the beginning hardly at all (Bernard, 1991; Russell, Spector, & Kelly, 1993).

Thus, the absence of an expected cognitive pattern can be a clue to feigned deficit. As already discussed, examination of cognitive patterns within an individual's test performance is a hallmark of cognitively based assessment methods. Wiggins and Brandt (1988) described a number of cognitive skills typically spared in amnesia, including semantic priming, word association task performance, and release from the effects of proactive interference. They suggested that impairment in these skills may serve as a basis for determining the presence of malingered deficit, again demonstrating the application of cognitive psychological research to clinical assessment.

In summary, cognitively based assessment has the potential to advance understanding of real-life, everyday behaviors. Traditional clinical neuropsychological methods, with a goal of delineating brain disorder, were not developed to be ecologically valid, and their relation to everyday functioning has been more difficult to establish. Similarly, cognitive neuropsychological methods, with the goal of developing theoretical models to explain normal cognition, also do not directly address real-world activity. However, by using cognitively based assessment methods and by placing more emphasis on cognitive skills that are relevant to daily living, there is an increased potential for facilitating an understanding of the impact of brain dysfunction on everyday skills.

COGNITIVE NEUROPSYCHOLOGY AND COGNITIVE REHABILITATION

The application of psychological principles to the treatment of brain-injured individuals has been a relatively recent development in neuropsychological practice (Sohlberg & Mateer, 1989; Wood & Fussey, 1990). Most early interventions were developed in response to perceived patterns of deficits in single cases of brain-injured patients, and the case study remains the primary method of reporting neuropsychological rehabilitation efforts. There is ongoing debate as to the efficacy of cognitive rehabilitation for the treatment of brain injuries, and more specifically, whether a developing technology of brain-injury rehabilitation can actually reduce the effects of injury on specific cognitive skills and on everyday functioning.

Cognitively based assessment appears particularly well suited to designing and testing intervention strategies for brain-injured individuals. For example, one proof of accuracy of a model of cognitive functioning would seem to be in its application to developing and testing a treatment plan for a brain-injured individual (Wood & Fussey, 1990). Luria (1980) and Rothi and Horner (1983) have suggested that rehabilitation of chronically injured patients would necessitate the use of intact cognitive modules to circumvent discretely affected abilities.

The present volume was designed to focus on neuropsychological assessment. However, in several of the presented case studies, contributors have conducted "therapeutic investigations," testing compensatory or substitutional strategies to bypass specific cognitive impairments. Mateer (1994) and Wilson and Patterson (1990) have suggested that intervention and follow-up are the logical endpoints of cognitively based assessment. The treatment of specific language disorders, attention deficits, executive problems, and memory disorders requires a thorough evaluation and understanding of residual impairment and cognitive integrity (Sohlberg & Mateer, 1989). The logical result of such thorough examination should be a nearly seamless transition to a cognitively based treatment plan.

There are examples of such interventions in the literature. Glisky, Schacter, and Tulving (1986) described a method of vanishing cues that made use of residually preserved procedural memory abilities, specifically priming effects, to train amnestic patients in job skills. By systematically reducing the strength and salience of the priming stimulus, they were able to demonstrate acquisition and maintenance of novel verbal information related to computer functioning over a several-month period. Cicerone and Wood (1987) described a method of shaping delay of gratification and impulse control in a residually brain-injured patient. Using a self-instructional procedure that made use of the patient's residually preserved verbal memory skills, they were able to teach a three-part problem-solving strategy that permitted him to rehearse social behaviors and to analyze the potential consequences of his behavior before actually responding.

Unfortunately, these studies are not representative of many cognitive rehabilitation treatment efforts. Instead, current approaches to cognitive rehabilitation are more likely to use discrete interventions that have little or no relation to deficit or to global outcome measures, including everyday functioning (Adams, 1994; Wood & Fussey, 1990). Despite criticism from a number of sources, many cognitive rehabilitation efforts continue to emphasize restitution of function, employing ill-conceived models of neural recovery, instead of emphasizing the substitutive models that cognitive neuropsychological examination would appear to complement (Wood & Fussey, 1990). Cognitive rehabilitation appears to offer an *in vivo* laboratory for testing the adequacy of the models provided by cognitively based assessment and the logical endpoint for the neuropsychological assessment process.

CONCLUSIONS: COGNITIVELY BASED ASSESSMENT IN CLINICAL PRACTICE

Cognitively based assessment defines an investigatory method that has the potential to shape a number of elements of clinical care. Within this approach, individualized assessment, the assumption of modularity and interdependence of cognitive functions, theory-based evaluation, and the testing of hypotheses generated by the evaluation process represent the essentials of sound clinical practice.

There is clearly more to a person's test performance than the score yielded on a particular instrument, although this may, in part, be attributed to insufficiently operationalized aspects of cognitive test performance, rather than because of the inherent complexity, uniqueness, or essentially qualitative nature of human performance, per se. The cognitive evaluation process must be more easily repeated, taught, and reported than it currently appears to be. To this end, the use of novel instruments and metrics, in general, and computerization, in particular, represent paths to better understanding the components of cognitive performance and their relationship to normal and abnormal brain functioning. Issues of stimulus control, cognitive efficiency, and repeatability are easily addressed using available technologies. Steps should be made to adapt cognitive measures to computerized administration.

The ultimate purpose of clinical neuropsychological assessment is to explain something important about the relationship between brain and behavior. The rejection of connectionist models of cerebral organization need not preclude the use of CNS function and structure as explanatory constructs for cognition. Improved CNS assay procedures, dynamic imaging, event-related testing, and real-time data acquisition and analysis all hold the promise of clarifying the relationship between behavior and neural functioning.

Cognitively based assessment and the rich information that it yields can be applied to complex and ecologically valid behaviors. There is a significant literature on the cognitive neuropsychology of self-awareness and on metacognition, and no reason at all that the real-world equivalents of executive functioning, including social judgment, impulse control, mental flexibility, and egocentricity, cannot be explored in as much detail, using similar methods.

The logical application of information gained via the cognitively based assessment is the remediation of cognitive impairment. The natural test of a cognitive model is the exploitation of other paths within the model to circumvent an impaired skill or cognitive process and return the brain-injured person to premorbid levels of functional integrity.

Acknowledgment

The author would like to thank Wendy A. Law, Ph.D., for very helpful input and comments during preparation of this chapter.

REFERENCES

Adams, K. M. (1994, February). *Efficacy of cognitive rehabilitation: Fact or fantasy?* Paper presented at the 22nd annual meeting of the International Neuropsychological Society, Cincinnati, OH.

Algina, J., & Swaminathan, H. (1979). Alternatives to Simonton's analyses of the interrupted and multiple-group time series designs. *Psychological Bulletin, 86,* 919–926.

Bashore, T. R. (1990). Age-related changes in mental processing revealed by analyses of event-related brain potentials. In J. W. Rohrbaugh, R. Parasuraman, & J. R. Johnson (Eds.), *Event-related potentials: Basic issues and applications* (pp. 242–275). New York: Oxford University Press.

Bates, E., Appelbaum, M., & Allard, L. (1991). Statistical constraints on the use of single cases in neuropsychological research. *Brain and Language, 40,* 295–329.

Benton, A. (1986). Reaction time in brain disease: Some reflections. *Cortex, 22,* 129–149.

Bernard, L. C. (1991). The detection of faked deficits on the Rey Auditory Verbal Learning Test: The effect of serial position. *Archives of Clinical Neuropsychology, 6,* 81–88.

Bihrle, A. M., Brownell, H. H., Powelson, J. A., & Gardner, H. (1986). Comprehension of humorous and non-humorous materials by left and right brain-damaged patients. *Brain and Cognition, 5,* 399–411.

Bub, J., & Bub, D. (1988). On the methodology of single-case studies in cognitive neuropsychology. *Cognitive Neuropsychology, 5,* 535–582.

Burchiel, K. J., Clarke, H., Ojemann, G. A., Dacey, R. G., & Winn, H. R. (1989). Use of stimulation mapping and corticography in the excision of arteriovenous malformations in sensorimotor and language-related neocortex. *Neurosurgery, 24,* 322–327.

Caplan, D. (1988). On the role of group studies in neuropsychological and pathopsychological research. *Cognitive Neuropsychology, 5,* 535–547.

Caramazza, A. (1984). The logic of neuropsychological research and the problem of patient classification in aphasia. *Brain and Language, 21*, 9–20.

Caramazza, A. (1986). On drawing inferences about the structure of normal cognitive systems from the analysis of patterns of impaired performance: The case for single case studies. *Brain and Cognition, 41*, 43–51.

Caramazza, A. (1992). Is cognitive neuropsychology possible? *Journal of Cognitive Neuroscience, 4*, 80–95.

Caramazza, A., & Badecker, W. (1989). Patient classification in neuropsychological research. *Brain and Cognition, 10*, 256–295.

Caramazza, A., & Badecker, W. (1991). Clinical syndromes are not God's gift to cognitive neuropsychology: A reply to a rebuttal to an answer to a response to the case against syndrome-based research. *Brain and Cognition, 16*, 211–227.

Caramazza, A., & McCloskey, M. (1988). The case for single-patient studies. *Cognitive Neuropsychology, 5*, 517–528.

Cicerone, K. D., & Wood, J. C. (1987). Planning disorder after closed head injury: A case study. *Archives of Physical Medicine and Rehabilitation, 68*, 111–115.

Coltheart, M. (1985). Cognitive neuropsychology and the study of reading. In M. I. Posner & D. S. M. Marin (Eds.), *Attention and performance XI* (pp. 3–37). Hillsdale, NJ: Lawrence Erlbaum.

Delis, D. C., Kramer, J. H., Kaplan, E., & Ober, B. A. (1987). *The California Verbal Learning Test*. New York: Psychological Corporation.

Fodor, J. A. (1983). *The modularity of mind*. Cambridge, MA: MIT Press.

Glisky, E. L., Schacter, D. L., & Tulving, E. (1986). Computer learning by memory-impaired patients: Acquisition and retention of complex knowledge. *Neuropsychologia, 24*, 313–328.

Goldstein, K. (1942). *Aftereffects of brain injuries in war*. New York: Grune & Stratton.

Grady, C. L., Haxby, J. V., Horwitz, B., Schapiro, M., Carson, R., Herscovitch, P., & Rapoport, S. I. (1990). Activation of regional cerebral blood flow (RCBF) in extrastriate cortex during a face matching task in patients with dementia of the Alzheimer's type. *Society for Neuroscience Abstracts, 16*, 149.

Gur, R. C., Jaggi, L., Ragland, J. D., & Resnick, S. M. (1993). Effects of memory processing on regional brain activation: Cerebral blood flow in normal subjects. *International Journal of Neuroscience, 72*, 31–44.

Heaton, R. K., & Pendleton, M. G. (1981). Use of neuropsychological tests to predict adult patients' everyday functioning. *Journal of Consulting and Clinical Psychology, 49*, 807–821.

Hoffman, D. A., Jacobs, R., & Gerras, S. J. (1992). Mapping individual performance over time. *Journal of Applied Psychology, 77*, 185–195.

Kane, R. L. (1991). Standardized and flexible batteries in neuropsychology: An assessment update. *Neuropsychology Review, 2*, 281–339.

Kane, R. L., Goldstein, G., & Parsons, O. A. (1989). A response to Mapou. *Journal of Clinical and Experimental Neuropsychology, 11*, 589–595.

Kane, R. L., & Kay, G. G. (1992). Computerized assessment in neuropsychology: A review of tests. *Neuropsychology Review, 3*, 1–117.

Kaplan, E. (1988). A process approach to neuropsychological assessment. In T. Boll & B. K. Bryant (Eds.), *Clinical neuropsychology and brain function: Research, measurement, and practice* (pp. 129–167). Washington, DC: American Psychological Association.

Kennedy, R. S., Wilkes, R. L., Dunlop, W. P., & Kuntz, L. A. (1987). Development of an automated performance test system for environmental and behavioral toxicology studies. *Perceptual and Motor Skills, 65*, 947–962.

LeBerge, D. (1990). Thalamic and cortical mechanisms of attention as suggested by recent positron emission tomographic experiments. *Journal of Cognitive Neuroscience, 2*, 358–372.

LeBerge, D., & Buchsbaum, M. S. (1990). Positron emission tomographic measurements of pulvinar activity during an attention task. *Journal of Neuroscience, 10*, 613–619.

Lee, G. P., Loring, D. W., Flanigin, H. F., Smith, J. R., & Meador, K. J. (1988). Electrical stimulation of the human hippocampus produces verbal intrusions during memory testing. *Neuropsychologia, 26*, 623–627.

Lesser, R. (1987). Cognitive neuropsychological influences on aphasia therapy. *Aphasiology, 1,* 189–200.

Lezak, M. D. (1978). Living with the characterologically altered brain injured patient. *Journal of Clinical Psychiatry, 39,* 592–598.

Lezak, M. D. (1983). *Neuropsychological assessment* (2nd ed). New York: Oxford University Press.

Lhermitte, F. (1986). Human autonomy and the frontal lobes. Part II: Patient behavior in complex and social situations: The "environmental dependency syndrome." *Annals of Neurology, 19,* 335–343.

Lhermitte, F., Pillon, B., & Serdaru, M. (1986). Human autonomy and the frontal lobes. Part I: Imitation and utilization behavior: A neuropsychological study of 75 patients. *Annals of Neurology, 19,* 327–334.

Luders, H., Lesser, R. P., Hahn, J., Dinner, D. S., Morris, H. H., Wyllie, E., & Godoy, J. (1991). Basal temporal language area. *Brain, 114,* 743–753.

Luria, A. R. (1973). *The working brain.* New York: Basic Books.

Luria, A. R. (1980). *Higher cortical functions in man* (2nd ed.). London: Basic Books.

Mapou, R. L. (1988a). An integrated approach to the neuropsychological assessment of cognitive function. In J. M. Williams & C. J. Long (Eds.), *Cognitive approaches to neuropsychology* (pp. 101–122). New York: Plenum Press.

Mapou, R. L. (1988b). Testing to detect brain damage: An alternative to what may no longer be useful. *Journal of Clinical and Experimental Neuropsychology, 10,* 271–278.

Mapou, R. L., Spector, J., & Kay, G. G. (in press). Neuropsychological and psychological assessment. In J. R. Rundell & M. G. Wise (Eds.), *American Psychiatric Press textbook of consultation-liaison psychiatry.* Washington, DC: American Psychiatric Press.

Margolin, D. I. (1991). Cognitive neuropsychology: Resolving enigmas about Wernicke's aphasia and other higher cortical disorders. *Archives of Neurology, 48,* 751–765.

Marshall, J. C., & Newcombe, F. (1984). Putative problems and pure progress in neuropsychological single-case studies. *Journal of Clinical and Experimental Neuropsychology, 6,* 65–70.

Marshall, R. C., & Tompkins, C. A. (1982). Verbal self-correction behaviors of fluent and nonfluent aphasic subjects. *Brain and Language, 15,* 292–306.

Mateer, C. A. (1994, February). *Efficacy of cognitive rehabilitation: Fact or fantasy?* Paper presented at the 22nd annual meeting of the International Neuropsychological Society, Cincinnati, OH.

McCarthy, R. A., & Warrington, E. K. (1990). *Cognitive neuropsychology: A clinical introduction.* New York: Academic Press.

McCloskey, M. (1993). Theory and evidence in cognitive neuropsychology: A "radical" response to Robertson, Knight, Rafal, and Shimamura (1993). *Journal of Experimental Psychology: Learning, Memory, and Cognition, 19,* 718–734.

Naugle, R. I., & Chelune, G. J. (1990). Integrating neuropsychological and "real-life" data: A neuropsychological model for assessing everyday functioning. In D. Tupper & K. Cicerone (Eds.), *Neuropsychology of everyday life* (pp. 57–73). Boston: Academic Press.

Newcombe, F., & Marshall, J. (1988). Idealization meets psychometrics: The case for the right groups and right individuals. *Cognitive Neuropsychology, 5,* 549–564.

Prigatano, G. P., & Schacter, D. L. (Eds.). (1991). *Awareness of deficit after brain injury.* New York: Oxford University Press.

Reitan, R. (1989). A note regarding some aspects of the history of clinical neuropsychology. *Archives of Clinical Neuropsychology, 4,* 385–391.

Robertson, L. C., Knight, R. T., Rafal, R., & Shimamura, A. P. (1993). Cognitive neuropsychology is more than single-case studies. *Journal of Experimental Psychology: Learning, Memory, and Cognition, 19,* 710–717.

Rothi, L. J., & Horner, J. (1983). Restitution and substitution: Two theories of recovery with application to neurobehavioral treatment. *Journal of Clinical and Experimental Neuropsychology, 5,* 73–81.

Russell, M. L., Spector, J., & Kelly, M. (1993, February). *Primacy and recency effects in the detection of malingering using the WMS-R logical memory subtest.* Presented at the 20th annual meeting of the International Neuropsychological Society, Galveston, TX.

Schacter, D. L. (1990). Toward a cognitive neuropsychology of awareness: Implicit knowledge and anosognosia. *Journal of Clinical and Experimental Neuropsychology, 12,* 155–178.

Shallice, T. (1979). A case study approach in neuropsychological research. *Journal of Clinical and Experimental Neuropsychology, 1*, 183–211.
Simonton, D. K. (1977). Cross-sectional time-series experiments: Some suggested statistical analyses. *Psychological Bulletin, 84*, 489–502.
Sohlberg, M. M., & Mateer, C. A. (1989). *Introduction to cognitive rehabilitation: Theory and practice*. New York: Guilford Press.
Sokol, S. M., McCloskey, M., Cohen, N. J., & Alimonosa, D. (1991). Cognitive representations and processes in arithmetic: Inferences from the performance of brain-damaged subjects. *Journal of Experimental Psychology: Learning, Memory, and Cognition, 17*, 355–376.
Spector, J., Kay, G. G., Geyer, C. A., Deveikes, J. D., & Sullivan, R. A. (1990, November). *Neuropsychological screening during trial balloon occlusion of the internal carotid artery*. Presented at the annual meeting of the National Academy of Neuropsychology, Reno, NV.
Starbuck, V. N., Kay, G. G., & Robinson, D. N. (1993). The N400 in recovery from aphasia [Abstract]. *The Clinical Neuropsychologist, 7*, 354.
Stokx, L. C., & Gaillard, W. K. (1986). Task and driving performance of patients with a severe concussion of the brain. *Journal of Clinical and Experimental Neuropsychology, 8*, 421–436.
Teuber, H.-L., & Rudel, R. G. (1962). Behavior after cerebral lesions in children and adults. *Developmental Medicine and Child Neurology, 4*, 3–20.
Thorne, D. R., Genser, S. G., Sing, H. C., & Hegge, F. W. (1988). The Walter Reed Performance Assessment Battery. *Neurobehavioral Toxicology and Teratology, 7*, 415–418.
Weinstein, E. A., & Cole, M. (1963). Concepts of anosognosia. In L. Halpern (Ed.), *Problems of dynamic neurology: Functions of the human nervous system* (pp. 254–273). Jerusalem: Jerusalem Post Press.
Whitaker, H., & Slotnick, H. (1988). Comments on "The case for single patient studies": Is (neuro)psychology possible? *Cognitive Neuropsychology, 5*, 529–534.
Wiggins, E. C., & Brandt, J. (1988). The detection of simulated amnesia. *Law and Human Behavior, 12*, 57–78.
Wilson, B. A., & Patterson, K. (1990). Rehabilitation for cognitive impairment: Does cognitive psychology apply? *Applied Cognitive Psychology, 4*, 247–260.
Wood, R. Ll., & Fussey, I. (Eds.). (1990). *Cognitive rehabilitation in perspective*. London: Taylor & Francis.
Woodcock, R. W., & Johnson, M. B. (1989). *Woodcock-Johnson Psychoeducational Battery-Revised*. Chicago: Riverside Publishing Co.
Zelinski, E. M., Gilewski, M. J., & Thompson, L. W. (1980). Do laboratory tests relate to self-assessment of memory ability in the young and old? In L. W. Poon, J. L. Fozard, L. S. Cermak, D. Arenberg, & L. W. Thompson (Eds.), *New directions in memory and aging* (pp. 519–551). New York: Lawrence Erlbaum.
Zurif, E., Gardner, H., & Brownell, H. (1989). The case against the case against group studies. *Brain and Cognition, 10*, 237–255.
Zurif, E. Swinney, D., & Fodor, J. A. (1991). An evaluation of assumptions underlying the single-ient only position in neuropsychological research—A reply. *Brain and Cognition, 16*, 198–210.

Index

ISBN 0-306-44869-6
90000
9 780306 448690

www.ingramcontent.com/pod-product-compliance
Ingram Content Group UK Ltd.
Pitfield, Milton Keynes, MK11 3LW, UK
UKHW050227160926
475607UK00005B/115
* 9 7 8 0 3 0 6 4 4 8 6 9 0 *